Computers and Medicine

Helmuth F. Orthner, *Series Editor*

Computers and Medicine

M. Michael Shabot   Reed M. Gardner
Editors

Decision Support Systems in Critical Care

With 136 Illustrations

Springer-Verlag
New York Berlin Heidelberg London Paris
Tokyo Hong Kong Barcelona Budapest

M. Michael Shabot, M.D.
Associate Director of Surgery
Director of Surgical Intensive Care
Cedars-Sinai Medical Center
Los Angeles, CA 90048-1865
and Clinical Associate Professor of
  Surgery and Anesthesiology
UCLA School of Medicine
Los Angeles, CA 90048, USA

Reed M. Gardner, Ph.D.
Co-Director, Medical Computing
LDS Hospital
Salt Lake City, UT 84143 and
Professor of Medical Informatics
University of Utah
Salt Lake City, UT 84112, USA

Series Editor:
Helmuth F. Orthner, Ph.D.
Professor of Computer Medicine
The George Washington
  University Medical Center
Washington, D.C. 20037, USA

Library of Congress Cataloging-in-Publication Data
Decision support systems in critical care / M. Michael Shabot, Reed M.
  Gardner, editors. — 1st ed.
    p.   cm. — (Computers and medicine)
    Includes bibliographical references and index.
    ISBN 0-387-97799-6. — ISBN 3-540-97799-6
    1. Critical care medicine—Data processing.   2. Medical
informatics.   I. Shabot, M. Michael.   II. Gardner, Reed M.
III. Series: Computers and medicine (New York, N.Y.)
    [DNLM: 1. Critical Care.   2. Decision Making, Computer-Assisted.
3. Medical Informatics.   4. Decision Support Techniques.   WX218
D2944 1993
RC86.7.D445   1993]
616'.028'0285—dc20
DNLM/DLC
for Library of Congress   93-11902

Printed on acid-free paper.

Production managed by Christin R. Ciresi; manufacturing coordinated by Vincent Scelta.
Typeset by Asco Trade Typesetting Ltd, Hong Kong.
Printed and bound by Edwards Brothers, Inc., Ann Arbor, MI, USA.
Printed in the United States of America.

9 8 7 6 5 4 3 2 1

ISBN 0-387-97799-6 Springer-Verlag New York Berlin Heidelberg
ISBN 3-540-97799-6 Springer-Verlag Berlin Heidelberg New York

Series Preface

This monograph series intends to provide medical information scientists, health care administrators, physicians, nurses, other health care providers, and computer science professionals with successful examples and experiences of computer applications in health care settings. Through the exposition of these computer applications, we attempt to show what is effective and efficient, and hope to provide some guidance on the acquisition or design of medical information systems so that costly mistakes can be avoided.

The health care industry is currently being pushed and pulled from all directions, from clinicians, to increase quality of care; from business, to lower cost and improve financial stability; from legal and regulatory agencies, to provide detailed documentation; and from academe, to provide data for research and improved opportunities for education. Medical information systems sit in the middle of all these demands. The generally accepted (popular) notion is that these systems can satisfy all demands and solve all the problems. Obviously, this notion is naive and is an overstatement of the capabilities of current information technology. Eventually, however, medical information systems will have sufficient functionality to satisfy most information needs of health care providers.

We realize that computer-based information systems can provide more timely and legible information than traditional paper-based systems. Most of us also know that automated information systems provide, on average, more accurate information because data capture is more complete and automatic (e.g., directly from devices). Medical information systems can monitor the process of health care and improve quality of patient care by providing decision support for diagnosis or therapy, clinical reminders for follow-up care, warnings about adverse drug interactions, alerts to questionable treatment or deviations from clinical protocols, and more. Since medical information systems are functionally very rich, must respond quickly to user interactions and queries, and require a high level of security, these systems can be classified as very complex and, from a developer's perspective, also as "risky."

Information technology is advancing at an accelerated pace. Instead of waiting for three years for a new generation of computer hardware, we are now confronted with new computing hardware every 18 months. The forthcoming changes in the telecommunications industry will be revolutionary. Within the next five years and certainly before the end of this century, new digital communications technologies, such as the Integrated Services Digital Network (ISDN) and very high speed local area networks using efficient cell switching protocols (e.g., ATM), will not only change the architecture of our information systems but also the way we work and manage health care institutions.

The software industry constantly tries to provide tools and productive development environments for the design, implementation, and maintenance of information systems. Still, the development of information systems in medicine is, to a large extent, an art, and the tools we use are often self-made and crude. One area that needs desperate attention is the interaction of health care providers with the computer. While the user interface needs improvement and the emerging graphical user interfaces may form the basis for such improvements, the most important criterion is to provide relevant and accurate information without drowning the physician in too much (irrelevant) data.

To develop an effective clinical system requires an understanding of what is to be done and how to do it, and an understanding on how to integrate information systems into an operational health care environment. Such knowledge is rarely found in any one individual; all systems described in this monograph series are the work of teams. The size of these teams is usually small, and the composition is heterogeneous, i.e., health professionals, computer and communications scientists and engineers, biostatisticians, epidemiologists, etc. The team members are usually dedicated to working together over long periods of time, sometimes spanning decades. Clinical information systems are dynamic systems; their functionality constantly changes because of external pressures and administrative changes in health care institutions. Good clinical information systems will and should change the operational mode of patient care, which, in turn, should affect the functional requirements of the information systems. This interplay requires that medical information systems be based on architectures that allow them to be adapted rapidly and with minimal expense. It also requires a willingness by management of the health care institution to adjust its operational procedures, and, most of all, to provide end-user education in the use of information technology. While medical information systems should be functionally integrated, these systems should also be modular so that incremental upgrades, additions, and deletions of modules can be done in order to match the pattern of capital resources and investments available to an institution.

We are building medical information systems just as automobiles were built early in this century (1910s), i.e., in an ad hoc manner that disregarded even existing standards. Although technical standards addressing computer and communications technologies are necessary, they are insufficient. We still need to develop conventions and agreements, and perhaps a few regulations, that address the principal use of medical information in computer and communication systems. Standardization allows the mass production of low-cost parts which can be used to build more complex structures. What are these parts exactly in medical information systems? We need to identify them, classify them, describe them, publish their specifications, and, most importantly, use them in real health care settings. We must be sure that these parts are useful and cost effective even before we standardize them.

Clinical research, health services research, and medical education will benefit greatly when controlled vocabularies are used more widely in the practice of medicine. For practical reasons, the medical profession has developed numerous classifications, nomenclatures, dictionary codes, and thesauri (e.g., ICD, CPT, DSM-III, SNOMED, COSTAR dictionary codes, BAIK thesaurus terms, and MESH terms). The collection of these terms represents a considerable amount of clinical activity, a large portion of the health care business, and access to our recorded knowledge. These terms and codes form the glue that links the practice of medicine with the business of medicine. They also link the practice of medicine with the literature of medicine, with further links to medical research and education. Since information systems are more efficient in retrieving information when controlled vocabularies are used in large databases, the attempt to unify and build bridges between these coding systems is a great example of unifying the field of medicine and health care by providing and using medical informatics tools. The Unified Medical Language System (UMLS) project of the National Library of Medicine, NIH, in Bethesda, Maryland, is an example of such an effort.

The automation of intensive care units in hospitals has advanced remarkably in the last 20 years. Two decades ago, we barely introduced patient monitoring and automatic alarms when vital signs reached a critical level. Our efforts to combine expertise from multiple disciplines such as physiology, biomedical engineering, computer science, biomathematics, and critical care medicine has resulted in state-of-the-art systems which utilize decision support technology based on experiences collected from numerous hospitals (e.g., the APACHE III System) and on rule-based expert system technology (e.g., intelligent respiratory monitoring for ventilated patients). Today, intensive care units (ICUs) are full of automated equipment. The problem, however, is not to collect data but to filter unnecessary redundancies that cause information overload. Today's decision support systems for ICUs are sophisticated clinical information systems drawing on many expert experiences. These systems are not only used for patient care but also for the efficient management of ICUs. The latter is important since ICUs are very expensive suites within a hospital.

The purpose of this series is to capture the experience of medical informatics teams that have successfully implemented and operated medical information systems. We hope the individual books in this series will contribute to the evolution of medical informatics as a recognized professional discipline. We are at the threshold where there is not just the need but already the momentum and interest in the health care and computer science communities to identify and recognize the new discipline called Medical Informatics.

Washington, DC   HELMUTH F. ORTHNER

Preface

Modern critical care is characterized by the collection of large volumes of data and the making of urgent patient care decisions. The two do not necessarily go together easily. For many years the hope has been that intensive care unit (ICU) data management systems could play a meaningful role in ICU decision support. These hopes now have a basis in fact, and this book will detail the history, methodology, current status, and future prospects for critical care decision support systems.

Computerized ICU data management is just 25 years old. As editors we are privileged to bring together a group of authors who are the pioneers, developers, system managers, and philosophers in this field, the individuals who transformed the dream into reality. Although this book is about intelligent systems, it is not about artificial intelligence per se. The state of the art in critical care and ICU data management does not yet permit the general application of artificial intelligence techniques, though it may in the future.

A number of commercially available ICU data management systems are beginning to reach the level of functionality at which decision support will be routinely available. In the current era of health care reform, prospective payment, and cost controls, multiple levels of decision support are required to practice auditable, cost-effective and medically effective critical care. This book will describe those levels, the successes and failures of past and present systems, and the practical aspects of bringing such systems to fruition in your own hospital.

Our hope is that this book will serve as an interesting and informative explanation of where we are in ICU decision support, how we got there, and where we are headed in the future. Please settle back and enjoy the trip.

M. MICHAEL SHABOT
REED M. GARDNER

The book is dedicated to my parents, Sam and Mona Shabot, who gave me everything, asked for nothing and provided the framework for my life.

M. Michael Shabot
July 1993

November 1993 will be a special month for me. This book will be printed and my mother will be 95 years young!! I dedicate this book to her. She has been a continual inspiration to me all of my life. She has encouraged each of her five children to be life-long learners. Learning and teaching have been a family value that I hope I can pass along to my children and to those I associate with. This specialized book about decision-making using computers is in large measure a result of the principles she taught me. When the going got tough at times it was her lively encouragement and spirit that encouraged me. Thanks mother.

Reed M. Gardner
July 1993

Contents

V. Conclusions

Contributors

H. SCOTT BJERKE, M.D.
Director of Surgical Critical Care, University of Nevada, Department of Surgery, 2020 W. Charleston Blvd., Las Vegas, NV 89102, USA

JUDY BLAUFUSS, R.N., CCRN
Director of Critical Care Nursing, LDS Hospital, Salt Lake City, UT 84143, USA

KAREN E. BRADSHAW TATE, PH.D.
Departments of Medical Biophysics and Computing, University of Utah, LDS Hospital, Salt Lake City, UT 84143, USA

TERRY P. CLEMMER, M.D.
Professor of Medicine, Director, Critical Care, University of Utah, LDS Hospital, Salt Lake City, UT 84143, USA

ROBERT O. CRAPO, M.D.
Pulmonary Division, Department of Medicine, University of Utah, LDS Hospital, Salt Lake City, UT 84143, USA

GEORGE A. DIAMOND, M.D.
Associate Director of Cardiology, Director, Stress Laboratory, Cedars-Sinai Medical Center, Los Angeles, CA 90048, USA

STUART B. DUBIN, M.D., PH.D.
Associate Director of Pathology, Director, Laboratory Information System, Cedars-Sinai Medical Center, Los Angeles, CA 90048, USA

THOMAS D. EAST, PH.D.
Associate Professor of Anesthesiology, Departments of Anesthesia, Medical Informatics and Internal Medicine, University of Utah, LDS Hospital, Salt Lake City, UT 84143, USA

REED M. GARDNER, PH.D.
Professor of Medical Informatics, University of Utah, Co-Director of
Medical Computing, LDS Hospital, Salt Lake City, UT 84143, USA

GISLE HANNEMYR
Norwegian Telecommunications Administration/NCC, P.O. Box 114,
Blinderin N. 0314, Oslo, Norway

JOHN J. HARRINGTON
Hewlett-Packard Company, Medical Products Group, Andover, MA
01810, USA

WILLIAM L. HAWLEY
Director of Clinical Engineering, LDS Hospital, Salt Lake City, UT
84143, USA

SUSAN HENDERSON, M.S.
Pulmonary Division, Department of Medicine, University of Utah, LDS
Hospital, Salt Lake City, UT 84143, USA

MICHAEL C. HIGGINS, PH.D.
Research Scientist, Hewlett-Packard Laboratories, Palo Alto, CA 94303,
USA

SAMUEL HOLTZMAN
Strategic Decisions Group, Menlo Park, CA 94025, USA

STANLEY M. HUFF, M.D.
Assistant Professor of Medical Informatics, University of Utah, LDS
Hospital, Salt Lake City, UT 84143, USA

RUSSELL K. HULSE, RPh, MBA
Associate Director of Pharmacy, LDS Hospital, Salt Lake City, UT
84143, USA

WILLIAM A. KNAUS, M.D.
Director of ICU Research, George Washington University Medical Center, Department of Anesthesiology, Washington, D.C. 20037, USA

KEITH G. LARSEN, RPh
Director of Pharmacy Computerization, Intermountain Health Care,
Inc., Salt Lake City, UT 84111, USA

BEVERLEY J. LEYERLE, R.N., CCRN
Clinical Project/Research Nurse, Department of Surgery, Cedars-Sinai
Medical Center, Los Angeles, CA 90048, USA

MARK LoBUE, M.A.
Systems Analyst, Department of Surgery, Cedars-Sinai Medical Center,
Los Angeles, CA 90048, USA

JAMES S. LOGAN, M.D.
National Aeronautics and Space Administration, Johnson Space Center, Houston, TX 77058-4399, USA

S. MEIYAPPAN
Department of Anesthesia, Thorax Center and Department of Anesthesia, Erasmus University, Postbus 1738, 3000 DR, Rotterdam, The Netherlands

ALAN H. MORRIS, M.D.
Professor of Medicine, University of Utah, LDS Hospital, Salt Lake City, UT 84143, USA

BRENT D. NELSON, M.S.
Department of Medical Informatics, University of Utah, LDS Hospital, Salt Lake City, UT 84143, USA

THOMAS A. ONIKI, M.S.
Department of Medical Informatics, University of Utah, LDS Hospital, Salt Lake City, UT 84143, USA

JAMES F. ORME, JR., M.D.
Associate Professor of Medicine, Associate Director, Shock Trauma ICU, University of Utah, LDS Hospital, Salt Lake City, UT 84143, USA

DAVID V. OSLTER
EMTEK Health Care Systems, 1501 W. Fountainhead Parkway, 190, Tempe, AZ 85285, USA

BRAD H. POLLOCK, M.P.H.
Division of Cardiology, Cedars-Sinai Medical Center, Los Angeles, CA 90048, USA

OMAR PRAKASH, M.D.
Professor of Anesthesia, Thorax Center and Department of Anesthesia, Erasmus University, Postbus 1738, 3000 DR, Rotterdam, The Netherlands

T. ALLEN PRYOR, PH.D.
Professor of Medical Informatics, University of Utah, Co-Director of Medical Computing, LDS Hospital, Salt Lake City, UT 84143, USA

ADAM SEIVER, M.D.
Clinical Instructor in Surgery, Stanford University, Chief, General Surgery, VA Medical Center, Palo Alto, CA 94304, USA

M. MICHAEL SHABOT, M.D.
Director, Surgical Intensive Care Units, Cedars-Sinai Medical Center, Clinical Associate Professor of Surgery and Anesthesiology, UCLA School of Medicine, Los Angeles, CA 90048, USA

CARL SIRIO, M.D.
University of Pittsburgh School of Medicine Department of Anesthesiology and Critical Case Medicine Pittsburgh, PA 15261, USA

DEAN F. SITTIG, PH.D.
Department of Medical Informatics, Vanderbilt University Medical Center, Nashville, TN 37232, USA

FRANK THOMAS, M.D.
Associate Professor of Medicine, Director of Life Flight, University of Utah, LDS Hospital, Salt Lake City, UT 84143, USA

DAVID A. TRACE, M.D.
Associate Professor of Medicine, University of Health Sciences, The Chicago Medical School, North Chicago, IL 60064, USA

C. JANE WALLACE, R.N.
Research Nurse, Shock Trauma ICU, LDS Hospital, Salt Lake City, UT, 84143, USA

LYNDALL K. WEAVER, M.D.
Associate Professor of Medicine, University of Utah, LDS Hospital, Salt Lake City, UT 84143, USA

MAX HARRY WEIL, M.D., PH.D.
Professor and Chairman, Department of Medicine, University of Health Sciences, The Chicago Medical School, North Chicago, IL 60064, USA

BLAIR J. WEST
Systems Programmer, Department of Medical Informatics, University of Utah, LDS Hospital, Salt Lake City, UT 84143, USA

JEFFREY W. WORK, M.D.
Division of Cardiology, Cedars-Sinai Medical Center, Los Angeles, CA 90048, USA

HSUEH-FEN W. YOUNG, M.S.
Department of Medical Informatics, University of Utah, LDS Hospital, Salt Lake City, UT 84143, USA

I
Fundamentals

Chapter 1
Medical Informatics and Decision Support Systems in the Intensive Care Unit: State of the Art

Terry P. Clemmer, Reed M. Gardner, and M. Michael Shabot

Introduction

Medical informatics involves the broad fields of management and use of biomedical information. Although based in medical computing, medical informatics incorporates a knowledge of the origin, nature, synthesis, and utility of the medical information itself. For medical informatics systems to be successful in improving health care, the skills of interested physicians, nurses, computer scientists, researchers, and other medical professionals must be combined in collaborative efforts.

Decision support systems represent a specific expression of medical informatics, embodied in systems which receive medical *data* as input and which produce medical *information* or even *knowledge* as outputs. Decision support systems incorporate an important ingredient—*medical knowledge*—to help caregivers interpret data and make better decisions. In the intensive care unit, patient care decisions are not only crucial, they must be made quickly and on the basis of a tremendous amount of data, frequently incomplete. This book fouses on the systematic conversion of raw *data* into *useful information, knowledge, and support for clinical decision-making*. Decision support systems can be as small as a palmtop computer or as large as multi-institutional networks of large-scale systems—the goals, methods, and principles of operation are the same.

Decision support systems embody up to three important operating principles. First, such systems *transform* raw data into information. Second, they can *combine* different kinds of information and re-present it to clinicians in the form of integrated displays and reports. Finally, decision support systems can utilize *inferencing* methods to detect associations

Adapted from an article published in the *Int J Clin Monit Comput* 8:237–250, 1991. Reprinted with permission of Kluwer Academic Publishers.

3

between different pieces of information, alerting clinicians to certain patterns of events, which may be serious or life-threatening. The ultimate output of this process is clinical decision support, which can be diagrammed as follows:

Product	Process
data	*transformation*
↓	
information	*combination*
↓	
integration	*inference*
↓	
decision support	

It is important to stress that these processes are knowledge-based; that is, the transformations, combinations, and detections performed on the incoming data are based on medical knowledge and expertise *that has been added to the system in advance*. Decision support systems do not require the use of artificial intelligence. Rather, they incorporate ordinary intelligence, expressed through software or configuration rules, for the distillation of information from data, integration from the information, and associations from the integrated information.

Sophisticated hardware and software developed without the collaborative effort described above, testing at the bedside, and integration into the clinical environment usually fail to become practical systems that enhance patient care. Basic research programs such as physiologic or pharmacologic modeling can be created in a laboratory, but they must be brought to the bedside for testing in order to influence patient care. This demands a close working relationship between the scientists in medical informatics and caregivers working in the clinical environment.

An integrated clinical information system provides many advantages for enhancement of direct patient care [1,2]. An integrated system facilitates retrieval of all the patient's information at a single location, saving time and enhancing the utilization of the system. Data review in unintegrated or disparate systems is slow, repetitious, and burdensome. The use of standardized screen and report formatting throughout the hospital simplifies the review and data entry process by allowing personnel in all areas to access data the same way regardless of where they are working. By having the data integrated, reports and displays can be created that facilitate the transfer of information to the user in such a manner that attention is focused on specific problems, thus strengthening medical decision-making by assuring that the data is complete, appropriately integrated, and properly presented [3–6].

In addition an integrated database allows for more sophisticated data-driven alerting, [7–11] quality assurance [12–16], and decision-making programs to be developed that reduce errors, improve care, and increase reliance on the system. It also facilitates research, enhances administrative uses, and allows some tasks to be accomplished that would be difficult or otherwise impossible [17].

However, an integrated patient data management system also presents many challenges to the developers. Indeed, these challenges are the genesis of the field of medical informatics. Among these challenges are 1) acquisition of data, 2) data quality control, 3) management of large quantities of data in a functional way, 4) standardization and transfer of data, 5) making the data useful to the clinician, 6) making the data useful to the researcher, and 7) logistical, cost, and confidentiality issues. These challenges will be addressed separately and in some detail in this paper. Many of these problems have not been resolved and present fertile areas for future medical informatics research.

Techniques Directed at Reducing Time and Effort for Data Entry

For a system to be usable, the cost and effort of inputing data must be minimized. Several techniques are used to facilitate data entry. Initially the direct interfacing of devices capable of generating digital signals is desirable. Many devices are readily adaptable to this concept and direct interface with bedside monitors and other hospital computers such as those in the clinical laboratory are now routine. Bar coding the input of patient identification, medications, and supplies could simplify or semi-automate this data entry. Other devices with outputs that can be directly interfaced include intravenous infusion devices, pulse oximeters, venous oximeters, ventilators, electronic urimeters, and gastric pH monitors [18–22]. Standard interfaces from medical device vendors and clinical information system vendors are now available, so these interfaces may be purchased rather than developed separately by each hospital.

Data derived from direct input is not without its difficulties however. *First*, there must be assurance that the device is identified with the correct patient from whom data is being collected or to whom the therapy is being delivered. Improper patient identification is still a major concern for every hospital. Automated data entry has its own form of identification errors that must be guarded against. These problems generally revolve around the human error of failing to tell the computer to which patient the devices are connected. When patients are disconnected and reconnected to as many as 15 different devices when being moved for special procedures or for transfer to other nursing units, the potential for error is large. *Second*, although the direct input of data eliminates many data entry errors, the quality of automated data is not guaranteed [19,20]. A blood pressure from a transducer may have erroneous signals for mechanical reasons, because of interference during blood drawing or line flushing, or because of sampling "non-representative" physiologic data while the patient is being stressed, placed in a different position, or responding transiently to a medication or procedure. Techniques to control data quality will be addressed in the following section. *Third*, the interface problems can be very challenging at times. The linking of different types of computers is not simple, and the same applies to many medical devices. Because of the lack of standardization, the interface problems of each computer, instrument, or device may have to be resolved individually.

The need to develop standards is clear, and the Institute of Electrical and Electronic Engineers (IEEE) is pursuing this so that in the future most devices will be compatible with a common Medical Information Bus (MIB). Such a bus will allow the host computer to access the information from many different types of instruments and also to communicate back to the device [6,19–24]. This communication allows the caregiver to know what the computer perceives it is monitoring or controlling. For example, the computer can flash the drug being infused on the LED display of the infusion pump, thus permitting the caregiver to confirm proper communication with the computer. Such two-way communication also helps with patient identification and in the future will be necessary for closed-loop control of devices. In addition, the standardization of device interfaces enhances the likelihood of obtaining timely and accurate data and reduces the possibility of technical and systems errors.

The other problem with direct interface is maintaining data capture while moving patients for procedures and following transfer to other nursing units. While the patient is located in one place, patient identification problems are reduced and a hardwired computer connection is possible. But while moving patients or during lengthy procedures in the operating room or radiology suite, continued monitoring and reliable data capture can be compromised. This presents new challenges, requiring either portable storage of information for later retrieval, telemetry of data, or at least the ability to change the patient's location quickly with proper identification being assured and as little interruption of data storage as possible. The availability of new portable monitors that store data and can later transfer the data into the integrated system is one approach to this dilemma. Another option is to provide computer interfaces in all operating rooms and special procedure areas, with software that will allow easy transfer of patient location.

A considerable amount of data cannot be directly obtained from bedside devices. This includes information about bolus medications, oral medications, nursing tasks, bedside patient assessments, and physical findings. If such data is entered into the computer in "free text" form, it is difficult to use the information for computerized alerting, quality assurance, decision support, and research purposes. Free text also carries with it the problems of typographical and spelling errors. Whenever possible, structured, list-driven data entry is desirable because it is faster and more uniform. This can be accomplished in several ways. The use of a mouse, trackball, light-pen, and touch screen are popular methods using a point-and-click system [25]. For speed, however, the ten-key pad may be the fastest, once personnel become familiar with the keyboard and menus [17]. Use of the keyboard allows the user to "stack" commands and drop quickly to the desired menu and location for charting. With point-and-click systems the user must wait for the screen to appear before pointing again and this may slow the process. Powerful graphic-based systems and innovative ways of entering numerical data with a trackball or mouse have made numerical entry with these systems as fast as the numeric keypad.

Regardless of which charting method is selected, access to the workstation is important in providing a friendly, usable system. In the Intensive Care Unit (ICU) it is desirable to have a workstation at each bed so that caregivers can chart directly into the computer, thereby eliminating the need to write the information on paper or chart from memory. This also keeps the personnel at the bedside, obviating the need to walk out to a workstation, and guarantees that a workstation will be available. In addition to the bedside workstation it is convenient to have other workstations at the central station for charting when the patient is resting, for review of data, and for administrative purposes. When data is recorded in a delayed fashion, frequent errors in data accuracy and timing have been shown to occur [19]. The advantages of real-time charting are accentuated when therapy is driven with computerized protocols that contain time-dependent decisions. If data is late or unavailable to the computer, then decisions will either not be made or will be made incorrectly from data entered earlier. This is an area where direct data acquisition from devices can be very valuable. The same limitation affects clinical decision-making, where data may be in a caregiver's head or pocket but not yet charted and available to the clinician at the time of decision-making. With an integrated system, information can also be accessed from other areas of the hospital, medical clinics, physicians offices, or even from home.

Techniques Used to Control the Quality of Data Entered

One of the most important problems in medical informatics is the entry of accurate data. Inaccurate data can result in compromises to patient care and loss of confidence in the system by the care team and even refusal to use the system. In addition, poor-quality data severely limits the ability to use the power of the information system because alerts, quality-assurance programs, and clinical decision-making cannot be effective if treatment recommendations are generated from fallacious data. Therefore, it is crucial to develop methods to enhance the quality and consistency of patient data entry.

The best control over the quality of the data is to *use it constantly*. The more the computerized data is used by the health care team, the greater the likelihood that errors will be found. Those who know the patient best are most likely to recognize errors when they are using the data to make decisions [26]. The care teams are also the most critical of inaccuracies, since their actions are determined by decisions made from the data and because they are legally and ethically liable for these actions. Therefore, they are demanding of the data and will insist on accuracy. It is desirable that everyone concerned with the care of the patient use the computer system properly and not just blindly enter or accept data.

If errors are identified, then it is imperative that a simple mechanism to correct the errors be available; otherwise, the error will be recognized and ignored for decision-making purposes yet not corrected in the patient record. This incorrect information will interfere with other valuable uses of the data, such as the alerting system, quality control, decision-making protocols, and research. The key then is to *use the data* and to *correct it* when errors are found. Modern systems provide "audit trails" of all changed or corrected data, so that prior entries and the time and identification of the person making the change are permanently recorded for legal purposes.

Another method of improving the quality of data is to create smart filters that will not allow the entry of data that is outside of credible limits. Certainly for physiologic data there are values that are impossible and keystroke errors resulting in such values should be rejected. Other data outside reasonable limits should require verification before being stored in the database.

When there is redundancy in the monitored data, it can be crosschecked for correlation. An example would be the heart rate from the ECG, the pulse rate from arterial blood pressure monitor, and the pulse from a pulse oximeter [19,20]. Thus an ECG artifact resulting in a rate markedly different from that of the other pulse monitors could be questioned. Other examples might include a hemoglobin value from a blood gas compared with one from a CBC, pH verification with the electrolyte panel, weights with, the intake and output record, respirations from the bedside monitor with data from the ventilator, PaO_2 with the fraction of inspired oxygen, Glasgow Coma Score with sedative and paralytic medications, etc.

Because hand entry of data is associated with many entry errors [19,20], automatic data entry is desirable but introduces problems of its own. One of the problems is that under normal conditions the caregiver unconsciously filters data and records only that which is perceived as representative of the patient's condition. For example, if a patient is turned or is on a bed pan, a transient rise in blood pressure will probably not be recorded. Instead, the caregiver will wait until the stress is over and the patient returns to baseline status before inputing vital signs. When a patient is coughing or fighting a ventilator, the caregiver will not report the peak airway pressure but will wait until the patient has passed this episode. With time-driven automatic data sampling, these episodes may not be avoided and artifact-ridden data may be stored that would not be useful for decision-making, quality-assurance, or research purposes. However, nurses' perceptions of representative data have frequently been shown to be in error [16]. One of the methods used to circumvent both of problems is to have the automated data verified or edited by the nurse or therapist. Another is to have the caregiver signal the computer when to sample the data and to consider these data of higher value for storage and decision-making purposes. Other mathematical filtering or averaging of data might be appropriate in some circumstances to eliminate transient fluctuations, but this approach risks missing clinically relevant data.

Another technique for controlling quality is to generate reports that become the legal medical record and have them reviewed by the caregiver for verification of accuracy [27]. Other reports routinely given to personnel responsible for statistical analysis and quality assurance simplifies the recognition of errors and problem areas in data quality. Once again the idea of using the computer data frequently is a key to acquiring quality data.

Managing and Storing the Data

The quantity of data available on any sick patient in the intensive care unit is phenomenal. With automatic data sampling it is possible to gather thousands of data points each day for each monitored parameter and each life support device. This presents the clinical and medical informatics team with the enormous challenge of determining what data is needed, how often it is necessary to sample, and what data should be stored [28]. If data is redundant, does it all need to be stored? If so, should duplicate data labels be used? If the redundant data is not identical, which data point takes priority? Which of the redundant data items should be used for decision-making, quality assurance, and alerts? These are fertile areas for research and are crucial to systems development. Currently these decisions are arbitrarily made with little or no scientific validation.

Some modeling can be used to help make such decisions. The rate of change of any given parameter will determine how often the signal must be sampled to detect significant change [28]. For example, the serum albumin changes very slowly, over hours or days, so sampling it every few minutes would be inappropriate. However, the heart rate may change in seconds; therefore, if all changes are to be detected, continuous beat-to-beat monitoring is necessary. Although the heart rate is monitored continuously for alarm purposes, does all the data need to be stored? Most manual and current computer systems store data at fixed time intervals. For example, vital signs may be measured and logged every hour. Perhaps it would be better to store data when significant changes are detected, but this would trigger data storage due to transient or artifactual changes caused by patient movement, medications, etc. Again, these are areas where more research is needed.

It is also important to determine what data is actually used by the care team to make decisions [29]. Although enormous volumes of data are generated in the ICU, relatively few items are used for decision-making and prognosis [30]. An example is the measurement of bulk respiratory data, including tidal volume, ventilation rate, blood gases, thoracic compliance, three different airway pressures, airway resistance, pressure volume curves, vital capacity, forced vital capacity, lung volumes, inspired oxygen concentration, and the chest x-ray [19–21,31,32]. But is all this data required to make decisions about the ventilator? What is really relevant and needed? How are decisions really made? Recent experience leads us to believe that only a few data items are actually being used in most clinical decisions [31,32].

Even if all this data is needed for immediate decision-making, does all of it need to be stored long-term? What kinds of questions are asked of long-term data? Our experience is that long-term data storage is very useful in answering questions that arise in the design of patient care protocols and guidelines. An example is the use of long-term data to develop a consultative blood ordering system [33]. The rapid expansion of inexpensive data storage systems may allow all data to be saved, but the sheer volume of data will be a hindrance when questions are asked of the database. Another issue pertains to how long such "long-term" data needs to be stored. Is immediate access required? How immediate is immediate (seconds, minutes, hours)? These are all questions that need consideration and answers as medical informatics systems are planned and implemented.

Standardization and Transfer of Data

For computer-stored data to be useful it must be searchable and retrievable. Therefore, it is critical that the data be in a standard format and coded in such a way that it can be easily identified, searched, retrieved, and used by various personnel for multiple purposes. Thus, blood oxygen tension, used by laboratory technicians, nurses, physicians, respiratory therapists, and researchers, must be coded in such a way that it can be used by everyone [34,35]. In institutions where there are many departments, divisions, and people, each with their own interests and capabilities, the danger of confusion, inappropriate duplication, and lack of coordination of data coding and storage is high and can be a major problem. Later, when the database is searched for information to generate alerts, quality assurance, severity scores, medical decision-making, or research, the task of having data in various places and in different formats creates major difficulties.

These problems are compounded when one tries to transfer data between computers [36–38]. Communications between different types of computers with different operating systems can be challenging [36–38]. The hospital business computer, designed and programmed to process financial data, is typically difficult to interface with clinical computer systems. However, such communication could be very valuable for automatic billing, administrative queries, and for research about the cost of health care delivery. The ability to transfer mainframe programs between institutions for collaborative research efforts today is nearly impossible because each system's coding, terms, and definitions are different. The need for standardization in this area is great and the speed with which progress is made in medical informatics will depend upon such standardization [2,39,40].

Clinical Use of the Information System

The proof of the success of the medical informatics department is its clinical acceptance and use of the system for patient care. The goal should be more than just facilitating the availability of data in a timely fashion for the clinician. A well designed system should improve patient care above and beyond what would be possible with the manual system. There are certain tasks computers do better than clinicians and the system should take advantage of this fact to enrich care.

Friendly, Fast, and Flexible

The time required for the physician and other health care personnel to interact with the computer is critical. The system must be fast, reliable, have minimal delays, and be user-friendly. With little or no training the user should be able to find the desired clinical information and generate reports. The menus or graphic screen design must be logical and easy to follow for the novice. Wherever possible the system should be flexible so that users can create their own menus or reports to satisfy special needs. This capability must be controlled, however, for the stability of the entire system.

The organization and display of workstation screens and printed reports can be crucial to the care of the patient and to the acceptance of the system by the clinical team. With an integrated database many options are available, and the data can be organized in different formats for different functions and purposes [41]. This is an area where collaboration with the clinical care providers is crucial because they are the primary users. Reports can be used to integrate data and emphasize specific areas of related information [42,43]. Certain data can be flagged to focus attention on problems [44]. Interpretations can be generated to help those who may be unfamiliar with the meaning of the data [3,5]. Graphs, tables, and charts can be used to show trends or to correlate information. The design of screens and reports is both an art and a science and is crucial to the success and utilization of the system [45,46]. Because it is difficult for clinicians to remember large volumes of prior data, the display of previous data along with current data is very useful. In the bedside setting it is routine to use this type of display for laboratory data and physiologic parameters. It is also valuable to cluster related data such as the active cardiovascular drugs next to the hemodynamic data so the clinician can visualize the level of drug support when interpreting cardiac performance [44]. Problems may arise, however, with various types of displays. For example, with graphical displays the user may encounter problems with resolution, the inability to interpolate digital numbers from the display, the handling of multiple scales and the overlap of data and time scales. The use of color displays may resolve some of these problems but significantly increases the cost of a hospital-wide system. Some users prefer graphs, while others want to see the data in digital format. There is no one "right" answer to this issue, and successful systems offer the user a choice of display methods. Again, close communication between the medical informatics team and clinical users is indispensable in resolving these conflicts.

Data-Driven Automatic Alerts and Alarms

One area where humans (clinicians!) have trouble is in handling an overload of data both from patients and advice from the literature [47]. When one parameter becomes available along with scores of other variables, it may be overlooked or improperly integrated with other information in the patient's database. The result is that a potentially dangerous situation may not be recognized. A computer, once programmed, will never tire from the task of processing every new piece of incoming data and comparing it to other available data and to its internal knowledge base. Thus an important role of the smart clinical information systems is to alert or warn caregivers about potentially dangerous situations. Alerts can warn of critical changes in laboratory and physiologic parameters, drug-drug interactions, drug-allergy combinations, and drug dosing errors. Such an alerting system must be automatic, and by definition it is data-driven. An integrated clinical information system with simultaneous access to the patient's laboratory data, allergies, height, weight, age, admitting diagnosis,

medications, and physiologic parameters allows for much more sophisticated alerting algorithms to be created [7–14,48,49].

A great deal of clinical computing experience is required to develop an
alerting system that is user-friendly, acceptable to the caregiver, and helpful without being obnoxious. The use of redundant information to avoid
false alerts can be helpful [7–14,50]. A careful evaluation and categorization of alerts by urgency level can make the system more acceptable. At
times the alerts may be channeled to pharmacists, nurses, or other paramedical professionals who can screen out or respond to minor or false
alerts [48,51]. If the system allows or requires that the physician personal-
ly enter orders into the computer, immediate feedback at the time of
ordering can be very helpful if done in a timely and nonobtrusive manner.

Stratifying the urgency of the alerts with different mechanisms
appropriate to the urgency can be used for feedback. For example, a life-
threatening alert should be more urgent than an "information only" alert.
An obnoxious sound or light that can only be turned off by recognizing
the alert is the most effective way to guarantee attention but is not
appropriate for alerts that do not require such immediate attention. A
less obnoxious method of presenting alerts to the caregiver is to pop up
an alert screen when the caregiver logs into the system. This method is
not as sure or timely but may be adequate for many non-urgent messages.
For minor alerts a report printed once a day might suffice.

Assuring Quality of Care

A well-designed alerting system allows the care provider to avoid potential errors before the institution of therapy and to avoid incompatible
orders [49]. Alerts and prompts also can be used to reduce costs by re-
minding physicians of more cost-effective medications or procedures that
would adequately satisfy the care need [14,15,33,52,53]. When total
parenteral nutrition (TPN) solutions are ordered such a program can alert
the physician incompatibilities or disallow specific combinations of calcium and phosphates, depending on pH [54]. The program also can also
block the addition of medications known to be unstable in the solution.
When antibiotics are ordered, the ordered dosage can be evaluated and
questioned on line if inappropriate for the size of the patient or because
of renal or liver dysfunction, as indicated by current lab values. Intravenous potassium orders can be questioned or denied if dangerous infusion rates are exceeded. When drugs that interact with others are
ordered, the physician can be reminded of potential problems. Such alerting systems have proven to be very effective with a physician compliance
of greater than 90%. [26,31,50]. Alerting and advising systems have also
been shown to rationalize the use of blood products and allow the
measurement of improvement in transfusion practice [33,52,53].

These same principles can be applied to cost containment efforts by advising physicians to use less costly antibiotics for a given diagnosis and available bacteriology results [10,11]. Reminders to stop medications have also proven to be very effective at reducing costs and improving the quality of care, especially in the area of prophylactic antibiotics [14,15]. Timely feedback to physicians of potentially dangerous situations such as metabolic acidosis, when coupled with suggestions on how to proceed with the patient evaluation and therapy, has been demonstrated to reduce the time the patient remains acidotic and to improve outcome [4].

Similar to the alerting system, real-time quality assurance reports can be used to improve the quality and cost of care. Most hospitals in the United States do quality assurance by defining criteria for quality and then determining compliance with a random chart review. If problems are found, educational or procedural mechanisms are used to improve quality. Following that intervention, another random chart review is performed to determine the success of the remedial measures. Using a computerized database, criteria for quality care can be explicitly described, programmed and monitored by the system in real time. When a breech in the quality "standard" is detected, an immediate report can be generated to quality assurance personnel, and the situation can be corrected immediately [55]. This allows real-time improvement in care along with the institution of educational and procedural steps. This monitor can be continued indefinitely and applied to every patient, not just those randomly chosen for review. Thus quality assurance can become a process control method, a vast improvement over manual, retrospective chart reviews.

Computer monitoring also can dramatically improve the identification of certain types of problems. For example, when adverse drug reactions were detected by a continuous computer surveillance program, the rate of detection of adverse reactions was 60-fold higher than when reported by hand [12,56]. These types of audits are only achievable with an integrated clinical information system.

The best measures of quality care are outcome and cost. However, the nonhomogeneity of patients, differences in severity of illness, and differences in disease expression make it impossible to measure quality with an outcome alone. A 1% mortality rate might be very acceptable for coronary artery bypass, but it would be far too high for inguinal hernia repair! To help normalize or stratify patients for outcome analysis, acuity scoring systems such as the Acute Physiologic and Chronic Health Evaluation (APACHE) [29,57,58], the Therapeutic Intervention Scoring System (TISS) [58,59], the Injury Severity Score (ISS) [60,61], and others [62] have been created. Scoring every patient by hand is laborious, time-consuming, and costly. With some effort these scores can be automated and stored as a part of the medical record, at which point statistical methods can be used to assess quality of care in a continuous fashion.

Another technique used to improve quality of care is to gather data prospectively from a specific group of patients for administrative, quality-assurance, and research purposes [42,43]. These patients can be automatically identified by computer screening and placed into specific data sets such as trauma, respiratory failure, or cancer registries. These standardized, prospectively gathered databases can then be analyzed for various purposes to provide a basis for quality control, research, and funding. Once again, if properly designed, a large portion of the database may be extracted from the integrated system, eliminating or reducing the need for hand entry.

The design and use of summary reports derived from the database can be very useful in quality control. Timely data on infectious complications, resource utilization, procedures performed, patient demographics, staffing patterns, and outcomes can be very valuable in identifying problems. Once problems are identified, administrative steps can be taken to improve the quality of patient care. [17,63]. It is very important to maximize the benefit/cost ratio. When cost reduction measures are implemented, the assessment of impact on care is critical to assure outcome has not been compromised. Again real-time reports generated from the database can be very valuable in optimizing and managing this process.

Standardization of Care

Most industries have found that standardization of processes improves quality and simultaneously decreases costs. There are many advantages to standardizing care in hospitals, and the computer lends itself nicely to this task. In hospitals where large numbers of a certain types of procedures are performed, such as coronary artery bypass, outcome improves [64]. Much of this improvement is due to the standardization of care that results from case frequency and repetition. Where care is delivered with standardized care protocols, mistakes are reduced. An example use in most intensive care units is in mixing intravenous infusion drugs. If mixed differently each time then administration of incorrect dosages is more common than if the concentration is set by policy and protocol. In addition, patient care is more uniform if all the care team members use the same principles and decision logic from shift-to-shift and day-to-day [65,66].

Standardization can reduce costs by reducing the inventory of required supplies and drugs and by reducing waste and personnel time. With standardization, quality-assurance programs will be strengthened, since it is easier to identify breeches in standards. Once standardization is accepted in the institution, changes that improve care are simplified and more readily accepted.

One of the major problems today is the difficulty in defining guidelines for the care for patients. For example, the process of care of a ventilator-dependent patient can be different depending on the disease being treated, the severity of illness, the hospital or ICU the patient is in, the types of ventilators available, and the practice pattern of the treating physician. Indeed, individual physicians can change their treatment style from day to day. For this reason it is difficult to know if one method of ventilator care is better than another or how to modify the process of care to improve outcome. Standardization of care facilitates the identification of areas where improvement can be made and allows for evaluation of the effectiveness of changes made in the standard [67–74].

One method used to bring standardization into the care environment is to use the computer to guide physician ordering. This has been used effectively in ordering more complex items such as TPN [54]. Using the patient's sex, age, height and weight, and Harris-Benedict equations, the computer can calculate the estimated caloric needs along with a precise mixture of proteins, lipids, and carbohydrates. In addition, factors such as the diagnosis, stress, and organ system dysfunction can be factored into the TPN mix, as determined by the nutritional experts who design the TPN mixing algorithm. The physician is given options for modifying the solution but begins at a standardized starting point that is tailored to the patient's needs. This saves the physician time and effort and reduces ordering errors. Electrolyte concentrations are then suggested based on the patient's latest laboratory data. The physician can select the suggested package or modify it. If the physician selects incompatible or dangerous concentrations, alerts are presented on the screen. Then standard nursing procedures and monitoring are automatically ordered, such as daily intake and output, weights, and every periodic urine glucose monitoring. Thus using the computer, subtle control of the delivery of care is provided through indirect expert guidance or critiquing. The number of calories, composition of nutrients, electrolytes, and nursing care related to the TPN are controlled and the inventory of products reduced [54]. Similar programs for antibiotic ordering [14,15] and blood banking [52,53] have also been developed.

Computer-assisted orders also can improve quality assurance measurements for specific information. An example is the indications for transfusion, which can be recorded for audit purposes and [52] evaluated later for appropriateness. Complications can be reviewed to check for logic errors and deficiencies in the ordering algorithm. In this way, computer-based standardization facilitates the identification of problems and allows for potential solutions to be proposed and validated.

Computer-guided TPN orders are flexible enough to allow the individual physician to maintain control and feel in charge. If designed properly these and similar orders can assist physicians and make their task easier, thus enticing compliance. A more severe type of control can be imposed for specific purposes but requires much more coordination and cooperation to introduce. For research purposes, detailed protocols have been developed that maintain tight control of the process of care [32,67–

74]. Acceptance of such control is limited and is usually resisted by the medical staff, who have been schooled in making decisions tailored to the needs of individual patients and their clinical situation. The proof of such variability in decision-making is lacking and many authors are challenging it by demonstrating inconsistencies in medical practice and decision-making [65]. It is due to this ideation that we are unsure of the benefit of much of the care we now deliver [66]. The use of computerized protocols permits measurement of the process of care in ways that will provide answers to many questions related to the efficacy of various treatments.

Research Uses of the Information System

If the initial obstacles of entering quality data into the information system and of proper coding and storage are overcome, the system becomes a powerful research tool for clinical investigators. The next challenge for clinical investigators is to develop mechanisms for the data in the integrated system to be converted to a format for review and statistical analysis. This can be accomplished in several ways, but one of the most satisfactory is to "download" the desired information into a separate research database, perhaps on a personal computer. The original decisions of coding and storage of data become vital to the process at this point. When research use of the information is contemplated, establishing a coding system is crucial in the system's design.

When designing clinical research projects, one objective is to reduce "noise" as much as possible. One method of accomplishing this task is to develop tight control of the process of care [70–74]. For example, the LDS Hospital group has used this methodology to determine if one method of caring for ventilator patients is superior to another. To answer such a question, both methods of care must be defined and performed in a randomized fashion. This control over the process of care provides the following advantages: 1) it reduces both random and non-random bias in the experiment, 2) it permits investigators to describe precisely in advance the methods of care, and 3) it allows others to verify the results by precisely duplicating the methods [31]. However, the cooperation of all involved physicians, nurses, and therapists is required, along with a commitment to abandon stylistic differences in care and to override the protocols only for valid and identifiable reasons [67,74].

Our experience with development and use of certain computerized protocols is that outcome is improved [68,73]. As the standardization process becomes mature, clinical personnel find it easier to care for patients and want to use the protocols for clinical care outside of the research study [67,72]. The LDS group has found that the computer database can be a powerful tool in running complex protocols and reduces the errors commonly made when paper flowchart protocols are used [26]. Whether it was operation of the protocols per se, or the process of developing the standardization protocols for ventilator care that improved outcome is not clear and will require further research.

Another unique capability of an enterprise-wide database is that all nursing and therapists tasks along with supplies, laboratory, x-rays, and clinical procedures are recorded in the database. From time-motion studies of each of these tasks, personnel time can be measured and the true costs of each task and procedure can be determined. It then becomes possible to calculate from the database the actual cost of caring for patients [75–78]. This allows research in the area of cost, charges, and reimbursement to be performed easily and with greater accuracy than was previously possible, thus adding a valuable dimension to clinical outcomes research efforts.

Logistics of Running and Integrated System

Hardware/Software Failures and Down Time

Nowhere in medicine is there greater need for timely and accurate data than in the ICU. Patients' physiological parameters are changing beat by beat and breath by breath. Fast system-response time and continuous availability are crucial issues that must be achieved before nurses, therapists, and physicians will "trust" and use computer systems. At LDS Hospital in Salt Lake City, the system is available 99.6% of the time. The 0.4% of the time it is not available (on average 5.77 minutes per day) about half the time is for planned downtime for hardware and software maintenance and the other half is for unplanned failures. These unplanned failures could be due to electrical storms, software bugs, hardware failures, etc. Every effort must be taken to minimize downtime. Redundant hardware, battery backed-up power supplies, carefully tested and "debugged" software, system disk backups, and a host of other steps must be taken to achieve reliability [79].

Confidentiality of Computerized Patient Records

Confidentiality of records is a "right" expected by patients in intensive care. Fortunately, public revelation of "confidential" medical data is seldom a problem, but could be in the future. The confidentiality of handwritten paper records is usually maintained by keeping the record in the ICU. Unfortunately the same factors that limit the usefulness of the traditional paper record also provides some measure of security to it. The computerized record can be made so totally secure and confidential that it is too difficult for clinicians to access to care for the patient. Therefore, a balance must be struck between confidentiality and reasonableness of access. Current methods used to allow "reasonable" access to patient records include—

1. Providing employees and physicians with "log-on" codes and requiring their use to review patient data. These codes automatically expire at frequent intervals (six months is typical) and must be changed.
2. Providing access to a limited data set for hospital employees who do not need to access all patient data. Only select management physicians and computer personnel have system wide access
3. Logging every access to clinical information.
4. Automatically logging out workstations left unattended for a predetermined interval.
5. Automatically detecting potential breaches in security (for example, multiple failed log-in attempts), with appropriate alerts to supervisory personnel.

How To Achieve an Integrated Medical Informatics System

The recent Institute of Medicine Report (IOM) states that "the patient record touches, in some way, virtually everyone associated with providing, receiving, or reimbursing health care services" [2]. With computer technology now ubiquitous in our society, there may be a temptation simply to try to connect a patient to a personal computer to do the task. Unfortunately, seemingly simple approaches of using "stand-alone" computers that do not interface with other systems and do not use a structured and integrated approach are doomed to failure. Data integration and communications are the keys to providing the health care professional with something they cannot now achieve with manual charting methods. There must be minimal changes in the user's environment as computers are introduced. Consistency in how data is acquired, the parameters recorded, the frequency of recording, and who records the data is crucially important. Many of the issues are not technological, but "sociological" [80]. A team spirit must exist so that the complex interactions that have been worked out over decades with manual methods can be implemented with computers. Cost of implementation must take into consideration not only the hardware and software costs, but the "people-ware" costs of training users, educating users as to the system benefits, and evaluating those benefits. Over time, the computer system may provide new and better ways of accomplishing patient care tasks that differ from the previous, manual methods.

Conclusions

The expectations of society for medical progress and increased use of computers for diagnosis and treatment are fueled by the increased use of computers in everyday life. Great strides have been made in the understanding of how to harness computer technology to help health care professionals take care of critically ill patients [81]. It seems clear that advances in the use of clinical computers in the hospital and in the ICU will be evolutionary rather than revolutionary. Parts of the health care system will require modification before optimally integrated systems will be widespread [82].

References

1. Leyerle BJ, LoBue M, Shabot MM. The PDMS as a focal point for distributed patient data. Int J Clin Monit Comput 1988; 5:155–161.
2. Dick RS, Steen EB (eds). The Computer-Based Patient Record: An Essential Technology for Health Care. Institute of Medicine. Washington DC. National Academy of Sciences Press, 1991.
3. Gardner RM, Cannon GA, Morris AH, et al. Computerized blood gas interpretation. Med Instrumentation 1974; 8:126.
4. Johnson DS, Ranzenberger J, Herbert R, Gardner RM, Clemmer TP: A Computerized Alert Program for Acutely III Patients. Nurs Administration 1980; 10(6):26–35.
5. Clemmer TP, Gardner RM, Orme JF, Jr. Computer support in critical care medicine. SCAMC 1980; 4:1557–1561.
6. Gardner RM. Computerized management of intensive care patients. MD Comput 1986; 3:36–51.
7. Bradshaw KE, Gardner RM, Pryor TA. Development of a computerized laboratory alerting system. Comp Biomed Res 1989; 22:575–587.
8. Tate KE, Gardner RM, Weaver LK. A computerized laboratory alerting system. MD Comput 1990; 7(5):296–301.
9. Kuperman GJ, Gardner RM, Pryor TA. HELP: A Dynamic Hospital Information System. New York: Springer-Verlag, 1991.
10. Pestotnik SL, Evans RS, Burke JP, Gardner RM, Classen DC. Therapeutic antibiotic monitoring: Surveillance using a computerized expert system. Am J Med 1990; 88:43–48.
11. Evans RS. The HELP system: A review of clinical applications in infectious disease and antibiotic use. MD Comput 1991; 8:282–288.
12. Classen DC, Pestotnik SL, Evans RS, Burke JP. Computerized surveillance of adverse drug events in hospital patients. JAMA 1991; 266:2847–2851.
13. Evans RS, Gardner RM, Bush AR, Burke JP, Jacobson JA, Larsen RA, Meier FA, Warner HR. Development of a computerized infectious disease monitor (CIDM). Comp Biomed Res 1985; 18:103–113.
14. Larsen RA, Evans RS, Burke JP, Pestotnik SL, Gardner RM, Classen DC. Improved perioperative antibiotic use and reduced surgical wound infections through use of computer decision analysis. Infect Control Hosp Epidemiol 1989; 10:316–320.
15. Evans RS, Pestotnik SL, Burke JP, Gardner RM, Larsen RA, Classen DC. Reducing the duration of prophylactic antibiotics use through computer monitoring of surgical patients. DICP, Ann Pharmacother 1990; 24:351–354.
16. Shabot MM, LoBue M, Leyerle BJ, Dubin SB. Decision support alerts for

clinical laboratory and blood gas data. Int J Clin Monit Comput 1990; 7:27–31.

17. Bradshaw KE, Sittig DF, Gardner RM, Pryor TA, Budd M. Computer-based data entry for nurses in the ICU. MD Comput 1989; 6(5):274–280.

18. Gardner RM, Tariq H, Hawley WL, East TD. Medical Information Bus: The key to future integrated monitoring (Editorial). Int J Clin Monit Comput 1989; 6:205–209.

19. Gardner RM, Hawley WH, East TD, Oniki T, Young HFW. Real time data acquisition: Experience with the Medical Information Bus (MIB) SCAMC 1991; 15:813–817.

20. Gardner RM, Hawley WH, East TD, Oniki T, Young HFW. Real time data acquisition: Recommendations for the Medical Information Bus (MIB). Int J Clin Monit Comput 1991; 8:251–258.

21. East TD, Yang W, Tariq H, Gardner RM. The IEEE medical information bus of respiratory care. Crit Care Med 1989; 17:580.

22. Shabot MM, LoBue M, Leyerle BJ: An automatic PDMS Interface for the Urotrack Plus 220 urimeter. Int J Clin Monit Comput 1988;5:125.

23. Shabot MM. Standaraized acquisition of bedside data: The IEEE P1073 medical information bus. Int J Clin Monit Comput 1989; 6:197–204.

24. Gardner RM, Clemmer TP, Morris AH: Computerized Medical Decision-Making—An Evaluation in Acute Care. Conference on Computers in Critical Care and Pulmonary Medicine (Lund, Sweden), June 1980.

25. Toong HD, Gupta A. Personal computers. Sci Am 1982; 247(12):87–105.

26. Henderson S, Crapo RO, East TD, Morris AH, Gardner, RM. Computerized clinical protocols in an intensive care unit: How well are they followed? SCAMC 1990; 14:284–288.

27. Brahams D, Wyatt J. Medicine and the law. The Lancet 1989; Sept 9, 632–634.

28. Gravenstein JS, DeVries A Jr, Beneken JFW. Sampling intervals of clinical monitoring variables during anesthesia. J Clin Monit 1989; 5:17–21.

29. Bradshaw KE, Gardner RM, Clemmer TP, Orme JF Jr, Thomas F, West BJ. Physician decision-making—Evaluation of data used in a computerized ICU. Int J Clin Monit Comput 1984; 1:81–91.

30. Knaus WA, Wagner DP, Lynn J. Short-term mortality predictions for critically ill hospitalized adults: Science and ethics. Science 1991; 254:389–394.

31. Sittig DF, Gardner RM, Morris AH, Wallace CJ. Clinical evaluation of computer-based, respiratory care algorithms. Int J Clin Monit Comput 1990; 7:177–185.

32. Sittig DF, Gardner RM, Pace NL, Morris AH, Beck E. Computerized management of patient care in a complex, controlled clinical trial in the intensive care unit. Comp Meth Prog Biomedicine 1989; 30:77–84.

33. Gardner RM, Laub RM, Golubjatnikov OK, Evans RS, Jacobson JT. Computer citiqued blood ordering using the HELP system. Comp Biomed Res 1990; 23:514–528.

34. Pryor TA, Gardner RM, Clayton PD, Warner HR. The HELP system. J Med Systems 1983; 7:87–102.

35. Pryor TA. The HELP medical record system. MD Comput 1988; 5:22–33.

36. McDonald CJ. The search for national standards for medical data exchange. MD Comput 1984; 1:3–4.

37. McDonald CJ. Interchange standards revisited. MD Comput 1990; 7:72–74.
38. McDonald CJ, Hammond WE. Editorial. Standard formats for electronic transfer of clinical data. Ann Intern Med 1989; 110:333–335.
39. Report to Congress: The feasibility of linking research-related data bases to Federal and Non-Federal Medical Administrative data bases. Agency for Health Care Policy and Research. April 1991. AHCPR Pub. No. 91-003.
40. Report to Congress: Progress of Research on Outcomes of Health Care Services and Procedures. Agency for Health Care Policy and Research. May 1991. AHCPR Pub. No. 91-004.
41. Gardner RM, Scoville DP, West BJ, Cundick RM Jr, Clemmer TP. Integrated computer systems for monitoring of the critically ill. SCAMC 1977; 1:301–307.
42. Sittig DF, Gardner RM, Elliott CG. Screening for adult respiratory distress syndrome patients: Use of the HELP hospital information system. J Clin Engin 1989; 14:237–243.
43. Evans RS, Burke JP, Classen DC, Gardner RM, Menlove RL, Goodrich KM, Stevens LE, Pestotnik SL. Computerized identification of patients at high risk for hospital-acquired infections. Am J Infect Control 1992; 20:4–10.
44. Gardner RM, Clemmer TP: Computerized protocols applied to emergency and acute care. J Emerg Med Serv 1987; 7(6):90–93.
45. Helander M (ed). Handbook of human-Computer Interaction. 2nd ed. Elsevier: North-Holland, New York, 1991.
46. Coie WG. Quick and accurate monitoring via metaphor graphics. SCAMC 14: 1900:425–429.
47. McDonald CJ. Protocol-based computer reminders, the quality of care and the non-perfectibility of man. N Engl J Med 1976; 295:1351–1355.
48. Hulse RK, Clark SJ, Jackson JC, Warner HR, Gardner RM. Computerized medication monitoring system. Am J Hosp Pharm 1976; 33:1061–1064.
49. Gardner RM, Clemmer TP, Larsen KG, Johnson DS: Computerized Alert System Use in Clinical Medicine. Proceedings of the 32nd Annual Conference of Engineering in Medicine and Biology (Denver, Colorado), pp 1–5, 1979.
50. Gardner RM, Hulse RK, Larsen KG. Assessing the effectiveness of a computerized pharmacy system. SCAMC 1990; 14:668–672.
51. Miller PL. Goal-directed critiquing by computer: Ventilator management. Comp Biomed Res 1985; 18:422–438.
52. Lepage ER, Gardner RM, Laub RM, Jacobson JT. Assessing the effectiveness of a computerized blood order "consultant" system. SCAMC 1991; 15:33–37.
53. Lepage EF, Gardner RM, Laub RM, Golubjatnikov OK. Improving blood transfusion practice: Role of a computerized hospital information system. Transfusion 1992; 32:253–259.
54. Larsen KG, Clemmer TP, Nicholson L, Conti MT, Peterson H: Computer support in monitoring of nutritional therapy. Nutritional Support Services 1983; 3(6):7–16.
55. Elliott CG. Computer-assisted quality assurance: Development and performance of a respiratory care program. QRB 1991; 17:85–89.
56. Evans RS, Pestotnik SL, Classen DC, Bass, SB, Menlove RL, Gardner RM, Burke JP. Development of a Computerized Adverse Drug Event Monitor. SCAMC 1991; 15:231–27.

57. Knaus WA, Draper EA, Wagner DP, Zimmerman JE, Branbaum ML, Cullen DJ, Kohles MK, Shin B, Snyder J. Evaluating outcome from intensive care in majormedical centers. Ann Intern Med 1986; 104:408–410.

58. Shabot MM, Leyerle BJ, LoBue M. Automatic extraction of intensity-intervention scores from a computerized surgical Intensive Care Unit flowsheet. Am J Surg 1987; 154:72–78.

59. Cullen DJ, Civetta JM, Briggs BA, et al. Therapeutic intervention scoring system: A method for quantitative comparison of patient care. Crit Care Med 1974; 2:57.

60. MacKenzie EJ, Steinwachs DM, Shankar BS, et al. An ICD-9-CM to AIS conversion table: Development and application. Montreal, Quebec, American Association for Automotive Medicine, Thirteenth Annual Proceedings, Oct 1986.

61. Baker SP, O'Neill B, Hadden W Jr, et al. The Injury Severity Score: A method for describing patients with multiple injuries and evaluating emergency care. J Trauma 1974; 14:187–196.

62. Horn SD, Sharkey PD, Buckle JM, Backofen JE, Averill RF, Horn RA. The relationship between severity of illness and hospital length of stay and mortality. Medical Care 1991; 305–317.

63. Kuperman GJ, Maack BB, Bauer K, Gardner RM. Impact of the HELP system on the LDS Hospital Medical Record. Top Health Rec Manage 1991; 12:76–85.

64. Berwick DM. The double edge of knowledge. JAMA 1991: 266:841–842.

65. Eddy DM. Clinical decision making from theory to practice: The challenge. JAMA 1990; 263:287–290.

66. Eddy DM. Clinical decision making from theory to practice: Anatomy of a decision. JAMA 1990; 263:441–443.

67. East TD, Morris AH, Clemmer TP, Orme JF Jr, Wallace CJ, Henderson S, Sittig DF, Gardner RM: Development of computerized critical care patients—A strategy that really works! SCAMC 1990; 14:564–568.

68. Morris AH, Wallace CJ, Clemmer TP, Orme JF Jr, Weaver LK, Dean NC, Butler S, Suchyta MR, East TD, Sittig DF: extracorporeal CO_2 removal therapy for adult respiratory distress syndrome patients: A computerized protocol controlled trial reanimation soins intensifs medecine d'urgence 1990; 6:485–490.

69. East TD, Bohm SH, Peng L, Wallace CJ, Clemmer TP, Weaver LK, Orme JF Jr, Hoffmann BH, Henderson S, Pace NL, Morris AH: A successful computerized protocol for clinical management of PC-IRV in ARDS patients. Chest 1992; 101:697–710.

70. East TD, Morris AH, Clemmer TP, Orme JF Jr, Wallace CJ, Henderson S, Sittig DF, Gardner, RM. Development of computerized critical care protocols—A strategy that really works! SCAMC 1990; 14:564–568.

71. East TD, Henderson S, Morris AH, Gardner RM. Implementation issues and challenges for computerized clinical protocols for management of mechanical ventilation in ARDS patients. SCAMC 1989; 13:583–587.

72. Henderson S, East TD, Morris AH, Gardner RM. Performance evaluation of computerized clinical protocols for management of arterial hypoxemia in ARDS patients. SCAMC 1989; 13:588–592.

73. Suchyta MR, Clemmer TP, Orme JF Jr, Morris AH, Elliott CG. Increased

survival of ARDS patients with severe hypoxemia (ECMO criteria). Chest 1991; 99:951–955.

74. Henderson S, Crapo RO, Wallace CJ, East TD, Morris AH, Gardner RM. Performance of computerized protocols for management of arterial oxygenation in an intensive care unit. Int J Clin Monit Comput 1992; 8:271–280.

75. Thomas F, Larsen K, Clemmer TP, Burke JP, Orme JF Jr, Napoli M, Christison E: Impact of prospective payment on a tertiary care center receiving large numbers of critically ill patients by aeromedical transport. Criti Care Med 1986; 14:227–230.

76. Thomas F, Fox J, Clemmer TP, Orme JF Jr, Vincent GM, Menlove RL: The financial impact of medicare diagnosis-related groups. Effect upon hospitals receiving cardiac patients referred for tertiary care. Chest 1987; 91(3):418–423.

77. Thomas F, Clemmer TP, Larsen KG, Menlove RL, Orme JF Jr, Christison EA: The severity, outcome, cost of care, and economic impact under DRG payment policies of trauma patients referred to a major trauma center. Trauma 1988; 28:446–452.

78. Clemmer TP, Orme JF Jr, Thomas FO, Peterson M, Merrow L, Peterson H: The impact of medicare prospective reimbursement system on nutritional support service patients: The importance of pass throughs. JPEN 1989; 13:71–76.

79. Gray J, Siewiorek DP. High-availability computer systems. Computer 1991; 24(9):39–48.

80. Lundsgaarde HP, Gardner RM, Menlove RL. Using attitudinal questionnaires to achieve benefits optimization. SCAMC 1989; 13:703–708.

81. Gardner RM, Shabot MM. Computerized ICU data management: Piftalls and promises. Int J Clin Monit Comput 1990; 7:99–105.

82. Rand T. Automated records aren't such a stretch. Healthweek September 9, 1991; 5(17):4–8.

Chapter 2
Computers in Critical Care: A Historical Perspective
David A. Trace and Max Harry Weil

Introduction

Computers were initially introduced to the bedside in conjunction with patient monitoring in the critical care environment [1]. In 1960, a decade prior to the introduction of minicomputers and two [2] decades prior to the introduction of conventional free-standing microprocessors, the potential of computer techniques was recognized. Computers were subsequently viewed as a means for facilitating patient data accumulation and computation [2,3]. Somewhat later their application was anticipated to include the control of bedside instrumentation. As such, they were conceived to be medical adaptations of the process control devices so widely used in industrial operations. This was with the intent to reduce the laborious monitoring, record-keeping, computational, and mechanical nursing routines performed at the bedside of patients who were critically ill. These patients—who required blood sampling, fluid infusion, urine and other body fluid measurements, and the use of more complex life-support systems including ventilators, pacemakers, cardiac assist devices, and dialysis—created formidable process control challenges for the bedside staff [4,5].

Incentives for the Use of Computer Systems

The incentives for computer use were present, therefore, in several domains. First, there was a very rapid expansion of technology at the bedside together with an increasing commitment to direct patient care by both physicians and nurses. During the earlier years, it was primarily patient monitoring of cardiovascular and pulmonary function which was to be facilitated by digital processing methodologies [6–8]. These came into routine use as analog operations in the early 1960s, e.g., the electrocardiogram, central venous and arterial pressures, and respiratory gas exchange [9–11].

With increasing bedside demands and therefore staffing requirements (both medical and nursing), perhaps the greatest anticipation of benefit was in the areas as alarms and automation (in order to reduce demands on staff). There was ever-increasing tension between the commitment to direct care of the patient at the bedside and the expansion of bedside technology. In parallel with the rapid expansion of coronary and intensive care units and the increased demand for skilled physician and nursing personnel, hospitals faced equally formidable staffing shortages due to the limited number of available nursing specialists to care for the critically ill. Administrators were often required to restrict not only the addition of new beds but also occupancy of already existing intensive care beds. Accordingly, budgets were readily provided for implementation of computer systems which were viewed as at least partial solutions to these personnel crises [12].

It was this situation that gave rise to the intense interest in computer-based methods which would provide automation. The most optimistic view was that it would increase efficiency and thereby reduce the impact of critical shortages of available personnel. The more tempered viewpoint was that the demand created by a remarkably rapid expansion of bedside technology could be met without further increases in personnel. By reducing the demands for manual record-keeping and especially the duplication of data recording from a diversity of hospital sites, early workers envisioned "total hospital automation" [13]. This included electronic telecommunication with the x-ray and other imaging departments, the central laboratory, pharmacy, dietary, medical records, and ambulatory care for scheduling, data transmission, billing, and inventory of equipment and supplies [14]. The early designers, system analysts, and programmers of centralized computer systems were optimistic that this would evolve on a par with the complex multi-site operation, control, and information systems introduced by large industry. Even more sophisticated options— including trend analysis of monitored and laboratory data [15], quantitation of severity of patient illness [16], and the inclusion of conventional medical records with textual, numerical, and graphic data—were proposed [17]. These had the additional promise of near optimal legibility and "user-friendly" format for review and interpretation by the clinicians [18–19]. The concept of computer-based automation at the bedside emphasized digital processing techniques for "intelligent" alarm setting by tracking multiple parameters. For instance, the traditional dependence on the electrocardiogram for alarms was to be complemented by the simultaneous acquisition of the arterial pressure pulse, such that erroneous cardiac arrest alarms would be minimized. If the pressure pulse was unchanged even though there was a fallacious "straight line" electrocardiogram, this did not constitute a high-level alarm indicating cardiac arrest.

Since the shortage of available critical care beds led to competition for admission (and discharge) of patients, there was early recognition that objective criteria were needed to guide physicians and nursing specialists in the triage process. Accordingly, there was and continues to be a high level of interest in severity measures and outcome predictors which might facilitate such triage [20,21] The objectivity of data acquired by digital systems was heralded as a potential advantage, not only for quality control and triage, but also for more precise historical documentation of the medical record, especially at the time of acute life-threatening crises such as respiratory or cardiac arrest [22].

In more recent years, the emphasis on cost containment also emerged as a major incentive for introducing computer technology to the bedside. In the past 30 years, the number of critical care beds has expanded to the extent that more than 10% of hospitalized patients are cared for in critical care units, which cost approximately three times more than general medical-surgical beds. Accordingly, as much as 30% of total hospital cost is currently accounted for by critical care services. Looking to the future, the entire in-patient service of acute care hospitals is emerging as one very large critical care service. If computers, in fact, would improve the efficiency of operation for this subset of patients, it would be likely to have a disproportionate effect on the costs of hospital operation [23,24].

In the light of these incentives, we will address the historical development of computers at the bedside and the extent to which these anticipated benefits have been realized. We will also review some of the historical development of the hardware and the software in relationship to both general and specific applications to bedside management. Based on our personal experience and the documented progress in the field, we shall briefly pinpoint not only the accomplishments but also the problems that have thwarted many of the optimistic predictions. Finally, we will conclude with what we hope will represent a balanced assessment of the practical place of computers at the bedside of the critically ill as of the time of this writing.

History

The earliest bedside computer was installed at the University of Southern California and the Los Angeles County Hospital in 1961 [1,25,26]. It was an IBM 1710 system, which served four beds in what was then known as the "shock ward" (Fig. 2.1). The shock ward was the predecessor to the intensive care units at that hospital. The system included a central processor which had 20 kilobytes of core storage. There was as yet no alphanumeric input capability but only a remote punch-card reader or, at the bedside, a total of 12 ten-position thumb wheels for entry of codes. This, of course, evolved in an era in which only machine language was available

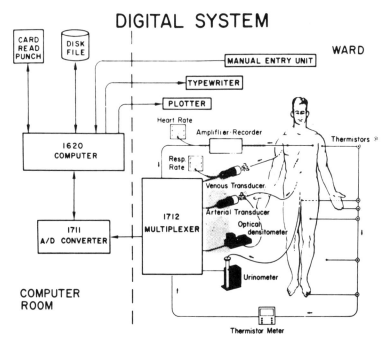

Figure 2.1. IBM 1710 ICU computer system in the Shock Ward of the Los Angeles County-University of Southern California Medical Center. This is the earliest recorded use of computers in the care of critically ill patients (1961). (Reprinted with permission from [25].)

and this long preceded the availability of current alphanumeric keyboards. A Sanborn physiological monitor system was the primary source of analog data. It included the electrocardiogram, the arterial pressure, the central venous pressure, the optical density of arterial blood for measuring dye concentrations in conjunction with cardiac output measurements, body and skin temperature measurements, a primitive urinometer for measuring the urine output, and provisions for either manual input of numerical data relating either directly to the patient (including age, height, weight, etc.) or manual input of laboratory data (Fig. 2.2) [27–29].

Analog signals were transmitted through appropriate amplifiers and signal conditioners to the computer's analog-to-digital converters. The system provided appropriate gain factors to allow for the input of signals ranging from 0.1 to 3.0 V under program control. The programs themselves were stored on a fixed disk. Special operations such as the measurement of cardiac output from a dye dilution curve were initiated by ward personnel through custom-made manual entry units and with the aid of of the thumb-wheel entries. The bedside operator was also able to

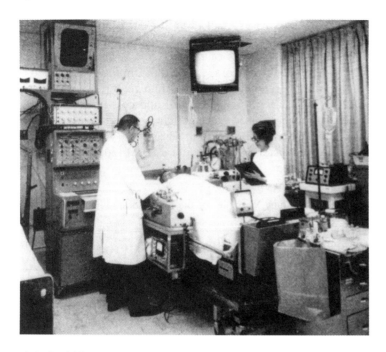

Figure 2.2. Bedside analog instrumentation, video displays, and closed circuit television monitor for teletype output.

instruct the computer to cycle at defined intervals of as little as one or as much as 60 mins for digitizing continuously monitored measurements. For practical purposes, the system was operated so as to digitize and display measurements at time intervals of 5 min. The maximum rate at which analog signals could be converted at that time was 200 samples per second, and this limited the time available for monitoring multiple parameters involving the high-frequency signals of the arterial pressure pulse and the electrocardiogram. Continuous monitoring of multiple parameters by digital methods was not yet developed.

Interpretive programs were then developed such that the "R" wave of the electrocardiogram could be identified by the magnitude of its slope. Diastolic and systolic pressures were recorded as minimal and maximal values. Intervals between such measurements integrated over a 10-sec period provided measurement of rate. Excessive noise or drift in either the electrocardiographic or the blood pressure signals were obviated by averaging values over five successive 2-sec intervals.

The cardiac output was computed by integration of the dye dilution curve. Blood gas and blood chemistry data were entered into the system through the same type of thumb wheel manual entry units except that the entry units were duplicated at a remote site in a laboratory adjoining the shock ward. The system was evolved such that more than 100 programs were developed which consisted of a total of approximately 100,000 instruction words. The capability of the system was limited by a maximum of 20,000 characters of core storage and a maximum of 2,000,000 characters of disk storage. Even though this system required a computer room which was equal in size to the ward itself and cost in excess of $500,000 (in 1961 dollars), its capability was less than one-hundredth of that of current midsize desktop microprocessors. The primary and display variables provided for by this system are listed in Table 2.1 [30].

Table 2.1. Primary Display Variables of the First Computerized ICU Data Management System

Primary measurement (channel)	Derived variable	Printout abbreviations
Arterial pressure	Systolic	SP
	Diastolic	DP
	Mean arterial	MAP
	Variotion between highest and lowest stystolic pressures in read interval	ΔS
	Pulse rate	PR
Venous pressure	Mean venous pressure	MVP
	Resiratory rate	PR
Electrocardiogram	Heart rate	HR
Temperature, rectal	Rectal temperature	RECT
Temperature, finger	Temperature of finger	FING
Temperature, toe	Temperature of toe	TOE
Temperature, thigh	Temperature of thigh	THIG
Temperature, arm	Temperature of arm	DEL
Temperature, air	Temperature of ambient air	AMB
	Cardiac output	CO
	Cardiac index/weight	CIW
	Cardiac index/area	CIA
Optical density of arterial blood	Work done by heart	WK
	Work done by heart per beat	SWK
		RES
	Resistance of circulatory system	CBV
	Central body blood volume	MCT
	Mean circulation time	ATC
	Appearance time	
Urine output	Urine output/hr	U60
	Urine output in last 5 min	U05

Modified from Rockweel MA Jr., Shubin H, Weil MH, et al. SHOCK III, A computer system as an aid in the management of critically ill patients. Communications of the ACM 1966; 9(5):355–357.

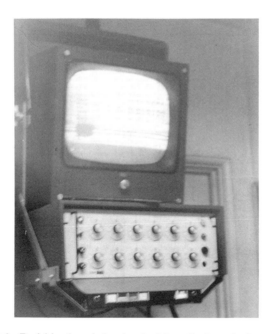

Figure 2.3. Bedside closed circuit television display of teletype output.

There was no bedside video display capability. In fact, the only source of data was a teletypewriter. A closed-circuit television system by which the typewriter output would be displayed on a television monitor was therefore, installed above the bedside (Fig. 2.3). Additionally, a digital plotter was included in the system for hard-copy display of graphic data. Such plotting was time-consuming and was time-competitive with real-time data acquisition.

Nevertheless, this prototype system demonstrated the feasibility of "on-line" acquisition, processing, and display of data from seriously ill patients (Fig. 2.4). It did prove useful for the clinical management of patients and especially so in a research unit in which reliability of data acquisition and the capability for increased frequency of data collection were major assets. It also demonstrated initial acceptance of computer systems in the critical care environment and established the capability of computer systems to identify trends in the clinical course. This was regarded as directly helpful for the management of a wide variety of life-threatening disease states [32]. For practical purposes, the computer generated what was equivalent to manually charted "time-lines" (Fig. 2.5); introduced the concept of continuous versus intermittent data acquisition; and, like in-flight data recorders, provided historical documentation for later review and disclosure of information which would otherwise have escaped detection (Fig. 2.6) [33].

At approximately the same time, hand-held calculators came into use

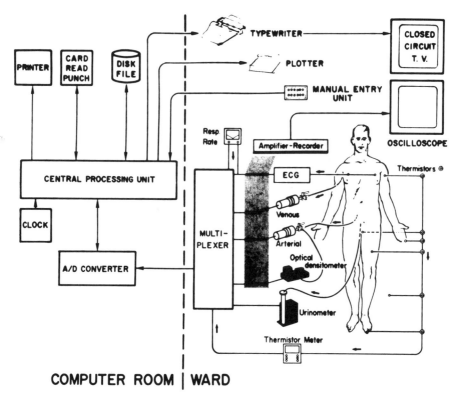

Figure 2.4. Schematic diagram of bedside and computer room equipment in 1966. (Reprinted with permission from [10].)

```
PATIENT 0522 BED 1 DATE 06-20-65

TIME    SP MAP    ΔS   HR   RECT TOE THIG
HRS     DP MVP    RR   PR   AMB  DEL FING
2380*
07-38 121 085   008 112 39.2 34.4 38.1
182.8 059 00.6 029 112 21.9 37.2 37.9
2381*
07-43 117 082   008 110 39.2 34.4 38.1
182.9 058 00.4 028 110 22.1 37.2 37.9
2382*
07-48 114 084   009 110 39.3 34.4 38.2
182.9 061 00.7 032 110 22.2 37.2 37.9
```

Figure 2.5. "Time line" printout of hemodynamic data. (Reprinted with permission from [27].)

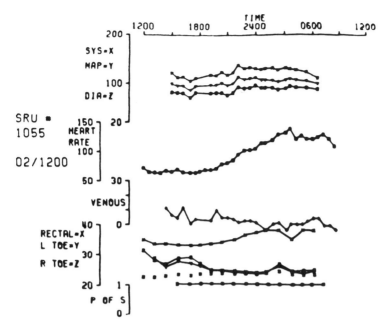

Figure 2.6. Graphical display of hemodynamic data. (Reprinted with permission from [12].)

in critical care units [34]. These were initially used for calculation of derived variables such as the cardiac output normalized against body surface area and peripheral resistance from measurements of cardiac output and mean arterial pressure. The options were rapidly expanded such that a large inventory of hemodynamic variables based on measurements of arterial, pulmonary artery, and central venous pressures; cardiac output and heart rate, including cardiac index, mean arterial pressure, stroke volume and stroke volume index, systemic vascular resistance and its index, pulmonary vascular resistance; and measurements of both left- and right-sided cardiac work and stroke work were indexed to the patient's body surface area [35]. Derived measurements on gas exchange from measurements of arterial and mixed venous blood gases and oxygen concentrations of inspired gas were also calculated [36]. Accordingly, arterial venous oxygen differences, oxygen consumption, oxygen extraction, and pulmonary arterial venous shunts were calculated, displayed and, in some instances, printed (Fig. 2.7). Measurements on serum and urine provided derived measurements of renal functions [37]. Nutritional prescriptions, based on caloric requirements and appropriate concentrations of glucose, nitrogen, and fat mixtures were calculated with the aid of such hand-held devices [38]. Programmable calculators were also used for calculation of doses, dilutions, and infusion rates of commonly used parenteral drugs, including vasopressor agents and aminoglycoside antibiotics [39]. For

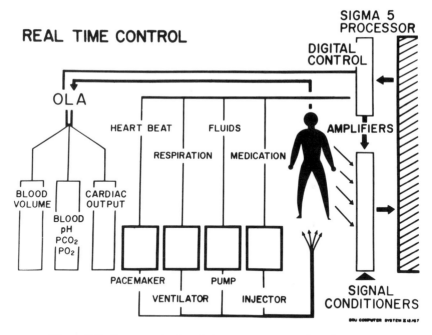

Figure 2.7. Computerized real time process control environment.

practical purposes, however, their benefit was restricted to the "massaging" of numbers which were manually entered. To that extent, they had a significant impact on decision-making but little direct impact on the monitoring process itself or on the efficiency of bedside data acquisition, alarms, or process controls.

External to the intensive care unit, there were early and impressive software developments for graphic analyses. Perhaps the most important of these was in electrocardiographic diagnosis [11,40]. These were subsequently applied to the monitoring of patients in coronary care units for dysrhythmia detection, diagnosis, and alarms. Heretofore, electrocardiographic alarms were based largely on electrocardiographically determined heart rates with analog systems in which alarms were triggered by increases or decreases in heart rate which fell outside of predetermined limits.

The expansion in the number and in the complexity of clinical laboratory tests in the 1960s and 1970s also prompted the use of process control and data management systems in the clinical laboratory [41,42]. Since this was a more conventional process control and data management operation which had much greater kinship to that of industry, laboratory automation advanced very rapidly (Fig. 2.7). This was to a large extent facilitated by the introduction of specialized digital microprocessors which made it possible to preprocess the output of analytical devices. The analytical devices were then linked to a central data acquisition system so that a comprehensive record of the results of laboratory analyses was generated and available for electronic transmission to remote sites, including the intensive care unit [43,44]. Because the instrumentation was now automated and, in many instances, required minimal operator skill, such devices became increasingly intelligent. They subsequently evolved as free-standing devices, which made it possible to bring them closer to the bedside. Indeed, computer-controlled, automated blood gas analyzers became commonplace in intensive care units, so that the bedside personnel could obtain immediate measurements without the constraint of transport of a specimen to the laboratory. Because the analyzers were provided with substantial "intelligence," the non-technologist operator would be prompted to perform the analysis correctly or otherwise confront error signals. With further expansion of the microprocessor technology, interpretations of measured data and especially blood gas values were available without dependence on a centralized host computer [45].

Specialized computer-based systems were also developed for the pulmonary function laboratory [46]. These subsequently found their way to the bedside for the purposes of pulmonary assessments (Fig. 2.8). Indeed they also became components of increasingly more elaborate mechanical ventilators. When these were endowed with "intelligence," they facili-

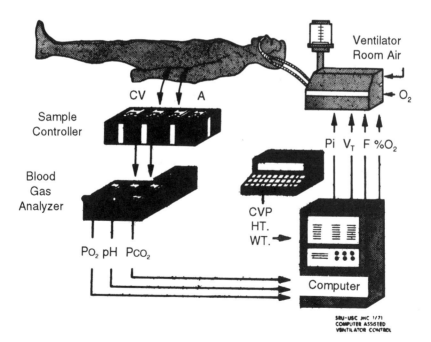

Figure 2.8. Computer assisted ventilator control.

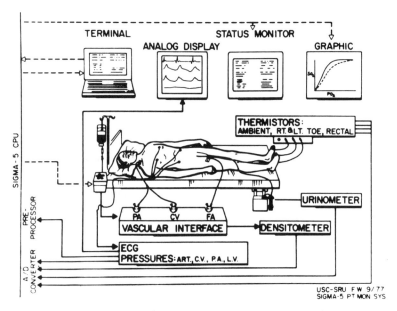

Figure 2.9. Second-generation ICU computer system for monitoring and data management (1977). (Reprinted with permission from [41].)

tated operation and alarms, thereby increasing the precision and safety of mechanical ventilation.

Since the control of volumes and infusion rates of blood and fluids and especially the simultaneous administration of several fluid mixtures involved risks and commanded much time commitment on the part of the nursing staff at the bedside, increasing automation of infusion systems was sought. Increasing precision in the rate of infusion; alarms which alerted the bedside staff to inappropriate operation of the pump or depletion of the fluid reservoir; and, more recently, a cumulative record which served a computer-generated intake-output record of fluids came to the fore with the development of automated infusion pumps (Fig. 2.9) [47–49].

In some instances, the separate operations of monitoring and recording of treatment were joined as part of a larger management system linked to medical informatics [50,51]. However, such systems are still evolving and, at this time, such integration remains a technically formidable challenge.

Hardware Development

With the rapid expansion of critical care medicine and both general and specialized intensive care units, a large market was created for both the conventional computer and for the more specialized medical electronics industries. As described above, there was rapid development of comprehensive monitoring systems with initial emphasis on electrocardiographic monitoring and, soon thereafter, hemodynamic monitoring. The typical system consisted of bedside electronic devices which included preamplifiers, amplifiers, and cathode ray oscilloscopes. The systems accepted the output from pressure transducers for analog display of the arterial pressure pulses. Prior to the 1970s and until the Swan-Ganz catheter was introduced, central venous pressure was usually monitored by a water monometer system [52]. After the balloon-tip catheter came into wide use in the mid-1970s, the monitoring systems were expanded to include additional channels for measurement of pulmonary artery and pulmonary artery occlusive pressures. Parallel developments for the cardiac catheterization laboratory and for intra-operative and postoperative cardiac surgical monitoring of hemodynamic variables accelerated development of the technology. The catheterization laboratory table, the operating table, and the intensive care bedside systems were often networked to central stations both for purposes of data display and alarms and for generation of a hard-copy record [53]. In larger centers, monitoring technicians evolved who would provide dedicated surveillance with the capability of responding very rapidly to an alarm. The alarms themselves would trigger the printing of a hard-copy record, especially the electrocardiogram. Accordingly, analog records of the electrocardiogram and subsequently of pressure pulses would be pasted into nursing notes to document events.

Until the microprocessor technology had fully evolved in the late 1970s, bedside instrumentation consisted of almost entirely analog devices. Their output was in many instances transmitted to a remote site, converted to a digital signal, and then processed by a mainframe computer. As lower-cost mini computer systems, emerged in the late 1960s, they became widely used as central processors. These "workstations" provided capability for both analog and digital displays, computations, and entry of alphanumeric text suitable for inclusion in the medical record. They also provided links to support services—namely, the laboratory, the radiology department, and the pharmacy—and provided data on patient location, vital data, scheduling, billing, inventory, and designation of clinical severity in answer to inquiries by family or hospital public relations personnel [54].

After microprocessor technology more fully emerged, analog systems became essentially obsolete. The bedside was then endowed with an "intelligent" device, and the capabilities for local alphanumeric input, computation, more elaborate and software-driven alarms, and expansion to accommodate other sensors—including those for temperature measurement, cardiac output measurement, expired gas measurements, multiple pressure measurements, infusion pumps, volume output measuring devices, and especially a urinometer—were implemented. External devices, including ventilators, external transvenous pacemakers, and even defibrillators, were subsequently integrated with the bedside system. The number of data items that could be measured at the bedside, then displayed and recorded has continued to expand. More recently, pulse oximetry, trancutaneous gas measurements, airway volumes and pressures, oxygen saturation of mixed venous blood, and even directly measured patient weight with load cells attached to the bed have been accommodated by the bedside microprocessor systems. The electronic capabilities for analog to digital conversion and the efficiency by which the system could accommodate high-frequency sampling were instrumental in the rapid development of this clinical technology [55].

Display capabilities were also greatly expanded. Initially, the clinician could only focus on two or three electrocardiographic or pressure pulses. With continuous scanning and greatly expanded local memory, it was possible to look at, recapture, and replay the entire sequence of events and thereby identify and document the events which preceded, accompanied, and followed an acute change in the status of the patient at the bedside. The displays themselves were enhanced by alphanumeric labeling of parameters, digital display of the numerical pressure values, frequencies, regularity, and even morphology of the analog display and capability for selecting continuous, intermittent, or alternative displays on a video screen.

The systems became more user-friendly. This, in part, evolved in parallel with giant strides in the development of sensors. For instance, the availability of electrocardiographic silver-silver chloride electrodes provided a major benefit in the reliability and fidelity of the electrocardiographic signal. There were comparable advances in pressure transducer technology, including the emergence of disposable high-sensitivity, high-fidelty, and miniaturized pressure measuring devices. Calibration became automated. Electrical calibration of such pressure transducers greatly reduced both the labor and the variability of pressure calibration, which previously required an external and cumbersome mercury manometer. Accordingly, many of the knobs and buttons at the bedside became obsolete. Indeed, the vast majority of operations of current systems provide for operation with either an alphanumeric keyboard or a keypad external to the computer and the preprocessing devices rather than knobs or switches.

The intelligence capabilities of the bedside system provided increasing options by which it could serve as an expert system. The bedside staff could be alerted to are electrocardiographic electrode or an arterial catheter "disconnect" rather than to a more general alarm. The monitored data, particularly when complemented by numerical text entered by the physicians, nurses, and technicians, could be reviewed and, in many instances, plotted to identify trends [56,57]. The system was increasingly adapted for estimation of severity of illness, including the APACHE (Acute Physiology And Chronic Health Evaluation) Score, which was implemented on-line [58]. Current efforts to develop software for medical decision-making, including diagnostic and therapeutic products, have substantial promise. The intensive effort in medical informatics to have data acquisition, alarms, and process-control operations are complement decision-making with quality controls is likely to yield increasing benefits. Equally impressive is the potential capability of expanding the systems' "intelligence" for diagnastic and treatment [55,59].

Limitations

The current status of medical practice, in part fostered by the remarkable capability of comprehensive physiological monitoring, makes it inappropriate to look to anatomical pathology as the ultimate arbitrator for determining causes of death. Sudden death, for instance, is unequivocally identified on the basis of such monitoring, whereas are anatomical explanation for the death may be substantially more remote, especially in the current epidemic of "sudden death" due to coronary artery disease. The moment-to-moment capability for identifying crises or for monitoring the effects of intervention through the use of modern digital systems leads to lower mortality. Admittedly, there continues to be debate regarding the actual benefits thereof with regard to meaningful survival for many of these patients. Yet, there is now consensus that at least in one domain, namely, in the case of the premature neonate, these techniques have had a remarkable impact on meaningful survival [60,61].

The greatest limitation in the present application of such systems is not the system itself, but rather the manner in which it is used. A remarkably large menu of parameters can be and are transduced, digitized, computed, displayed, and even intelligently interpreted. However, the severity and course of life-threatening illness is almost always contingent on only a small number of parameters, typically two or three [62,63]. What is to be measured, therefore, is contingent on competent understanding of the nature of the underlying disease state or injury. Accordingly, the plethora of measurements that the clinician is currently able to monitor is likely to prove counterproductive if they are not used selectively.

As yet, clinical diagnosis and management is contingent on conventional methods of medical observation and measurements other than those that are provided directly by the monitoring system. For instance, underlying causes, be they infectious endocarditis or other life-threatening infections; auto-immune processes; traumatic injuries to the head, abdomen or extremities; or immediately life-threatening endocrinopathies must be identified by conventional methods of history, physical examination, imaging, and highly select and generally not directly monitored laboratory data. Accordingly, if the clinician regards the system as the ultimate resource without dedication to continuing clinical examination, the benefits are likely to be small. Equally important, if the clinician's time and effort are committed disproportionately to the evaluation of the data which can now be so easily generated in such large volumes by a comprehensive patient monitoring system remote from the patient, there will be proportionately less time available for essential clinical evaluation. It is for this reason that the remarkable historical developments of bedside computer systems reviewed in this chapter should be viewed in context. These systems supplement and facilitate bedside decision-making and management, but their appropriate exercise will require vigilance lest they be viewed as alternatives rather than selective contributions to medical and nursing care.

References

1. Weil MH, Shubin H, Rand WM. Experience with a digital computer for study and the improved managment of the critically ill. JAMA 1966; 198:147–152.
2. Turner WA, Lamson BG. Automatic data processing in hospitals: A powerful new tool for clinical research. Hospitals 1964; 38:87.
3. Spencer W, Vallbona CA. Application of computers in clinical practice. JAMA 1965; 191:917.
4. Wilber SA, Derrick WS. Patient monitoring and anesthetic management: A physiological communications network. JAMA 1965; 191:893–898.
5. Jensen RE, Shubin H, Meagher PF, et al. On-line computer monitoring of the seriously ill patient. Med Biol Engin 1966; 4:265–272.
6. Warner HR. Some computer techniques of value for study of circulation in computers. In Stacy RW, Warman B(eds):Biomedical Research 1965. New York and London: Academic Press, 1980; p 239.
7. Hara HH, Belville JW. On-line computation of cardiac output from dye dilution curves. Circulation Res 1963; 12:379.
8. Dammann JF Jr., Wright DJ, Updike OL Jr. Physiological monitoring: Its role and contribution to patient care. Sixth National Biomedical Sciences Instrumentation Symposium 1968; 5:17–27.
9. Rand WM, Weil MH, Shubin H. Automated measurement of cardiac output by use of a digital computer. Physiologist 1966; 9:272.
10. Shubin H, Weil MH. Efficient monitoring with a digital computer of cardiovascular function in seriously ill patients. Ann Intern Med 1966; 65:453–460.
11. Warner HR, Gardner RM, Toronto AF. Computer-based monitoring of cardiovascular functions in post-operative patients. Circulation 1968; 7 (suppl 2):II–68–II–74.
12. Shubin H, Weil MH, Palley N, et al. Monitoring the critically ill patient with the aid of a digital computer. Comput Biomed Res 1971; 4:460–473.
13. Weil MH, Shubin H. Automation of medical facilities: A challenge to industry. IEEE Trans Biomed Engin 1971; 18:74–75.
14. Weil MH, Shubin H, Martin R, et al. Automated techniques for the bedside of the critically ill. In Laughlin JS, Webster EW (eds): Advances in Medical

Physics. The Second International Conference on Medical Physics, 1971; pp 91–98.

15. Shubin H, Palley N, Weil MH. Computer surveillance of the seriously ill patient. J Assoc Adv Med Instrument 1972; 6:48–51.

16. Osborn JJ, Beaumont JO, Raison JC, et al. Measurement and monitoring of acutely ill patients by digital computer. Surgery 1968; 64:1057–1070.

17. Lindberg DH. Electronic retrieval of clinical data. J Med Educ 1965; 40:753.

18. Weil MH, Shubin H, Stewart D. Patient monitoring and intensive care units. In Dickson JF, Brown JHV (eds): Future Goals of Engineering and Biology and Medicine. New York: Academic Press, 1969; p 232–246.

19. Shubin H, Weil MH, Palley N, et al. Automated system for monitoring the critically ill. Circulation 1970; 42:198.

20. Shubin H, Weil MH, Liu VY, et al. Selection of metabolic, respiratory and hemodynamic variables for evaluation of status in critically ill patients. In Advances in Automated Analysis. Tarrytown, New York: Technicon International Congress, Mediad Inc., 1979, pp 23–27.

21. Knaus W, Zimmerman J, Wagner G. APACHE: acute physiology and chronic health evaluation: A physiologically based classification system. Crit Care Med 1981; 9:591–597.

22. Gibbs RF. The present and future medicolegal importance of record keeping in anesthesia and intensive care: The case for automation. Journal of Clinical Monitoring 1989; 5:251–255.

23. Osborn JJ. Computers in critical care medicine: promises and pitfalls. Crit Care Med 1982; 10(12):807–810.

24. Gomez JV, Haddad AG, Mentz WM, et al. An interactive patient data base for intensive care trend analysis. IEEE 1983; 163–166.

25. Rockwell MA, Shubin H, Weil MH, et al. Shock 111. A computer system as an aid in the management of critically ill patients. Communications of the ACM, 1966; 9(5):355–357.

26. Weil MH, Shubin H, Cady LD, et al. Use of automated techniques in the management of the critically ill. In Bekey GA, Schwartz MD (eds): Hospital Information Systems. New York: Marcel Dekker, Inc., 1972; pp 333–381.

27. Shubin H, Weil MH, Rockwell MA. Automated measurement of arterial pressure in patients by use of a digital computer. Med Biol Engin 1967; 5:361–369.

28. Shubin H, Weil MH, Rockwell MA. Automated measurement of cardiac output in patients by use of a digital computer. Med Biol Engin 1967; 5:353–360.

29. Palley N, Weil MH. A computerized system for routine cardiac output measurements. IEEE 1970; 31.

30. Joly H, Trotter J, Weil MH, et al. Real time entry and display of clinical data in an intensive care unit. Meth Inform Med 1971; 10:133–138.

31. Weil MH, Shubin H, Carrington JH, et al. Physiological and biochemical monitoring and the application of automated methods to the care of the critically ill. In Advances in Automated analysis. Tarrytown, New York: Technicon International Congress, Mediad Inc., 1972; pp 1–14.

32. Afifi AA, Rand WM, Palley NA, et al. A method for evaluating changes in sets of computer monitored physiological variables. Comput Biomed Res 1971; 4:329–339.

33. Lewis E, Deller S, Quinn M, et al. Continuous patient monitoring with a small digital computer. Comput Biomed Res 1972; 5:411–428.
34. Kenny G. Programmable calculator: A program for use in the intensive care unit. British Journal of Anaesthesia 1979; 51:793–796.
35. Shabot MM, Shoemaker WC, State D. Rapid bedside computation of cardiorespiratory variables with a programmable calculator. Crit Care Med 1977; 5(2):105–111.
36. Powles AR, Hersher, Rigg J. A pocket calculator program for noninvasive bedside assessment of cardiorespiratory function. Comput Biol Med 1980; 10:143–147.
37. Bar Z. A computer program for bedside renal function studies. Crit Care Med 1981; 9(4):340–341.
38. Edwards F. Computer-assisted planning of hyperalimentation therapy. Crit Care Med 1982; 10(8):539–543.
39. Neu J, Mahoney C, Wilson AD, et al. Calculator assisted determinalion of dilutions for continuous infusion ICU medications. Crit Care Med 1982; 19(9):610–612.
40. Bonner RE, Wortsman D, Schwetman HD. Computer diagnosis of electrocardiograms. Comp Biomed Res 1968; 1:366.
41. Weiner F, Weil MH, Carlson RW. Computer systems for facilitating management of the critically ill. Comput Biol Med 1982; 12:1–15.
42. Shinozaki T, Deane RS, Mazuzan JE. A devoted mini-computer system for the management of clinical and laboratory data in an intensive care unit. IEEE 1982; 267–269.
43. Gardner RM, West BJ, Pryor TA, et al. Computer-based ICU data acquisition as an aid to clinical decision-making. Crit Care Med 1982; 10(12):823–830.
44. Warner HR, ed. A computer based information system for patient care. In Bekley GA, Schwartz MD (eds): Hospital information systems. New York: Marcel Dekker, 1972; p 293–332.
45. Shabot MM, Carlton PD, Sadoff S, et al. Graphical reports and displays for complex ICU data: A new, flexible and configurable method. IEEE 1985; 418–421.
46. Gardner RM, Crapo RO, Morris AH, et al. Computerized decision-making in the pulmonary function laboratory. Respir Care 1982; 27:799–816.
47. Westenskow DR, Bowman RJ, Ohlson KB, et al. Microprocessors in intensive care medicine. Med Instrument 1980; 14(6):311–313.
48. Chaffee M, Weil MH, Rystrom L. Automated withdrawal and infusion through intravascular catheters. J Assoc Adv Med Instrument 1972; 6:162–163.
49. Macneil A, Michelson S, Weil MH. A desk top medical decision assistance system. Crit Care Med 1981; 9:266.
50. Siegel JH, Cerra FB, Moody EA, et al. The effect on survival of critically ill and injured patients of an ICU teaching servie organized about a computer-based physiologic CARE system. Trauma 1986; 20(7):558–579.
51. McDonald CJ. Protocol-based computer reminders, the quality of care and the non-perfectability of man. N Engl J Med 1976; 295:1351.
52. Swan HJC, Ganz W, Forrester J, et al. Catheterization of the heart in man

with the use of a flow-directed balloon-tipped catheter. N Engl J Med 1970; 283:447–451.

53. Siegel JH, Coleman B. Computers in the care of the critically ill patient. Comput Urol 1986; 13(1):101–117.

54. Pollizzi JA. The design of a "functional" database system and its use in the management of the critically ill. IEEE 1983; 167–170.

55. Michaels DF. Hardware-software framework of microcomputerized real-time biomedical instrumentation: Near-term future. SCAMC 1987; 809–816.

56. Bradshaw KE, Sittig DF, Gardner RM, et al. Improving efficiency and quality in a computerized ICU. SCAMC 1988; 12:763–767.

57. Sittig DF. Computerized management of patient care in a complex, controlled clinical trial in the intensive care unit. SCAMC 1987; 11:225–232

58. Wong DT, Knaus WA. Predicting outcome in critical care: the current status of the APACHE prognostic scoring system. Can J Anaesth 1991; 38(3):374–83.

59. Leyerle BJ, Nolan-Avila LS, Shabot MM. Implementation of a comprehensive computerized ICU data management system. IEEE 1985; 386–387.

60. Chance GW. Neonatal intensive care and cost effectiveness. Can Med Assoc J 1988; 139(10):943–6.

61. Joyce T, Corman H, Grossman M. A cost-effectiveness analysis of strategies to reduce infant mortality. Med Care 1988; 26(4):348–60.

62. Afifi AA, Chang PC, Liu VY, et al. Prognostic indexes in acute myocardial infarction complicated by shock. Am J Cardiol 1974; 33:826–832.

63. Shubin H, Weil MH, Afifi AA, et al. Selection of hemodynamic, respiratory, and metabolic variables for evaluation of patients in shock. Crit Care Med 1974; 2:326–336.

Chapter 3
Physician Decision-Making: Evaluation of Data Used in a Computerized ICU

Karen E. Bradshaw, Reed M. Gardner,
Terry P. Clemmer, James F. Orme, Jr.,
Frank Thomas, and Blair J. West

Introduction

Intensive Care Units (ICUs) have become an integral part of many hospitals throughout the world. Their concentration on treatment of critically ill patients requires pertinent physiologic data to be readily available for medical personnel so that quick and accurate decisions can be made in life-threatening situations. In recent years, development of instrumentation and techniques aided by computer technology has made an unprecedented amount of physiologic data available to clinicians in the ICU. Physiologic monitoring of all kinds originated and developed due to the feeling that more patient data would result in better patient care [4,5]. It was thought additional data would improve the timeliness and appropriateness of medical decisions, reduce the number of of oversights, and facilitate training of those specializing in intensive care [1]. However, so much data is becoming available that it will soon be difficult to assimilate and use it effectively [6]. Important factors may become obscured or forgotten in the midst of numerous less important ones [1]. Devices which permit monitoring of new physiologic signals have generated an exploration of additional indices and models for patient care that are constantly being evaluated and may or may not become permanent fixtures on the medical scene. All these factors cause confusion and uncertainty in both the medical community and the instrumentation industry [6].

Because of their speed and information-processing capabilities, computers have been increasingly employed in the ICU environment to aid in management of patient data. At LDS Hospital, computers are employed in six ICUs to the extent that the units are almost completely compu-

Adapted from an article published in the *Int J Clin Monit Comput* 1:81–91, 1984. Reprinted with permission of Kluwer Academic Publishers.

terized [3]. Quantitative physiologic data, laboratory results, drug and IV information, and demographics are all integrated into the patient's computer record. Only some observational data, such as that obtained from physical examination, and free text nurse and physician comments on patient status, are excluded from our computer records [3].

At the LDS Hospital, computing capabilities have not been limited to data storage and retrieval, but have also been applied to the problems of data management to facilitate effective use of the patient database. Goals in this area include development of an organized, compressed, prioritized presentation of important information and the refinement of the computerized database to make it as efficient as possible. Steps taken to realize these goals include the development of the ICU Rounds Report, and a study of the use of patient data by physicians in decision-making in the ICU.

Methods

Background

This study was conducted in the Shock-Trauma Intensive Care Unit at LDS Hospital. The unit admits about 550 patients per year and the average length of stay is 4.5 days. Annual mortality rate during 1982 was 14%. The patient population consists of trauma victims (30%), patients with post operative complications (50%), and patients with medical problems such as diabetes, renal failure, or cardiac arrest (20%). The majority of the patients (65%) come to the unit from within the hospital. Of the patients included in this study, 88% were hemodynamically monitored with arterial and/or pulmonary artery catheters. The unit is staffed by four house officers, two medical students, a critical care fellow, and three full-time staff physicians who specialize in critical care. The nurse to patient ratio is usually 1 to 2.

At the time this project commenced, patient data was accumulating in the computer system at an approximate rate of 8 Kbytes per patient per day, and was accessed through a series of computer reports. For each 12-hour shift, the computer compiled cardiac output reports, blood gas reports, several laboratory reports, and shift reports containing drug, IV, input/output, temperature, and cardovascular data [3]. Seven-day reports were also available showing the patient's course in temperature, blood pressure, drugs. fluid input/output, weight, and nutrition [3].

ICU Rounds Report

The ICU Rounds Report was developed to provide an organ-system-oriented report of important patient data, including hemodynamic, re-

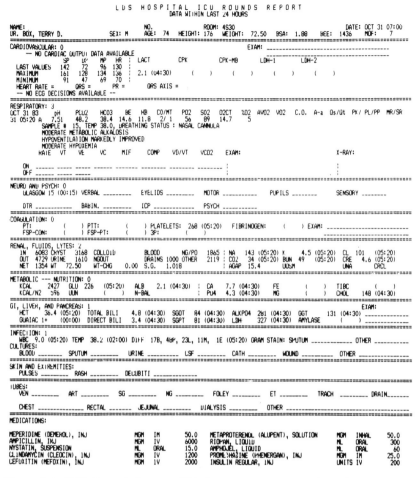

Figure 3.1. ICU Rounds Report. This is an organ-system-oriented computer report designed to present important items of patient data concisely. Space has been left to allow the addition of pertinent information not contained in the computer record.

spiratory, clinical laboratory, blood gas laboratory, medication, and nutritional information. The unit's specialists in critical care medicine chose the items included in the report as being the most useful in assessing patient status.

The top of the report (Fig. 3.1) contains the patient's demographic data, including name, patient number, room number, date, attending physician, sex, age, height, weight, body surface area, estimated basal energy expenditure (BEE), and a multi-organ failure score (MOF) which gives an indication of the seriousness of the patient's condition. The rest of the report is then organized by organ system. There is space on the report to record observational data which is not available from the computer re-cord (dotted lines). If an item (such as a laboratory result) is normally stored on the computer, but that particular test or procedure has not been done for a patient during the last 24 hours, the corresponding space is left blank. Recent additions to the report include microbiology and x-ray results.

Patient Data Usage Study

The most easily observed decision-making situation in the Shock-Trauma ICU occurs during morning physician teaching rounds. At this time, pertinent data on each patient being cared for in the unit is reviewed, and plans are formulated for the patient's care during that day. The initial part of the study evaluated the use of patient data in physician decision-making in the rounds setting. During December 1982 and January 1983, patient data used in rounds was recorded for 30 patients. Fourteen patients in the study were reviewed more than once, with each review taking place on a separate day. For this time period, patient data usage for 63 patient evaluations was recorded.

Review of patient data was by organ system in a format similar to the ICU Rounds Report. Because of this, the Rounds Report became a con-venient form for recording the items of patient data used in formulating plans for patient care. The items used were checked off on the report as they were reviewed. Items not present on the rounds report were written in the margin.

To evaluate data gathered, all the patient data available for decision-making was divided into six categories (Table 3.1). For each patient eva-luation, the data used were tabulated in the appropriate category. The

Table 3.1. Patient Data Categories

1. Bedside monitor	Heart rate, blood pressures, cardiac output, cardiac rhythm, respiratory rate, temperature
2. Laboratory	Electrolytes, white count, differential, cultures coagulation, lactate, enzymes, drug levels, hematocrit-hemoglobin, metabolic/nitrogen balance
3. Blood gas	pH, PCO_2, HCO_3, BE Hb, COHb, PO_2, $SatO_2$, O_2 content, FiO_2, AVO_2 diff., venous O_2, A-a gradient $\dot{Q}s/\dot{Q}t$
4. Drugs—input/ output IV	Medications, intravenous feeding, fluid balance urine output, energy balance
5. Observations	Cardiac exam, respiratory parameters (weaning), neuro-psych, weight, weight change, GI exam, gram stains. skins & extremities
6. Other	History, ECG, X-ray, EEG, CT scan, etc.

number of items used in each category was summed over the entire patient population. Each category total was converted into a percentage of the total amount of data used in all of the patient evaluations. Patients were then divided into three subgroups based on their hemodynamic monitoring status. These subgroups were 1) no invasive monitoring, 2) arterial catheter monitoring, and 3) arterial and pulmonary artery catheter monitoring. One patient with only pulmonary artery catheter monitoring was not included in the analysis. Each subgroup was analyzed to determine what percentage of total patient evaluation data each data category represented. The percentage of data used per category was compared with the corresponding average percentage of data used for the total population. The computerized patient database was also analyzed to determine what percentage of patient data storage each category represented. The average percentage of data used per category was compared with the corresponding percentage of data stored in the computer. This ratio was used to evaluate the efficiency of data storage and to point out areas in which the computerized patient database could be improved.

The second phase of the study evaluated the use of patient data outside of rounds (in "on-site" or bedside decision-making), and repeated the evaluation of data usage in rounds done in phase I. The evaluation of on-site data usage was included to provide a more complete picture of patient data usage in physician decision-making. It was decided that the most workable plan for looking at patient data usage on-site was to devise a checklist to be marked by physicians after a decision was made to indicate which items of patient data had been used in making the decision. Our goals in the development of this checklist were to include all items of patient data frequently used in physician decision-making, to make it as concise as possible and to organize it so that data items used by the physician could be easily found and tabulated. Additional research was then undertaken to provide the necessary information to meet these goals.

The first step was to identify the patient problems about which a nurse most frequently consulted a physician. This was accomplished through the use of another checklist, the Nurse–Physician Interactions sheet (Table 3.2). This sheet was based on a list, compiled by the ICU nursing staff, of reasons that a nurse might consult a physician concerning patient status. The list was put into the organ system format used in the ICU Rounds Report. A section on the right of the sheet provided space for the nurse to mark the reasons for which they had consulted a physician during a shift. The nurse's name, the date, and the shift were entered at the top to insure that a sheet would be filled out by each nurse on duty so that the information gathered would be as complete as possible.

Nurses in the Shock-Trauma ICU filled out these sheets for a ten-day period. During this time, 19 patients were treated in the ICU for a diverse set of problems considered by the ICU staff to be typical.

Over 1960 nurse–physician (RN-MD) interactions were recorded dur-

Table 3.2. Nurse–Physician Interactions Checklist

NURSE:	DATE:	SHIFT:

Please check the appropriate reason each time you consult with a physician in regard to a patient. Possible reasons are listed by organ system in format similar to the Rounds Report. If the reason is not listed, please record it under "Other."

SYSTEM	REASON–CHANGES IN:	FREQUENCY
Cardiovascular	BP	_____
	HR	_____
	CO/CI	_____
	Rhythm	_____
	Chest pain	_____
	Lactic acid	_____
	Swan PW	_____
	PA	_____
	RA	_____
Respiratory	ABGs	_____
	Lung auscultation	_____
	Lung compliance	_____
	Respiratory pattern	_____
	Supplemental O_2	_____
	Vent 1 FiO_2	_____
	2 mode	_____
	3 rate	_____
Neuro	Level of consciousness	_____
	Pupils	_____
	Motor activity	_____
	EEG	_____
Coagulation	PT	_____
	PTT	_____
	Platelets	_____
Renal, fluid, and lytes	Urine output	_____
	Specific gravity	_____
	SMA 6	_____
	IV rate	_____
	IV fluid	_____
Nutrition, GI, liver, and pancreas	TPN	_____
	NG output	_____
	NVD problems	_____
	Amylase	_____
Infection	CBC	_____
	Temp	_____
	Cultures	_____
	Wound—drainage, odor, color, etc.	_____
Skin and extremities	Pulses	_____
	Rash	_____
	Decubiti	_____

(Contd)

Table 3.2. (Cont)

NURSE:	DATE:	SHIFT:

Please check the appropriate reason each time you consult with a physician in regard to a patient. Possible reasons are listed by organ system in format similar to the Rounds Report. If the reason is not listed, please record it under "Other."

SYSTEM	REASON–CHANGES IN:	FREQUENCY
Tubes	IV site problems	_____
	Line placement probs	_____
	Feeding tube position	_____
	Foley problems	_____
Other	Patient's family	_____
	_____	_____
	_____	_____
	_____	_____
	_____	_____
	_____	_____
	_____	_____

ing the ten-day period. The number of interactions triggered by each of the 72 items of patient data listed on the sheets was totaled, and the eight most frequent items, constituting 45% of the total RN–MD interactions, were found. The problems included changes in blood pressure, urine output, blood gases, level of consciousness, IV rate, pulmonary wedge pressure, IV fluid, and heart rate. It was felt that a reasonably comprehensive list of patient data used in on-site decision-making would be obtained by taking the data used in the decision logic for dealing with the eight most frequent problems and combining them with items of patient data found on the rounds report. The end result of this process was the ICU Patient Data Checklist (Table 3.3). Patient history was not included on the checklist because it was felt that any decision on patient care would require such knowledge; and therefore, its use in any given situation could be assumed.

Both the on-site and the second rounds data usage evaluations were conducted in October 1983. For the study of on-site patient data usage, the ICU's physician and nursing staffs were oriented on the use of the Patient Data Use Checklist by the ICU director and head nurse, and asked to cooperate in marking them for one month. It had been decided earlier that the most feasible plan was to ask the house staff to fill out a form directly after they made each decision concerning a patient. It was feared that if forms were not filled out at this time, or if a number of decisions made over a specified period of time (8, 12, or 24 hours) were lumped together, the physicians would be unable to recall their thought processes accurately. Data gathered both inside rounds and on-site was evaluated in

Table 3.3. ICU Patient Data Use Checklist

Instructions:
1. Please put patient's name on this checklist.
2. Check the reason you were asked to see the patient.
3. Check each data item that you took into consideration in making your decision concerning this problem. Where multiorgan system evaluation is applicable, please check items in each system.
4. For *each* data item you considered that is not listed, place a check mark by "Other."

Patient   Name: _____

Reason for seeing patient
BP ___ Urine Output ___ Mental status ___ Blood Gases ___ PW Pressure ___ HR ___ Other _____

Patient data items used:

Cardiovascular
HR ___ BP ___ CO ___ CI ___ SVR, PVR ___ PW, CVP ___ PA ___ CPK ___ ECG ___ Cardiac Exam ___ Lactate ___
Rhythm ___ Drugs ___ Mechanical Problem ___ Other _____

Respiratory
Spontaneous Rate ___ V_T ___ V_T ___ pH ___ PCO_2 ___ PO_2 ___ Compliance ___ $\%O_2$ ___ X-ray ___ Lung Exam ___ Chest
Exam ___ Drugs ___ Other _____
Rate ___ Mode ___ V_T ___ Peak Pressure ___ Plateau Pressure ___ PEEP ___ Mechanical Problem ___ Other _____

Coagulation
PT ___ PTT ___ Platelets ___ Drugs ___ Other _____

Neuro & Psych
Glasgow ___ Verbal ___ Eyelids ___ Eye Movements ___ Corneals ___ Motor ___ Pupils ___ Sensory ___ DTR ___ Babinski
___ ICP ___ PSYCH ___ Pain ___ Drugs ___ Other _____

(Contd)

Table 3.3. (Contd)

Renal, Fluid & Lytes
In ___ Out ___ Urine Out ___ NG Out—Wt-Chg ___ S.G. ___ Na ___ K ___ Cl⁻ ___ HCO₃ ___ BUN ___ Cre ___ AGAP
___ UNaUO_sm ___ IV Fluids ___ Drugs ___ Mechanical Probs ___ Other ___

GI, liver & pancreas
Hct ___ Guaiac ___ Bili ___ SGOT ___ SGPT ___ AlkPO₄ ___ LDH ___ GGT ___ Amylase ___ Exam ___ Drugs ___ Other ___

Infection
WBC ___ Temp ___ Diff ___ Sputum Gram Stain ___ Chills, Sweats ___ Drugs ___ Other ___
Cultures:
Blood ___ Urine ___ Sputum ___ Other ___

Skin & extremities
Pulses ___ Edema ___ Skin Color ___ Skin Temp ___ Drugs ___ Other ___

Tubes
Ng ___ Drains ___ Other ___

Metabolic & nutrition
TPN Rate ___ Serum Glucose ___ Serum Ketones ___ Urine Glucose ___ Urine Ketones ___ Drugs ___ Other ___

Table 3.4. Patient Data Use Study Results

	Lab	Drugs input/ output & IV	Observations	Beside monitor	Blood gas lab	Other
A. % of data reviewed in rounds—63 patient evaluations (Dec 82–Jan 83)	33	22	21	13	9	2
B. % of data reviewed in rounds— 58 patient evaluations (Oct 83)	29	24	21	12	10	3
C. Average % of A and B 121 patient evaluations	31.5	24	21	12.5	9.5	2.5
D. % of data used on on-site (35 decisions) (Oct 83)	18	13	22	22	20	5
E. % Change in data usage between C and D	−13.5	−10	+ 1	+ 9.5	+10.5	+2.5
F. % of data in computer record	8.5	36	6.8	32.5	7.8	8.4

the same way as data from the December 1982–January 1983 phase of the
study described above.

Results

The results of each phase of our study of data usage in decision-making
are shown in Table 3.4 and summarized in Figure 3.2 During December
1982 and January 1983, use of patient data in physician decision-making
during rounds was recorded for 63 evaluations of 30 ICU patients. The
percentage of data used in each of the six categories of patient data is as
shown in Table 3.2, row A. Patient data use in rounds during October
1983 was recorded for 58 evaluations of 30 ICU patients. Percentage of
data use per category for this this time period is listed in B. Results from
both study periods were combined to give the average percentage of data
use per category. These averages are found in C. In the on-site phase of
the study, 35 ICU Patient Data Use check-lists, filled out during one
month, reflected items of patient data used in 35 decisions relating to patient care. The results of this phase of the study are shown in D. The difference in data usage between rounds and on-site decision-making was
calculated and is listed in E. Row F shows the composition of the computerized patient database. Figure 3.2 shows use of patient data in each
of the six data categories for both settings looked at in the study.

The distribution of data usage in rounds over the total patient population for the bedside monitor and combined laboratory (laboratory and
blood gas laboratory) categories is shown in the graphs in Figure 3.3A
and B along with the mean, median, and standard deviation for each.

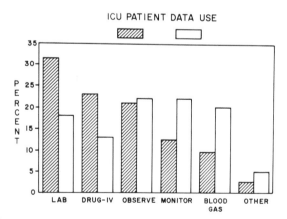

Figure 3.2. ICU patient data use. This graph shows the average percentage of patient data used in physician decision-making from each of the six patient data
categories in both the rounds and on-site decision-making settings.

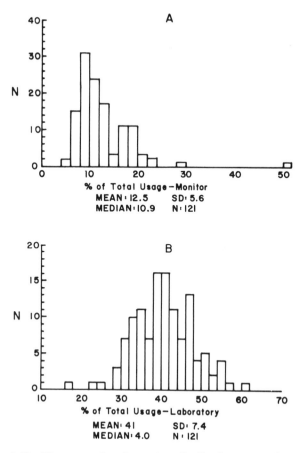

Figure 3.3. A,B: These graphs show the distribution over the total patient population of the percent of patient data used in physician decision-making from, the bedside monitor (A) and combined laboratory (B) (laboratory and blood gas laboratory) data categories in the rounds setting.

Figure 3.4 compares patient data use in rounds for the three hemody-namic patient monitoring subgroups with the average figures for the total patient population. Also shown is the number of patients which belong to each subgroup. This type of figure was not presented for the on-site data because of its different structure and the small sample size.

Discussion

From the study of data usage in physician decision-making, the adequacy of our computerized database and data collection system was analyzed. Data usage was compared to data storage in the computer to pinpoint

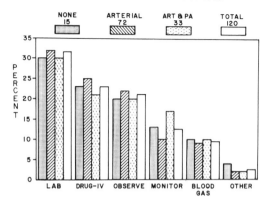

Figure 3.4. Data usage in rounds by patient monitoring status. This graph compares use of patient data from the six patient data categories for three subgroups of patients with the average use calculated for the total patient population. The subgroups of patients were 1) no invasive hemodynamic monitoring (NONE), 2) arterial catheter monitoring (ARTERIAL), and 3) arterial and pulmonary artery catheter monitoring (ART & PA). TOTAL was used to designate results for the total patient population.

areas that could be improved for each category (Table 3.4, rows C, D, and F).

The most widely used patient data in the rounds decision-making setting was laboratory results. Clinical, blood gas, and microbiology laboratory results made up approximately 40% of all patient data reviewed during both the periods in which rounds data usage was recorded (Table 3.4). Our preliminary work on-site indicated that laboratory data usage was about 38% (18% + 20%) of total usage, with a large drop in the use of clinical and microbiology laboratory data (to 18%) and an almost equally large increase in the use of blood gas laboratory data (to 20%). The total laboratory data occupied only 16.3% of the computerized database. Because of the high usage-to-storage ratio for laboratory data, it was felt that optimization of the speed and ease of data retrieval was the indicated improvement to be made.

The second most widely used categories of data during rounds were observations and drugs, input/output, and IV (Table 3.4). The amount of data usage in both the rounds and on-site settings for the observations category was about the same. Comparison of data usage with data storage for this category shows a favorable ratio. However, much of the observational data used by physicians in decision-making is not currently entered into the computer record. We are therefore proposing to add more entries from the observations category to the computer data base. There was a large drop in the use of data from the drugs, input/output, and IV category in on-site decision-making (Table 3.4E). This suggested that data stored exceeds data used by 13% to 23%. One mitigating factor was that in rounds, the actual amount of patient data used for this category was somewhat higher than 22%, because in rounds, all medications were looked at as a group and were counted as only one data item. On-site. this effect was lessened because drugs were listed as an item of data under each organ system on the Patient Data Use Checklist, so that if, for example, a physician looked at both cardiac drugs and antibiotics in making a decision, these would be marked and counted as two separate data items. It would probably have given a more correct picture if each drug had been considered as a separate item, in which case the percentage of use would have been more in line with the storage space occupied. For the drug, input/output, and IV category, we want to optimize the amount of data stored while still meeting medical decision-making, long-term, and legal requirements relating to the patient record.

Data obtained from bedside monitors during rounds made up only about 13% of total data used in decision-making while occupying 32.5% of the computer record. On-site. this usage increased to 22%, which still left a gap of over ten percentage points between the amount of data stored and the amount of data actually used. This finding indicates an area in which data storage should be reevaluated and optimized so that medical and legal requirements for the patient database can be efficiently met.

The final category, including history, x-ray, and ECG, represented between 2.5% to 5% of the data used and took up 8.4% of the computerized data-base. It is important to remember that each of the items in this category contained a great deal of information about the patient which was not being broken down into individual components, but rather was viewed as a conglomerate. Items in this category are required parts of the patient record, so that medical and legal requirements are satisfied.

Of the two decision-making settings studied, it was only in the rounds setting that sufficient information was gathered to draw quantifiable conclusions. Physician decision-making in rounds in our ICU utilizes the computerized patient database to a greater extent than does on-site decision-making. This is due to the ready availability of some patient data types at the bedside (on-site) without the need to access the patient's computer record (an example is "real time" data from the bedside monitor). The use of patient data in rounds followed the same general pattern regardless of the hemodynamic monitoring status of the patient (Fig. 3.4). The greatest difference in data utilization occurred in the bedside monitor category with a high of 17% (Art & PA) and a low of 10% (Arterial) of total patient data reviewed. The percentage of patient data use from each data category varied from patient to patient, as shown in the graphs in Fig. 3.3 for the bedside monitor and laboratory categories. It is important to realize that a data category can make up a very large percentage of total patient data reviewed even though only a small number of items in the category were looked at by physicians, if the total number of patient data items reviewed is also small. Such is the case for the patient in which 50% of total data used was from the bedside monitor category. These factors taken together led to our choice of average percentage of patient data use per data category taken over the total patient population (Table 3.4C) as the most useful figure for evaluating our computerized patient database.

It was estimated that physicians made over 5,000 decisions on patient treatment on-site during the month's time that they were asked to mark Patient Data Use Checklists. The estimate was based on the number of nurse–physician interactions recorded over the course of ten days and assumed that a decision resulted from each interaction. Of these 5000 decisions, use of patient data in the decision-making process was recorded only 35 times. Among reasons for there being such a small amount of on-site data was the fact that paperwork is not a top priority for physicians, especially in an ICU setting where a patient's condition may deteriorate rapidly and necessitate immediate therapeutic action. However, the members of the ICU house staff stated that they were using the Patient Data Use Checklist to record data usage in the majority of their decisions. It appears from this observation that many decisions on patient care are made so automatically that a physican may not even recognize that a decision is being made. To rectify this, it is necessary either to continue the data collection process for a much longer period of time, or to devise some other method of looking at data usage in on-site decision-making.

In this study, it was recognized that the frequency with which a data item is used by a physician in decision-making does not correspond on a one-to-one-basis with the importance of the data item in influencing the physician's decision. Definitive attempts to rank data items in the order of importance in patient treatment were beyond the scope of this preliminary study, and were only indicated generally in the results by the frequency with which an item was looked at. Also, it was not possible to equate frequency of use with proven value of use or with any proven effect of knowledge of an item of patient data on the patient's outcome. Unfortunately, data collection and utilization procedures are often implemented in medical care before their real value or effect is known, and they may then become standard practice regardless of this knowledge. We regard this study as preliminary work in which we have only been able to take certain "snapshots" of the total data utilization in decision-making process by which patients are treated in a specific ICU. Much work remains to be done to bring the total picture into view.

It has been pointed out that conventional paper medical records are bulky, disorganized, unstructured, and redundant, and that retrieval of patient information is slow [2]. It has also been shown that fixed format patient records organized as flow sheets, such as the ICU Rounds Report, can be accessed in one-fourth the time of a conventional record [2]. The design of the ICU Rounds Report has overcome many of the problems associated with conventional paper medical records, and has been accepted and utilized by clinicians.

It is hoped the implementation of the ICU Rounds Report, along with improvements in the patient database, will facilitate physician decision-making by making the most important items of patient data rapidly and readily available. Beyond this, it should be pointed out that the results obtained from this study show several areas in which our emphasis in patient data collection and storage needs to be changed to make best use of available resources. Notable among these is data collected from the patient's bedside monitor, which is collected and stored in much greater volume than it is subsequently used. This does not discount the importance of the bedside monitor in reflecting the current hemodynamic status of a patient at bedside, but rather forces us to evaluate how much of this information is really useful after the fact. Since monitoring equipment may well represent the most costly component in equipping an ICU, it is important to evaluate which physiologic parameters must be monitored for effective patient care. Our study also shows that it is desirable to have monitors which are capable of transmitting their physiologic data to a computerized database. This data, when selectively stored and combined with other types of data in an optimized database, allows the physician to get an overall picture of patient status to facilitate effective medical decision-making.

Summary

New instrumentation, techniques, and computers have made such large amounts of information rapidly available to ICU clinicians that there is now a danger of information overload. To help with this problem at LDS Hospital, a computerized system was implemented in the Shock-Trauma ICU. This ICU is almost totally computerized with each patient's physiologic, laboratory, drug, demographic, fluid input/output, and nutritional data integrated into the patient's computer record.

In the ICU, physician decision-making takes place in two situations: during rounds and on-site. For this study, data usage in decision-making was evaluated in both of these environments. The items of data used in decision-making were tabulated into six categories: 1) bedside monitor, 2) laboratory, 3) drugs, input/output and IV, 4) blood gas laboratory, 5) observations, and 6) other. Comparisons were made between the portion of the computerized database occupied by a category and its use in decision-making.

Combined laboratory data (clinical, microbiology, and blood gas) made up 38–41% of total patient data reviewed and occupied 16.3% of the database. Observations made up 21–22% of the data reviewed and occupied 6.8% of the database. Drugs, input/output, and IV data usage ranged from 13% to 23%, but occupied 36% of the database. Bedside monitor data usage was 12.5% to 22% and occupied 32.5% of the database. The "other" category, used 2.5% to 5% of the time, made up 8.4% of the database.

These results indicate that patient data collection and storage must be evaluated and optimized. This evaluation, along with implementation of the computerized ICU Rounds Report developed for optimal data presentation, will help physicians to evaluate patient status and should facilitate effective decisions.

Acknowledgments

This study was supported in part by GM 23095.

References

1. Booth F: Patient monitoring and data processing in the ICU. Crit Care Med 1983; 11:57–58.
2. Fries JF: Alternatives in medical record formats, Med Care 1974; 12:871–881.
3. Gardner RM, West BJ, Pryor TA, Larsen KG, Warner HR, Clemmer TP, Orme JF: Computer-based ICU data acquisition as an aid to clinical decision-making. Crit Care Med 1982; 10:823–830.
4. NIH Consensus Conference-Critical Care. JAMA 1983; 250:798–804.
5. Osborn JJ: Computers in critical care medicine: promises and pitfalls. Crit Care Med 1982; 10:807–810.
6. Stafford TJ: Wither monitoring? Crit Care Med 1982; 10:792–795.

Chapter 4
Development of Decision Support Systems

T. Allan Pryor

Use of decision support systems within a hospital are becoming almost a necessity. As Hospital Information Systems (HIS) usage has grown in the hospital the requirements of such a system to assist in the decision processes of the medical personnel has simultaneously grown. The fact that data is now available on the computer has stimulated those with access to that data to demand increased software to utilize the data in their decision support requirements. These requirements have come not only from the medical staff, but include the nursing, administrative, and ancillary staff as well. In response to those requests system developers have used both the power of the PC for quickly developing decision support programs and attempted to upgrade existing HISs to incorporate decision support software. Because of the need to integrate all decision support programs with an integrated hospital database, we at LDS Hospital have chosen to develop an HIS which is knowledge driven for the express purpose of being a decision support system which also performs all of the traditional HIS functions.

The HELP system [1–4] at LDS Hospital differs greatly from other hospital information (HIS) and decision support systems currently available. It differs first from traditional HIS systems in that it incorporates decision support mechanisms in every HIS application. It also differs from the expert systems reported in the literature in the breadth of decision domains and methods which it handles. Expert systems such as DXPLAIN [5], MYCIN [6], and Internist [7] are limited to a single decision model and application. These programs use a particular model for implementing expert logic and attack a single decision problem such as diagnosis. The HELP system, on the other hand, is a system where multiple decision support models and applications can coexist. Therefore, there is

Adapted from an article published in the *Int J Clin Monit Comput* 7:137–146, 1990. Reprinted with permission of Kluwer Academic Publishers.

no single decision support model which exclusively defines the HELP decision support methodology. Within HELP the use of decision support is not limited to a single application. As explained below HELP is designed to support the entire application needs of a hospital—i.e., administrative, clinical, and financial.

Decision Support Uses

In design of the HELP system we first investigated where decision support was used within the hospital. This investigation was necessary to ensure that the design we chose to implement the system would provide the necessary tools for easy creation of decision support software in every required application. We discovered that unlike a traditional program design a decision support HIS must allow the expert to manage the knowledge of the system. This investigation also lead us to define six major generic uses of decision support in the hospital which are

1. Alerting
2. Interpretation
3. Assisting
4. Critiquing
5. Diagnosing
6. Managing

Understanding these generic decision needs leads to the development of a flexible HIS which allows creation of decision supported applications which serve the entire user population of an HIS.

Alerting decision support is defined as automatic notification of the appropriate personnel of a time critical of action-oriented decision. The most common clinical example where alerting decision support is incorporated is medication ordering systems [8]. In these systems alert criteria are evaluated at the time the order is entered into the system, and an alert is generated if the criteria of the alert are met. The alert generally is in the form of a message on the terminal to the ordering person before subsequent orders may be entered. This alert may indicate a drug interaction, an allergy contraindication, or some important clinical laboratory interaction/contraindication. For example, an alert may be generated when ordering a potassium-sparing drug in a patient whose laboratory values already indicate the patient has a low potassium value. In this instance the alert may suggest the need to order potassium concurrently with the potassium-sparing agent. Beyond the use of alerting decision support in pharmacy systems, the same alerting techniques can be extended to include notification of the nurse on any abnormal trends sensed from nurse-charted data, management alerts which could notify nursing of failure to complete some required task, or alerts for notification of hospital administration of a DRG cost overrun on a patient, etc. One of the features of most alerting systems is their ability to monitor data in the background and create alerts as the appropriate criteria are met. Bradshaw [3] describes and evaluates such a background laboratory alerting system. Alerting systems have easily been the most used mode of decision support in the hospital. Virtually every hospital information system today probably has some simple or sophisticated alerts in one or more of its applications.

Interpretation refers to assimilation of data resulting in a conceptual understanding of the data. The mode of decision support has also been widely used for many years in the hospital. The most common application of interpretation found in hospital computers systems today is the computerized interpretation of the ECG. Early in the development of the HELP system, ECG interpretive system was developed [9]. Several commercial companies, including Hewlett-Packard and Marquette Electronics, offer ECG interpretive systems. With these systems the ECG is not only recorded by the instrument but is analyzed to determine both the morphological and rhythm status of the patient. A report is then generated which provides the actual wave-forms, measured values from the waveforms, and the clinical interpretation of the waveforms. Another example of an interpretive decision support use is the interpretation of blood gas data [10]. As with the ECG systems the interpretive blood gas programs report to the physician not only the measured values from the blood, but an interpretive report of the meaning of those values. Many of today's instruments used in hospitals are equipped with microprocessors which accomplish some level of interpretation of the data they are processing.

Assisting decision support is decision support used to speed or simplify some human interaction with the computer system. Assisting decision support usually incorporates predictive knowledge about the task to be performed. Clinically assisting decision support is commonly used in systems to enter physician orders. For those systems which are intended for use by the physician to enter his/her own orders, assisting decision support is a necessity if the program is to be sufficiently efficient for use by the busy physician. In this example the assisting decision support would use predictive knowledge to suggest the appropriate order parameters for a given patient and order. This could be in the form of a fixed standing order list, calculated parameters of the order such as patient-specific dose rates for a given drug, fixed or patient-specific protocols for care of the patient, etc. In each of these examples the assisting decision makes use of logic available to the application to reduce the number of steps normally taken in the ordering process. This reduction usually translates to a system which is then sufficiently rapid to make it viable for the use by the time conscience physician. Prokosch [2] has reported on the use of an assisting decision support system to aid in physician ordering of medications. Likewise predictive knowledge can be easily built into the nurse-charting applications, again making those computer tasks simpler and more efficient. While many systems provide for some sort of fixed default/predictive knowledge/tables in the ordering process, the use of more complex assisting logic is still primarily a research effort.

Critiquing decision support is defined as the computerized analysis of human suggested decisions to verify the appropriateness of the decision. This form of decision support has been widely suggested in reviewing physician-entered clinical orders or patient management plans. This form of decision support is distinguished by the formulation of the order or plan. In the critiquing mode it is assumed that no decision support was provided to suggest the order/plan, but merely to use the knowledge base to evaluate the order/plan and report to the user the result of that computerized evaluation. One example of critiquing decision support by Miller [11] is the management of ventilator settings on a respirator. In this example the physician enters into the critiquing program a suggested set of respirator settings. The program using its critiquing logic evaluates the suggested settings against the patient's computer stored findings and the rules of the critiquing logic. The results of the critique are then presented to the physician for review and action. The results could be agreement with the initial suggested plan or present reasons why such a plan may be detrimental to the patient. Under the later conditions the program would suggest more appropriate settings with some justification of its reasoning. Except in the simplest form of critiquing medication orders similar to the alerting mode, critiquing decision support remains a research issue.

Diagnostic decision support is the use of decision support to generate diagnostic suggestions about the patient/system. This form of decision support has probably received more attention in the literature than any other form of decision support. With these programs the user generally enters some initial signs, symptoms, and laboratory values from which the program begins hypothesizing diagnoses. In order to conclude on a diagnosis, the programs generally begin a dialogue with the user to gather the most pertinent data which it believes is necessary to conclude an appropriate diagnosis. While the logic of the different diagnostic programs vary, one of the most distinguishing features between them is the number of diseases they consider. Programs such as DXPLAIN [5] may consider several thousand diseases, while another program may be limited to only pulmonary diseases. In general the utility and accuracy of the programs is commensurate with the number of diseases it considers. As the number of diseases rise, the speed of the program generally decreases and the ease of use of the program declines. Because of the complexity of these programs, the authors have explored their use in teaching environments where the student may interact extensively with the program to gain experience in the diagnostic process. Warner [12] has described such a system called ILLIAD. Diagnostic decision support can be used to create applications not only for traditional patient diagnosis, but where models exist for understanding any other aspect of the hospital environment, the decision support can be applied to help the user understand the state of any system in the hospital.

Finally, management decision support is the automatic generation of action-oriented decisions designed to improve the system state. Management decision support differs from critiquing decision support in that with management, decisions suggest treatment plans, whereas in critiquing support the computer is reacting to treatment plans entered by the physician. With management decisions the roles of the computer and physician have changed. The physician takes the role of critiquing the computer rather than the computer critiquing the physician. Clinically management decisions have taken the form of simple or complex protocols encoded in the computer. Using the logic of these protocols, the computer can monitor the state of the patient and make suggestions regarding subsequent treatment. With the exception of some small closed-loop medication administration systems, the suggestions of the computer are always reviewed by the user before implementation of the computer logic. The use of management decision support in nursing is also being investigated by several researchers. In particular the automatic creation of nursing care plans is being developed at several institutions. In this application the computer working off the patient's diagnosis would automatically suggest to the nursing staff a care plan which could be accepted or modified by the nurse. The level of sophistication of management decision systems is dependent on the amount of patient-specific logic contained in the programs. While those with fixed protocols are easy to implement, without tailoring the protocols to the individual patient, they may be too simple to serve as valuable assistance. Sittig [13] reports on an extensive protocol management system used in the ICUs to assist in the management of patients with adult respiratory distress syndrome.

System Design to Implement Decision Support Uses

As noted, our research into the use of decision support in the hospital led us to believe that 1) there is need for widespread use of decision support in the hospital, and 2) the system must permit the expert to manage the decision support logic in his domain. To research these goals HELP, therefore, was designed as a knowledge-driven HIS which executes expert defined and maintained knowledge modules (frames). This required, therefore, developing for HELP a set of knowledge tools which the expert could use for definition and maintenance of their decision logic. These knowledge tools would provide access to the knowledge base in a form that is easily understood and controlled by the expert and implemented in an efficient lower level machine executable form. Two primary knowledge tools were developed. The first was a knowledge editor to

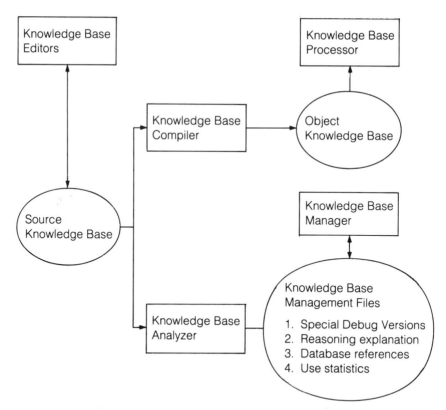

Figure 4.1. Block diagram of the knowledge frame generation process. Source frames are first created using special knowledge editors. These frames are then compiled into object code using a special purpose frame compiler to a general query language on HELP. The object knowledge base consists of modular randomly accessible frames of knowledge ready for execution by the HELP knowledge editor. The knowledge base manager is used to analyze the contents of the frame for maintenance, use and explanation purposes.

create and maintain the logic, and the second was a knowledge compiler to generate the machine executable programs. With this design we hoped to create a system which is both maintainable by the expert and efficient for the user. Figure 4.1 portrays this process. As outlined in the figure, the expert interfaces with the knowledge base through general or domain-specific knowledge editors for creation/maintenance of the source knowledge frames. The knowledge frames are then compiled into a general purpose query language for execution on the computer. The compiled knowledge frames reside in the object knowledge base and can be randomly executed when needed in the decision support applications of the HIS. Because all of the knowledge frames exist independently in a common knowledge file, a single knowledge frame may be shared/executed by several HIS applications.

To assist the expert in creation/maintenance of his expert logic we had to design a decision support language (frame language) which would be used to write the knowledge frames. The knowledge editors were created to also enhance the ability of the domain expert to manage his/her expert logic. In designing our frame language the first goal was to make the language simple enough to be understood by non-computer experts and yet complete enough to perform the logic required by the decision support applications. The language had to support four major feature/functions which were deemed necessary in programming a complete decision support application. These features are 1) the ability to interface knowledge variables to the HIS database, 2) the ability to define data acquisition methodologies, 3) the ability to define data/decision reporting requirements, and 4) the ability to write the actual decision logic. Given these requirements we developed a frame structure where the frame slots are segmented into the following components: 1) frame management knowledge slots, 2) attribute knowledge slots, and 3) declarative/procedural knowledge slots.

Figure 4.2 illustrates the slots defined for frame management knowledge. The slots of the knowledge segment allow us to track the source, validity, utility and type of the knowledge represented in the frame. Figure 4.3 is an example of a frame where the slots have been instantiated with the particular values illustrated in the figure. As seen in Figure 4.3 not all of the available slots need be instantiated in a frame. While most of the slots are self-explanatory, the frame type, gold standard, validation level, and utility slots require some explanation. The frame type slot defines the intended primary use of the frame. Several frame types have been declared. They include management frames, diagnostic frames, data acquisition frames, and report frames. The gold standard slot contains knowledge about any gold standard which could be used to measure the accuracy of the frame. The gold standard slot could refer to another

Frame Management Knowledge

Author:
Title:
Frame Type:
Create/Update Data:
References:
Gold Standard:
Validation Level:
Utility:
Comments:

Figure 4.2. The slots in the knowledge frame used for management purposes.

Title:	Aminophyllin bolus in asthma (continuous drip in separate frame) (7.126.3)
Author:	Peter Haug
Type:	Management
Message:	"Suggest asthmatic treatment begin with an aminophyllin IV bolus of <dosage> mg."
Utility:	5/9
Reference:	Washington Manual of Medical Therapeutics

Figure 4.3. The knowledge management slots from a typical decision frame.

frame, a particular test, a discharge diagnosis, etc. That is any criteria which could be used by a knowledge management system to validate the knowledge of this frame. The validation slot contains knowledge concerning the level of validation through which the frame has been tested. For example, is this logic only the best guess of the knowledge engineer who wrote the frame or does the logic come from some literature reference or has the logic been tested in a controlled study, etc. The utility slot is used to record the importance of the decision medically. That is, how clinically significant is the result of the logic of the frame.

The attribute knowledge of the frame contains knowledge about the relationship of the attributes/variables and the decision of the frame and knowledge about the database where the attributes/variables resides. We have also included as attribute knowledge, knowledge about the screen presentation of the attributes. This knowledge is in the form of window definitions for presentation/acquisition of the attributes/variables. Included in the attribute knowledge of the frame knowledge about attribute statistics such as sensitivity/specificity, ad hoc scores, allowed values, etc., are also included. For some decision frames (e.g., medication order prediction frames) attribute knowledge is sufficient to contain all the necessary knowledge of the frame. Figure 4.4 is the attribute knowledge segment of a frame intended to suggest treatment with aminophyllin. In this example the underlined phrases represent individual elements which would be found in the patient's database. The attributes/variables such as aminophyllin-allergy represent the attributes/variables which in this instance would be used in the declarative knowledge section of the frame.

The declarative/procedural knowledge of the frame contains the rules, equations, and procedural flow of the frame. Control of terminal and/or database acquisition of the attributes/variables is contained in this section of the frame. In the example of Figure 4.5 the logic statement contains a simple decision rule. The Ask slot contains control logic for the acquisition of variables which are needed for subsequent execution of the frame. In this example the patient is to be asked about his/her reaction to asthma medications. The Evoke slot describes the logic necessary for automatic execution of this frame. In this example if the patient has at any time dur-

Declare Variables: asthma **which is** <u>REACTIVE AIRWAY DISEASE (ASTHMA),</u>

> aminophyllin_allergy **as an expression containing** theophyllin
> **which is** <u>THEOPHYLLINES</u> **and** theophyllin_containing_meds
> **which is** <u>THEOPHYLLINES IN COMBINATION WITH OTHER AGENTS</u>
> **and** drug_sensitivity **which is** <u>DRUG SENSITIVITY</u>
> **if** drug_sensitivity **exists and** (theophyllin exists or
> theophyllinp_containing_meds **exists**),
>
> asthma_med_reaction **which is** <u>HAVE YOU EVER HAD A REACTION TO A MEDICATION GIVEN FOR ASTHMA?</u>
>
> current_aminophyllin **as an expression containing** theophyllin
> **which is** <u>THEOPHYLLINES</u> **and** theophyllin_containing_meds
> **which is** <u>THEOPHYLLINES IN COMBINATION WITH OTHER AGENTS</u>
> **and** current_med **which is** <u>CURRENT</u> and home_med **which is**
> <u>HOME MEDICATION</u>
> **if** (theophyllin **exists or** theophyllin_containing_meds **exists**) **and**
> (current_med **exists or** home_med **exists**),
>
> weight **which is** <u>WEIGHT,</u>
>
> arterial_pO2 **which is** <u>PO2,</u>

Figure 4.4 The attribute knowledge from a typical decision frame. The underlined text correspond to the actual database variables.

ing his/her hospital stay noted the fact that he/she has a probability of asthma GE 0.70 stored in his/her computerized medical record, then this frame would automatically be processed by the system to determine the need for aminophyllin treatment. In the case of background or data-driven execution of the frame the resulting decision of the frame will be stored in the patient's computerized record.

We designed the syntax for the frame slots with the goal of insuring that the frame will be able to accomplish all the tasks necessary in implementation of a complete decision support application. Some of the features supported by the frame language syntax include 1) reference to the HELP database, 2) sophisticated screen presentation, and 3) support of different decision support models.

Logic: **If** asthma **GE** 0.70 **and Not Exist** aminophyllin_allergy **and Not Exist** current_aminophyllin **and Not** (asthma_med_reaction **EQ** yes) **Then** dosage = 5 *weight
       Else Stop.

Ask: Patient (asthma_med_reaction) **Hierarchical.**

Evoke: **If** asthma **GE** 0.70.

Figure 4.5. The declarative/procedural knowledge of a frame of suggesting use of aminophyllin.

Database syntax in the HELP frame language allows the frame developer to retrieve complex variables easily from the patient database, reference other relational files supported by HELP, and record results of data entry and/or decisions in the patient database. Screen presentation syntax allows the use of multiple windows within a frame. This syntax is interfaced to a PC-based window package which actually manages the windows and terminal data entry. Thus, the frame writer may easily define presentation attributes, allowed data entry ranges, validation procedures, and help screens within the context of the frame language. Finally, syntax is available in the frame language for easy implementation of simple logic rules, Bayesian decisions, and other mathematical models. This ability of the frame system to support multiple decision models and screen presentations gives to the system a flexibility not supported in most decision support systems. While this adds complexity to the language, the knowledge-specific editors provide a user-friendly mode of interaction with the frames in those areas where a common model is desired for an entire application.

Development of the Decision Support Applications

Development of the decision support applications now becomes a process of either writing new frames or utilizing existing frames in a new context. Most new applications, in fact, are a combination of the two methods. That is, existing frames are combined with new frames to constitute a new decision support application. Since the frame library is a common resource to all application developers, its scope and utility continue to grow as the new applications (frames) are added to the system. Of importance in this design concept is that not only are the source representations of the frames kept in the common library, but the object (executable) representations of the frames are kept in a common frame object library. Thus, maintenance of applications using shared frames is automatic with the modification of the shared frames. For example, a frame which monitors blood pressure trends and is used by both the application for automatic monitoring of blood pressure from bedside monitors and the nurse-charting application for manual entry of blood pressure are automatically updated to new criteria when the blood pressure trends frame is changed to incorporate newer criteria.

To enhance the productivity of the application developers, several knowledge frame tools are available. The first is a general purpose frame editor. This editor is designed to permit the developer to write frames in the frame language easily. It is syntax dependent and requires the user to be conversant with the syntax of the frame language. With this tool or a text editor, source knowledge frames can be created and transmitted to the frame compiler for compilation into the frame object representation.

We have also written a series of special purpose frame compilers intended for use by domain experts who are not familiar with programming techniques. An example of such a special purpose editor is our general questionnaire editor. This editor permits the user to create data acquisition frames used with terminal data entry applications. The editor, through menus presented to the user, creates a frame with sophisticated windowing and permits definition of decision logic for evaluation of the entered

```
TITLE:  NEURO MENU                              [1 : 1 : 2];
MESSAGE:
AUTHOR:  I-0 0 0 0 0 0 0 0 - NANCY                      -I;
FRAME TYPE:   DATA ACQUISITION;
MAINTENANCE
VARIABLE DECLARATIONS:
ORIENT        ;LOC        ;MOVE          ;GENBEHAV       ;DATABASE
    MOVES WHICH IS I-28  01  01  02  03  04-I;
    GENERAL WHICH IS  I-28  01  01  02  03  05-I;

WINDOW: NEURO                   (type (MC), minmax ( 0,  5),
    heading ("NEUROLOGICAL MENU", NORMAL),
    location ( 2,  0), control (NP),
BEGIN
FIELD:  ORIENT        (order (, 0),
    text ("Orientation", NORMAL),
    location ( 1,  2), input (N),
    default ( ),
    select (SN), control (NS),
    field help ( " ", " " ) );
FIELD:  LOC
    text ("Loc", NORMAL),
    location ( 2,  2), input (N),
    default ( ),
    select (SN), control (NS),
    field help ( " ", " " ) );
FIELD:  MOVE                    (order (,0) ,
    text ("Movement and strength", NORMAL),
    location ( 3,  2), input (N),
    default ( )
    select (SN), control (NS),
field help ( " "," " ) );
FIELD:  GENBEHAV                (order (, 0),
    text ("General behavior", NORMAL),
    location ( 4,  2), input (N),
    default ( ),
    select (SN), control (NS),
    field help ( " ",   " ") ) ;
END;
 LOGIC:  ACQUIRE NEURO;
Pack;
 FOLLOWUP:   ALERT: =4;
    IF NOT $ EXIST ORIENT OR NOT $ EXIST LOC OR NOT $ EXIST MOVE OR
    NOT $ EXIST GENBEHAV OR NOT $ EXIST DATABASE THEN BEGIN
    STACK (ALERT, MOVES, GENERAL);
    EXIT FALSE;
    END;
    IF $ EXIST ORIENT THEN CALL 28 . 1 . 10;
    IF $ EXIST LOC THEN CALL 28 . 1 .  11;
```

Figure 4.6. A frame data acquisition which includes windowing syntax in the frame language.

data. Figure 4.6 is a typical frame created by this tool. The user does not need to know the syntax of the window/field statements, but is responsible for creation of Acquire, Diagnostic, and Follow-up logic. Acquire logic is that logic executed by the frame prior to presentation of the data acquisition screen. Diagnostic logic is that logic executed by the frame immediately following the completion of the data acquisition for purposes of validating and/or error checking of the entered data. Follow-up logic is that logic executed by the frame to complete the decision function of the frame. Additional editors have been written for entry of medication requisition frames, general standing orders, etc.

In order to mover conveniently to this knowledge-frame-based application model, we have interfaced the executable frame system to all existing languages running on HELP. Therefore, applications on HELP can evolve to completely frame-based applications. For example, the pharmacy application may initially use the decision frames only for evaluation of medication contraindications by calling the appropriate frames following the entry of the medication order from the traditional non frame written pharmacy program. It can then evolve to calling predictive ordering frames from the same program by merely replacing the code in the pharmacy program for entry of the medication order with a call to a set of frames to assist in the medication order. This process allows to easy enhancement of our existing applications without requiring a complete rewrite of the application as a frame-based application.

All of the decision support applications on HELP are undergoing the transformation to this newer architecture of frame-based decision support. As we continue the transformation we anticipate newer syntax/features to be added to the frame language. Effort is also underway to develop frame management programs which will assist us in the maintenance and understanding of the use of the knowledge frames as a model for a generalized decision support system.

Summary

Use of hospital information systems (HIS) is no longer limited to administrative functions. The addition to these systems of decision support capability is now a necessity. Development of the decision support modules requires a different software architecture than that employed by most HIS systems today. This paper describes the generic uses of decision support throughout the many hospital applications. Several levels of decision support are outlined with examples to illustrate the many areas where decision support is useful. At LDS Hospital in Salt Lake City, Utah, we have developed an HIS using a new software architecture which supports the creation of decision support applications. This system uses a frame structure to represent knowledge. Examples of the frames and their syntax is presented. Using the frame tools which are provided, an application developer can easily develop and test decision support modules which interact directly with the clinical user and the patient database.

References

1. Pryor TA, Gardner RM, Clayton PD, Warner HR. The HELP System. J Med Systems 1983; 7:87–101.
2. Prokosch HU, Pryor TA. Intelligent Data Acquisition in Order Entry Programs. Proceedings of the Twelfth Annual Symposium on Computer Applications in Medical Care. 1988:454–458.
3. Bradshaw KE, Gardner RM, Pryor TA. Development of a Computerized Laboratory Alerting System. Comput Biomed Res 1989; 6:575–587.
4. Pryor TA, Clayton PD, Haug PJ, Wigertz O. Design of a Knowledge Driven HIS. Proceedings of Eleventh Annual Symposium on Computer Applications in Medical Care, 1987; 60–63.
5. Barnett GO, Cimino JJ, Hupp JA, Hoffer EP. DX plain: An evolving diagnostic-support system. JAMA 1987; 258:67–74.
6. Shortliffe EH. Computer Based Medical Consultion: MY. CIN. New York; Elsevier 1976.
7. Miller RA, Pople HE, Myers JD. Internist-1, and experimental computer-based diagnostic consultant for internal medicine. New Engl J Med 1982; 307:468–476.
8. Hulse RD, Clark SJ, Jackson JC, Warner HR, Gardner RM. Computerized medication monitoring system. Am J Hosp Pharm 1976; 33:1061–1061.
9. Pryor TA, Lindsay AE, England W. Computer analysis of serial Electrocardiograms Compent Biomed Res 1973; 6:228–234.
10. Gardner RM, Cannon GH, Morris AH, et al. Computerized blood gas interpretation and reporting system. Res Care 1985; 30:695–700.
11. Miller PL. Medical plan-analysis by computer: Critiquing the pharmalogical management of essential hypertension. Comput Biomed Res 1984; 17:25–40.
12. Warner HR, Haug PJ, Bouhaddou O, Lincoln M, Warner H Jr., Sorensen D, Williamson JW, Fan C. ILLIAD As An Expert Consultant to Teach Differential Diagnosis. Proceedings of Twelfth Annual Symposium on Computer Applications in Medical Care, 1988; 371–376.
13. Sittig D. Computerized Management of Patient Care in a Complex, Controlled Clinical Trial in the ICU. Proceedings of the Eleventh Annual Symposium on Computer Applications in Medical Care, 1987; 225–229.

Chapter 5
Decision Analysis: A Framework for Critical Care Decision Assistance

Adam Seiver and Samuel Holtzman

Over the next five years, computer-based systems will replace the paper chart in many critical care units [1]. Powerful, easy-to-use bedside workstations will acquire, store, and display a comprehensive set of patient data, including the patient's history and physical exam, physiological variables, laboratory results, and radiographic images. Using such a system, the clinician will have vastly better access to facts about his or her patients than he now has, using the existing manual charting methods. However, having ready access to facts leaves the clinician with the difficult task of choosing what to do. It is natural to expect that the computer should provide assistance here, as well. Reed Gardner [2], President of Computers in Critical Care and Pulmonary Medicine has said: "The ultimate goal of a medical computer system is, after all, to assist physicians in making medical decisions."

Systems that provide clinical decision assistance will significantly affect clinical practice. However, to be truly useful, these systems will need to be based on sound principles. Decision analysis offers a rigorous framework for designing and implementing computer-based systems that offer decision assistance. In this paper, we begin by examining existing critical care decision-making practices. Next, we present the decision analysis approach to decision-making, including key decision-analytic concepts and techniques. We then introduce intelligent decision systems— computer-based systems that automate decision analysis. Following this, we discuss how decision analysis can be applied in the critical care environment given this environment's special decision-making features. Finally, we briefly describe a pilot intelligent decision system, *Orchestra*, that we are developing for ventilator management.

Adapted from an article published in the *Int J Clin Monit Comput* 6:137–156, 1989. Reprinted with permission of Kluwer Academic Publishers.

Current Critical Care Decision Practices

Let's start by looking at a typical scenario that illustrates current critical care decision practices.

Mr. A is admitted to the surgical intensive care unit in shock. The physician decides to institute monitoring with radial and pulmonary artery lines. After several attempts, the physician determines that the radial artery line cannot be placed percutaneously. She considers a percutaneous femoral artery line, but assesses the risk of thrombosis as too high. Finally, she succeeds at inserting the catheter through a radial artery cut-down.

One hour after admission, approximately 20 physiological variables are being measured continually. The physician studies the bedside flowsheet and notes that the patient has a mean arterial pressure of 125 mmHg and a very high systemic vascular resistance.

The physician decides to use a nitroprusside infusion to reduce afterload while maintaining preload with a crystalloid infusion. Accordingly, before leaving, the physician writes the following orders for the nurses:

1. Bolus with saline to keep wedge pressure at 10–15 mmHg.
2. Titrate nitroprusside to keep mean arterial pressure at 80–90 mmHg.

When the physician returns four hours later, she notes with satisfaction that the patient's resistance has decreased, that the wedge pressure is 15 mmHg, and that the mean arterial pressure is 85 mmHg.

Twelve hours later, however, the patient has received three liters of saline, is nauseated from the nitroprusside and is *still in shock*.

At first glance, the patient management illustrated in the scenario appears satisfactory and its ineffectiveness at 12 hours seems surprising. However, when we review the case in greater detail, we can discover at least four different decision-making defects that contribute to this ineffectiveness: 1) sparse alternatives, 2) information overload, 3) superficial objectives, and 4) ineffective delegation of decision-making.

Sparse Alternatives

Sparse alternatives lead to missed opportunities. In the scenario, the patient is admitted to the intensive care unit for resuscitation, and the physician is unable to place a radial artery line percutaneously. At that point, she considers her alternatives: percutaneous femoral artery line versus radial artery line placed by cut-down. She decides to perform a cut-down. However, has the physician considered all the pertinent alternatives? Perhaps *no line* is a reasonable alternative, and other monitoring technologies could be substituted. For example, arterial pulse oximetry and end-tidal carbon dioxide monitoring can reduce the need for arterial blood gases. Blood pressure can be measured automatically with self-inflating cuffs. Mixed venous oximetry can provide corroborating evidence about perfusion. These alternative technologies can be substituted singly or in combination. Critical care decision-making suffers when the decision-maker considers only a narrow range of options.

Information Overload

Information overload can put the patient in danger. In the scenario, the physician must interpret the large amount of patient data organized in time-oriented fashion on the flowsheet reproduced in Table 5.1. She correctly notes that the mean arterial pressure, 125 mmHg, and the systemic vascular resistance, 4,232 dyne sec cm^{-5}, are quite high. However, because of the large array of numbers confronting her, she fails to note that the pulmonary artery occlusion pressure (the wedge pressure), which is recorded as 13 mmHg, is 12 mmHg higher than the pulmonary artery di-

Table 5.1. The flowsheet for the Patient in the Scenario Overwhelms the Clinician With a Large Array of Data.

Variable	Time							
	7	8	9	10	11	12	13	14
Temperature	34.5	34.5	34.6	34.6	34.6	34.6	34.6	34.6
Respiratory rate	8	8	8	8	8	8	8	8
Tidal volume	1200	1200	1200	1200	1200	1200	1200	1200
PaCO$_2$	33	27	30	28	32	32	32	35
PaO$_2$	67	62	65	69	62	70	75	71
pH	7.48	7.57	7.53	7.55	7.50	7.50	7.49	7.45
ETCO$_2$	25	18	20	18	22	22	22	21
SaO$_2$	0.94	0.93	0.93	0.93	0.93	0.93	0.93	0.90
SvO$_2$	0.45	0.36	0.42	0.55	0.56	0.55	0.55	0.52
HR	101	102	101	101	102	104	105	103
Radial systolic	180	170	150	118	120	117	117	116
Radial diastolic	100	68	68	69	70	71	71	71
Radial mean	125	101	94	85	86	85	85	85
Pulmonary systolic	40	42	43	42	40	42	41	41
Pulmonary diastolic	1	2	3	3	4	3	4	4
Pulmonary mean	14	15	16	16	16	16	16	16
Central venous	17	18	18	17	18	18	18	18
Wedge	13	14	15	15	16	15	16	16
Resistance	4232	3867	3153	2071	2021	2080	2156	2070
Cardiac output	2.1	1.7	1.9	2.6	2.7	2.6	2.5	2.6

* Note that the pulmonary artery occlusion pressure, the wedge, is greater than the pulmonary artery pressure—easily overlooked evidence that the wedge is inaccurate.

astolic pressure, which is recorded as 1 mmHg. The physician should know that, usually, this situation indicates that the wedge pressure value is wrong, but she fails to take advantage of this knowledge because she is distracted by the large amount of other numbers she needs to consider. Thus, she erroneously concludes that the patient needs afterload reduction. In fact, the patient simply needs volume. Although the physician prescribes saline to maintain preload, this only compensates for the preload-reducing effects of the nitroprusside and the patient remains in hypovolemic shock.

This example illustrates the problem that has been well articulated by Roger Bone: "Possibly the most serious danger . . . is that of drowning a physician in a flood of numbers. The presentation of more data that can be assimilated can contribute to incorrect clinical decisions" [3].

Superficial Objectives

Superficial objectives can lead to misguided action. In the scenario, the physician returns after four hours to evaluate the patient's response to therapy and notes that the patient's resistance has decreased, that the wedge pressure is 15 mmHg, and that the mean arterial pressure is 85mmHg. She feels the therapeutic goals are being accomplished. In fact, the patient remains in shock: cardiac output is low, and there is inadequate perfusion to meet the patient's oxygen needs. From the point of view of survival, the patient has not been adequately resuscitated. This illustrates how clinicians often choose superficial objectives that do not promote ultimate objectives, a problem that William Shoemaker has frequently discussed: "The traditional approach usually assumes that normal values are the appropriate therapeutic goals . . . Therapy should restore physiological defects not just to their normal values but to their optimal value" [4].

Ineffective Delegation

Ineffective delegation of decision-making erodes the quality of patient care. One compelling feature of critical care delivery is that it must be sustained 24 hours a day, 365 days a year. Therefore, those individuals with ultimate responsibility or with valuable expertise simply cannot be continuously present at the patient's bedside. For example, the attending surgeon or the pulmonary specialist have responsibilities in the clinics, in the operating room, in the wards, in the office, and in other critical care units. (And health providers also need time for their personal lives.) While a few critical care units now provide in-house intensive coverage around the clock, collaborative decision-making—particularly between physicians and nurses—is essential to high-quality care. In a prospective study of treatment and outcome in 5,030 patients in intensive care units at 13 tertiary care hospitals, death rates (adjusted for severity of illness) significantly diminished when there was improved interaction and coordination between the intensive care unit staff [5].

Currently, two mechanisms exist for accomplishing this coordination: 1) implicit orders, and 2) standing orders. Implicit orders are unwritten guides to decision-making. For example, there is generally no written rule in critical care units that states that if a ventilated patient becomes unstable, the fractional inspired oxygen concentration should be increased to 100% while the patient is resuscitated. However, the staff is expected to know enough to increase the oxygen concentration based on training and experience. Likewise, the staff is expected to know that when a surgical patient has a urine output that is less than 0.5 cc kg per hour, it must manage the possibly poor renal perfusion by addressing overall perfusion (usually with volume, occasionally with inotropes) by calling the physician, or by performing both actions.

When all ICU team members are in constant contact and when the team shares a large body of patient experience, unwritten orders are effective, because all members implicitly know what to do and why. However, constant staff turnover and shift-work fragment this background of understanding and severely disrupt coordination based on group intuition.

For example, Mr. Jones, a new nurse, may not know that Mr. A's urine output should be maintained at 50 cc per hour. If Ms. Smith, the nurse during the preceding eight hours, does not convey that fact during report at change of shift (a not-too-infrequent occurrence), Mr. A may be left dangerously oliguric overnight. In short, implicit orders are susceptible to breaking down under the stress of realistic staffing conditions.

Standing orders are used to fill the gaps that may occur with implicit orders. For example, the physician could obviate unreported oliguria in Mr. A. by writing the following orders:

1. Measure urine output every hour.
2. Call physician for urine output less than 50 cc/hr.

Standing orders aim to decrease errors of *omission*, but they often promote serious errors of *commission*. *Excessive testing* is one consequence of standing orders. For example, to ensure that anticoagulation therapy is closely monitored, the physician might write the order:

Send blood to laboratory for partial thromboplastin time every four hours.

Such an order will ensure that the laboratory tests are sent off regularly, even if the physician is not physically present to make the request. Unfortunately, the lab ordering system does not always recognize when these orders become obsolete. Joseph Civetta studied testing for coagulation in his unit and found. "[There was] repetitive testing of coagulation parameters in many patients who showed no evidence of a coagulation disorder" [6]. Civetta advocates eliminating standing orders for laboratory tests, but this requires developing a better mechanism for delegating decision-making.

Another consequence of delegating decision-making with standing orders is *tail chasing*. Tail chasing was illustrated in the scenario when the physician left her standing orders:

1. Bolus with saline to keep wedge pressure at 10–15 mmHg.
2. Titrate nitroprusside to keep mean arterial pressure at 80–90 mmHg.

In following these orders, the nurses gave the patient 3 liters of saline; however, the patient remained in shock, despite the fact that the basic defect was hypovolemia. Administering nitroprusside decreased both the mean arterial pressure and the wedge pressure, which, in turn, caused the nurse to infuse a bolus of saline. This action brought the wedge pressure back up to the desired value, but it also increased the preload and, thus, the mean arterial pressure. As a result, the nurse increased the nitroprusside dosage, which decreased the wedge pressure, which necessitated further saline, and so on. The increased venous capacitance caused by the nitroprusside prevented the massive saline infusion from correcting the hypovolemic defect. These positive feedback situations can be created whenever the management of therapies with counteracting effects (e.g., nitroprusside and dopamine, crystalloid infusion and diuretics) is ineffectively delegated.

The four defects revealed in the scenario—sparse alternatives, information overload, superficial objectives, and ineffective delegation—are symptomatic of a single underlying defect: faulty decision-making. Each of these problems may be viewed as the result of the critical care staff committing to an action that is inconsistent with either what they can do, what they know, or what they really want. Decision analysis provides a framework for avoiding these inconsistencies and for thereby improving the quality of critical care decision-making.

Decision Analysis Approach to Decision-Making

Decision analysis comprises the philosophy, methodology, and professional discipline for ensuring high-quality decision-making. While Professor Ronald A. Howard of Stanford University coined the term "decision analysis" in 1964 [7], the roots of decision analysis date back to the work of two great mathematicians, P.S. Laplace [8] and D. Bernoulli [9]. sional application of decision analysis possible; and since 1965, decision analysis has been regularly taught at the graduate level at Stanford University and at many other universities. Decision analysis is now a growing professional field, with a two-decade success record.

Science is a *descriptive* discipline: it studies what *is* by describing it. And engineering is a *prescriptive* discipline: it creates what *should be* by designing it. Decision analysis is a *normative* discipline: it is a prescriptive discipline guided by a set of *norms*—that is, principles of right action.

Decision analysis focuses on bringing clarity of action to difficult decisions. By an *action*, we mean the irrevocable allocation of valuable resources. By a *decision*, we mean the commitment to irrevocably allocate valuable resources. Decision analysis can address a wide range of decisions, but it is particularly well suited for decisions involving complexity, dynamics, and uncertainty.

Because of its cost (typically tens or hundreds of thousands of dollars) and the long time necessary to carry out an analysis (around 100 person-hours), professional decision analysis has been almost exclusively applied within business and industry. However, in an academic setting, decision analysis has also been successfully applied to many medical decisions [10]. Later in this paper, we will discuss how (through the use of intelligent decision systems) professional-level decision analysis can be made much less costly and faster for use in a clinical setting.

Using decision analysis effectively requires understanding its *philosophy*, *procedures*, and *tools*. The decision analysis philosophy fundamentally defines high-quality decision-making in the form of key concepts and distinctions. The procedures of decision analysis constitute an extensive array of techniques to capture and reason about all aspects of a decision. The tools of decision analysis greatly facilitate the decision-analytic process and make it efficient and easy to use.

In decision analysis, *decision theory* provides the general and sound framework for recommending a course of action—*given a decision model*. Decision theory takes as an input a mathematical model of a decision problem and provides as an output a prescription for action. Decision theory can therefore be viewed as a conditional statement, as shown in Figure 5.1.

Decision analysis is based on decision theory much like medicine is based on biology. Just as physicians must devote considerable time and effort to formulating a medical problem in biological terms and to interpreting any biological conclusions in terms that are meaningful for patient care, so decision analysts must devote the time and effort to formally

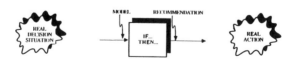

Figure 5.1. Decision theory is a conditional statement.

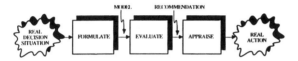

Figure 5.2. Formally capturing real decision situations and interpreting formal recommendations are major tasks in decision analysis. (Reprinted by permission of Strategic Decisions Group.)

capture the decision as a decision model and then to interpret the formal recommendations resulting from applying decision theory to the model.

Given this situation, we can thus view the practical use of decision theory as a three-stage process (Figure 5.2) whose three stages are *formulation* (i.e., developing the formal decision model), *evaluation* (i.e., computing a recommendation from the model), and *appraisal* (i.e., interpreting the formal recommendation).

However, this strictly sequential approach to using formal decision methods has a major short-coming—it does not account for the likely disagreement between the decision-maker and the method's recommendation. In fact, such disagreement is almost certain to occur. Given that the decision-maker requires assistance to gain new insight into his problem, we can assume he is having difficulty dealing with his decision. Therefore, formally analyzing the decision will probably expose many of the inconsistencies and lack of focus that made the decision difficult in the first place. Moreover, such disagreement is very beneficial, because it exposes important flaws in either the decision-maker's understanding of his decision (i.e., how he preceives and interprets it) or his logic.

A simple way to deal with the possible unacceptability of a formally obtained recommendation—in fact to take advantage of it—is to extend the sequential process by explicitly adding a *feedback* path, as shown in Figure 5.3. Such a closed-loop decision process allows the decision-maker to react to any surprising element of the formal prescription by reevaluating and possibly modifying his formulation. Alternatively, if after developing enough insight he agrees with the suggested strategy or if he determines that his disagreement results solely from logical error, he may choose to follow the formal recommendation. Hence, by producing

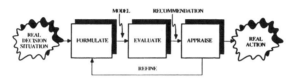

Figure 5.3. By producing a sequence of increasingly refined decision models, decision analysis generates the insight necessary for action. (Reprinted by permission of Strategic Decisions Group.)

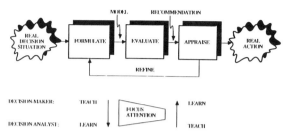

Figure 5.4. Decision analysis is a carefully engineered conversation that develops insight by focusing attention on the key aspects of the decision at hand. (Reprinted by permission of Strategic Decisions Group.)

a sequence of increasingly refined decision models, we can help the decision-maker develop the insight necessary for action.

The closed-loop decision process described in Figure 5.3 can be viewed as a blueprint for a conversation, which is illustrated in Figure 5.4 It involves two key participants—the decision-maker and a decision analyst. During the formulation stage of the process, the decision-maker *teaches* the details of the decision at hand to the decision analyst, who *learns* by building an appropriate decision model. These activities are reserved during the appraisal stage, where the decision analyst *teaches* the decision-maker the implications of the formal recommendation for action obtained during the evaluation stage. Most of the insight developed in the closed-loop decision process shown in Figure 5.4 results from this interchange of information and new knowledge between the decision-maker and the decision analyst. Moreover, the formal machinery embodied in the evaluation stage guides and focuses this interchange. This attention-focusing effect assits the decision participants in producing an increasingly simple, yet representative, model of the decision as the process progresses.

Key Decision Analysis Concepts

As the above discussion makes clear, the *decision-maker* plays a central role in decision analysis. The decision-maker either owns the resources to be allocated or is acting in the best interests of their owner. An *expert* is a source of information and alternatives, but he is *not* a source of recommendations. And a *decision analyst* is an expert on process—not content—who guides the conversation toward clarity of action.

We must also be precise about our use of decision terms in medicine. *Diagnosing* consists of thinking about the patient's condition. *Decision-making* consists of thinking about what to do, given a possibly uncertain and incomplete diagnosis. *Treating* consists of action—of doing something to the patient whether that action is diagnostic, therapeutic, or both. Given these definitions, it would thus be incorrect to say: "I have decided that the patient has appendicitis" One can *decide* on "appendectomy," but one *diagnoses* "appendicitis."

Decision-making has three fundamental components: *alternatives* (what you *can do*), *preferences* (what you *want*), and *information* (what you *know*). Key concepts related to each are now considered in turn.

Alternatives

Alternatives should encompass a wide range of possible action, generally both inside and outside strictly medical dimensions. For example, changes in a patient's personal lifestyle and work activities are an important component of radiation therapy and must be part of the definition of that alternative. Alternatives must also account for the patient's specific circumstances. For example, the patient's economic situation, the presence or absence of a living will, and the presence or absence of relatives willing to donate organs are all special constraints that may expand or restrict the set of possible options.

Decisions are often difficult to make because there is no *dominating alternative*. A dominating alternative is an alternative that would be recommended to the vast majority of the patients with a particular set of findings or diagnosis. For example, appendectomy is the dominating alternative for appendicitis. In contrast, there is no dominating alternative for infertility due to blockage of the fallopian tubes. Celiotomy, in vitro fertilization, and doing nothing are all reasonable options. In such cases, doctors must know more about the problem—principally about the patient's preferences—before they can identify the best alternative [15].

Preferences

Preferences directly represent the desires of the decision-maker, who (as noted earlier) either owns or acts on behalf of the owner of the recources to be allocated. In medicine, preferences almost always concern the patient's length of life (lifetime), personal and work life (lifestyle), overall well-being (comfort), and financial and other economic resources such as health maintenance contracts (wealth). Achieving clarity of action requires explicitly quantifying the trade-offs that the patient wants made among these fundamental attributes.

Measuring preferences is particularly challenging in making medical decisions, because possible outcomes are often unfamiliar to those who will bear them. For example, the patient undergoing radiation therapy for the first time probably has little experience that can allow him or her to translate descriptions of the possible complications into personal terms. Implicit guardianship is often another complicating factor. When the patient cannot make choices for himself or herself, whose preferences should be used? We believe that the preferences used should be those of the patient—the person whose resources are at stake—or, if these are unavailable, those of someone (i.e., a guardian) who understands the patient well enough to act on his or her behalf with his or her best interests in mind. In many circumstances—but not always—this individual would be the bedside physician. Frequently, however, there are multiple stakeholders: the patient, family members, physicians, nurses, and governmental agencies. And even when the source of the preferences is clear, ethical concerns may still make trade-offs difficult. Because of these challenges, decision-analytic methods are the most robust and humane way to deal with difficult preferences, because these methods are explicit, comprehensive, and incisive.

It is important not to confuse direct (primary) preferences with indirect (secondary) preferences. For example, while a patient has an *indirect* preference on his or her mean arterial pressure, he or she has a *direct* preference on survival. In medicine—as in most human endeavors—indirect preferences are a useful means of delegation. However, making decisions requires being aware of primary preferences to avoid pursuing objectives that have become obsolete. For example, keeping the mean arterial pressure normal may be *desirable*, but it is secondary to keeping the patient *alive*.

Information

Information—knowledge about the possible consequences of pertinent actions—is essential to decision-making. In decision analysis, information, both certain and uncertain, is treated explicitly. This information can take one of two forms: structural and parametric. *Structural* information specifies relations among decision elements. For example, the relationship between FIO_2 and PIO_2 given by the alveolar gas equation is structural. *Parametric* information specifies decision elements individually. For example, the value of the cardiac output is parametric.

Decision analysis treats uncertainty explicitly. Consequently, decision-analytic recommendations effectively reflect the decision-maker's uncertain situation. In particular, decision analysis can yield optimal recommendations that would be discarded if uncertainty were ignored. These recommendations are often referred to as "hedging" alternatives. For example, consider a patient who has just suffered a myocardial infarction and is demonstrating second-degree atrio-ventricular block. If we know for sure the patient will develop fixed, complete heart block, we should put in a permanent pacemaker. And if we know the patient will *not* develop complete heart block, no pacemaker is indicated. In fact, however, we have only incomplete knowledge about whether the patient will develop fixed, complete heart block, so we hedge by placing a transvenous pacemaker. This alternative is inferior to the permanent pacemaker if heart block is present and inferior to no pacemaker if heart block is absent. However, the hedging alternative is preferable to both if heart block is *uncertain*.

In capturing uncertain information, decision analysis uses the rigorous methods of probability. Specifically, decision analysis views probability from the perspective of its inventors (i.e., P.S. Laplace and D. Bernoulli): probability is a state of *information*, *not* a state of *nature*. For example, imagine a 35-year-old man who presents to the emergency department with mild chest pain. An EKG is performed and blood work is drawn. You are the physician called to the emergency department to evaluate the patient. What is your probability that the patient has had a myocardial infarction? Based on what you know—mild chest pain, young patient—you would presumably assess this probability to be quite low. However, suppose you discover during your interview with the patient that his father and grandfather both died suddenly at age 35. Now your index of suspicion has increased, and you assess a higher probability. Next, the technician hands you your copy of the EKG, which shows only nonspecific ST-T wave changes. Perhaps now your suspicions are lessened and you decrease your probability of a myocardial infarction. Finally, the laboratory work is returned—the creatinine phosphokinase (CPK) is quite high with a significantly elevated myocardial band (MB) fraction. Now your probability has significantly increased and myocardial infarction has become your diagnosis. Throughout all this diagnostic effort, the patient—the state of nature—has, of course, not changed. What *has* changed is your state of information. You revise your probability assessment to accommodate the changes in your state of information. In other words, there is no single "correct" probability—it depends on what you know.

Because uncertainty is involved in most important decisions, we must distinguish the quality of decisions from the quality of outcomes. An example illustrates the point. Suppose you were offered the opportunity to buy a ticket to a lottery for $1 that offered a 1-in-1,000 chance of winning $100 million (tax free). While this investment would be outstanding for most individuals, it involves a 99.9% chance of a bad outcome! Suppose you invested and lost—would purchasing the ticket have been a good or bad decision? Would you invest again in an identical deal? The point is that because the consequences of actions may be uncertain, it is possible to make a good decision and get a bad outcome. (All other combinations of good/bad decision and good/bad outcome are, of course, also possible—including making a bad decision and getting a good outcome.)

The clinical approach to appendicitis provides a medical example that illustrates the difference between the quality of outcomes and the quality of decisions. For example, a 20-year-old man presents with nausea, epigastric pain localizing in the right lower quadrant, and point tenderness at McBurney's point. There is fever and leukocytosis. As a result, the patient undergoes an appendectomy. Most surgeons would consider this a good decision. However, suppose the appendix is found to be normal during the operation. Was it still a good decision to operate? From a decision-analytic perspective, performing the appendectomy would be considered a good decision, because it was consistent with the decision-maker's alternatives, preferences, and knowledge *at the time the decision was made.*

A logical consequence of this distinction is that we should focus on high-quality decision-making, not on high-quality outcomes. Decision analysis shows us that the quality of decisions and the quality of outcomes should be measured separately. However, most individuals' performance is measured in terms of their outcomes, not their decisions. Unfortunately the price of rewarding outcomes and not decisions is *bad decisions.* Defensive medicine illustrates this effect. For example, a 30-year-old man is admitted for hernia repair. A detailed history and physical examination are unremarkable except for the hernia. Intraoperatively, the patient has a massive myocardial infarction and dies. The surgeon is sued for not obtaining a preoperative electrocardiogram. Now the surgeon obtains a pre-operative electrocardiogram for all his patients–regardless of indications. Having been sued because of a bad outcome that resulted from an extremely rare event, the surgeon thus makes bad decision-making a routine part of his practice.

Decision Models in Decision Analysis

A *decision model* is a formal representation of a decision problem. A good decision model captures the decision at hand explicitly, succinctly, and unambiguously. Because it is explicit, all important aspects of the decision are available for review. Because it is succinct, only important aspects are represented. Because it is unambiguous, all model elements are clearly defined.

Influence diagrams are the foremost way of representing decision models in modern decision analysis [11]. Influence diagrams are easy to understand, mathematically well defined, very general, and compact. In general, influence diagrams have significant theoretical and practical advantages over another commonly used decision representation language-decision trees. In addition to representing probabilistic independence effectively, enforcing a clear distinction between informational and probabilistic relationships, and preventing loss of information from asymmetries, influence diagrams grow linearly (as opposed to exponentially) with the size of the problem they represent and, thus, can be used to model much larger decisions than trees can model. These technical advantages are enhanced by the fact that the mathematical concept of influence, conditional as well as informational, is very close to its intuitive counterpart.

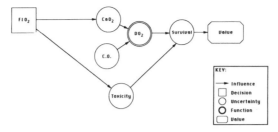

Figure 5.5. Influence diagrams can represent FIO$_2$ adjustment decisions. The choices for FIO$_2$ (ranging from 21% to 100%) are represented by the rectangular decision node. The physiological and clinical variables that mediate the effect of FIO$_2$ on survival are represented by the oval chance nodes (which may be uncertain, e.g., toxicity; or deterministic, e.g., DO$_2$). The patient's preference for survival is represented by the value node. FIO$_2$, fractional inspired oxygen concentration; CaO$_2$ oxygen content arterial blood; C.O., cardiac output; DO$_2$, oxygen delivery. (Reprinted by permission of Strategic Decisions Group.)

As defined by Howard and Matheson [12], an influence diagram is a singly connected, acyclic, directed graph with two types of nodes—decision and chance—two types of arrows or arcs—conditioning and informational—and typically a single sink node of type chance (Figure 5.5). The acyclic, singly connected nature of influence diagrams implies that sets such as predecessors and successors of a node are defined in the usual manner.

Decision nodes are usually represented by a rectangle or a square and denote variables under the decision-maker's control. *Chance nodes*—usually represented by an oval or a circle—denote probabilistic variables. A special form of a chance node is a deterministic node, which is usually represented by a double-ringed oval or circle. The value of a deterministic node is known exactly if the value(s) of its predecessor node(s) are specified. *Conditioning arrows* are always directed toward a chance node and denote probabilistic dependence. *Informational arrows* are always directed toward a decision node and denote available information. An influence diagram usually (although not necessarily) has a single chance node with no successors (i.e., a sink node), which is called the *value node* and which represents the decision-maker's direct preferences. Chance nodes without direct chance predecessors (i.e., chance source nodes) are called *border nodes*.

Figure 5.5 shows a simple influence diagram that represents the FIO$_2$ adjustment decision. The possible choices for the FIO$_2$ (e.g., 21% to 100%) are represented by the square decision node. The fractional inspired oxygen concentration affects the oxygen content of arterial blood (CaO$_2$) and the potential for oxygen toxicity. These are treated as probabilistic relationships and represented as chance nodes with conditioning arcs arising from the FIO_2 decision node. Cardiac output (CO) is represented as a chance border node. Oxygen delivery (DO_2) is represented as a deterministic node, because it is known for certain given CaO_2 and cardiac output—in other words, it is the product of the values of these predecessors of DO_2. Survival depends probabilistically on oxygen toxicity and oxygen delivery. Finally, we declare survival to be the only significant attribute of the possible outcomes by attaching the value node to survival alone.

Figure 5.5 shows the structure of the FIO_2, adjustment decision and in particular highlights the trade-offs and the key relationships. An influence diagram, however, can represent a decision completely, not just in terms of its structure. A full description of a decision problem requires that the diagram contain at least one decision node directly or indirectly influencing a value node and that consistent, detailed specifications exist for each node in the diagram. For decision nodes, the set of possible outcomes corresponds to the set of decision alternatives; for chance nodes, this set of outcomes corresponds to the sample space of the variable being represented. Furthermore, for chance nodes, a detailed description should also include a probability measure over the set of possible outcomes. An important, yet subtle, fact about probabilistic specifications of chance nodes is that they must be consistent with the set of direct predecessors of the node and their respective outcomes.

A structurally complete influence diagram whose nodes and relations have not been specified in detail is said to be defined at the level of *structure*. A diagram developed in all the necessary detail is defined in terms of both its *structure* and its *parameters*. An influence diagram is *well-formed* when it has been consistently defined both structurally and parametrically. Algorithms exist for computing the optimal policy from a well-formed influence diagram representing a decision [13,14] and for deducing other important inferential results (e.g., value-of-information, value-of-control, and other sensitivity measurements).

Intelligent Decision Systems

As mentioned earlier, decision analysis is not widely used in medicine, because it is too expensive and too slow. Professional decision analysis has been almost exclusively applied in business and industry. By automating the decision analysis process, intelligent decision systems make decision analysis inexpensive and fast. Therefore, intelligent decision systems open the door for the wider medical application of decision analysis.

A *decision system* is a system that makes recommendations for action and is typically implemented on a computer. An *intelligent decision system* is a decision system that delivers expert-level decision analysis assistance [15]. As part of this assistance, the intelligent decision system

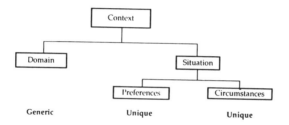

Figure 5.6. A decision context is composed of both generic and unique elements.

may provide access to a substantial knowledge base in the domain of the decision.

Intelligent decision systems arise from the use of artificial intelligence technology to automate the formulation and appraisal skills of professional decision analysts in a well-defined decision arena. Intelligent decision systems are made possible by our ability to indentify and analyze in advance the common aspects of the decisions we face.

We refer to all the elements that are relevant to a decision as the *decision context* As shown in Figure 5.6 the decision context can be hierarchically decomposed into its *domain* and its *situations*. The domain consists of the generic subject matter with respect to which the decision is being made. The situation consists of the *preferences* and the *circumstances* pertinent to the decision at hand. Preferences refer to a statement of the satisfaction the decision-maker receives from particular states of the world. Circumstances are the information, constraints, and alternatives in a decision that are unique to a specific decision-maker.

Expert systems technology makes it possible to bring specialized domain knowledge to a decision problem. Decision analysis makes it possible to incorporate circumstances and preferences into decision-making. Intelligent decision systems facilitate the incorporation of all elements— domain, preferences, and circumstances—into the decision. Therefore, intelligent decision systems are ideal for making high-quality decision-making assistance widely available. In an important sense, expert systems increase the *quantity* of decisions (a useful feature when good decision-making relies on the knowledge of a few key individuals whose expertise can thus be made widely available). In contrast, decision analysis increases the *quality* of decisions. By combining both technologies, intelligent decision systems can make *high-quality* decisions available in *quantity*.

Figure 5.7 shows a plausible architecture for an intelligent decision system [15]. This architecture consists of four interconnected parts: a general-purpose inference engine, a set of data structures, a corresponding set of specialized procedures, and user interface (or front end).

The general purpose inference engine (illustrated on the top left corner

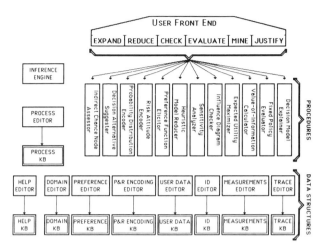

Figure 5.7. An architecture for an intelligent decision system. KB, knowledge base; ID, influence diagram.

of Figure 5.7—viewed from the side) interprets the knowledge bases throughout the system. In technical terms, its function is to implement efficiently a useful portion of the first-order predicate calculus and associated syllogisms.

The operation of the system revolves around a set of nine data structures. These structures, depicted as double-lined boxes along the left and bottom margins of Figure 5.7 can be accessed through structure-specific editors. Editors allow all interactions with the data to occur with consistent syntax and semantics at a high level, which allows the rest of the system to be independent of the physical implementation of the data structures and helps ensure their reliability and integrity.

The data structures in this architecture are manipulated by a set of specialized procedures. Figure 5.8 depicts a set of 12 such procedures, which are representative of those that should be part of an intelligent decision system. However, a somewhat different set may be better suited in any given implementation. The leftmost five procedures shown deal with decision-model development. In particular, the indirect chance node assessor, the decision alternative suggester, and the preference function elicitor develop the influence diagram model both structurally and parametrically. The probability distribution encoder and the risk attitude encoder further develop the model parametrically.

An important part of the proposed architecture for an intelligent decision system is an interface program to interact directly with the user. This program facilitates the use of the procedures and data structures that constitute the intelligent decision system and adapts the system's interaction to the indentity and expertise of each individual user.

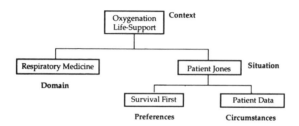

Figure 5.8. The Oxygenation Life-Support decision context has a domain—Respiratory Medicine—and a situation defined by the patient's preferences and data.

Applying Decision Analysis to Critical Care

In applying *decision* analysis to critical care, we must allow for special features of critical care decision-making, which include *delegated responsibility* and *distributed expertise*. Delegated reponsibility governs critical care physician and nurse decision-making. Fundamentally, the patient is the decision-maker, because it is primarily the patient's resources—his or her life and limb—that are at stake. In the critical care setting. the patient delegates decision-making responsibility to the physician, either *explicitly* when the patient is well enough to communicate or *implicitly* when the illness prevents such communication. The physician commits to action by providing a decision strategy. For example, the physician may decide that the patient should be placed on mechanical ventilation and receive hemodynamic life support. The nurse interprets and implements the physician's strategy into specific actions, such as adjusting the settings on the ventilator and the rates of infusion of the cardiac drugs.

Distributed expertise refers to the fact that different members of the critical care team are experts about different things. For example, the critical care physician specialist is most likely to be familiar with life-support technology and the pathophysiology of critical illness. The patient's attending physician is more likely to be familiar with the longitudinal nature of the patient's illness, having had the opportunity to interview the patient pre-operatively and to follow the patient from admission on the ward to the operating room to the intensive care unit. The nurse has the best perspective on the patient's minute-to-minute circumstances. A nurse is physically present at the bedside 24 hours per day and is the first to be aware of changes in the patient's condition, as reflected in his or her history, physical exam, monitored observations, and laboratory measurements.

As noted above, we can distinguish within each decision a generic domain and a unique situation. The situation is further divided into preferences and circumstances. Thus, for example, within the context of oxygenation life-support decisions, we identify a body of knowledge applicable for all patients—respiratory medicine (Figure 5.8). Every oxygenation life-support decision, however, will be made for a specific patient, and it is that patient's preferences and circumstances that define the situation. The patient's preferences may be very easy to describe (e.g., survival at all costs), or they may be difficult to capture, (e.g., subtle trade-offs between a desire to survive and a desire to die with dignity). The patient's circumstances not only include the unique constraints governing what can be done for the patient, but also the structural and parametric information about the patient, which correspond to data and diagnoses now typically recorded in the medical chart.

We can use the taxonomy of the decision context to accommodate the features of delegated responsibility and distributed expertise in critical care decision-making. Delegating decision-making corresponds to assigning responsibility for elements of the decision context. When the patient delegates to the physician, he or she assigns the physician the authority to determine each of the elements of the decision context. The physician may, in turn, wish to assign responsibility for the domain to a consultant critical care specialist and responsibility for the circumstances to the nurse who is continually present at the bedside. And he or she may wish to reserve responsibility for delineating the patient's preferences based on his or her personal contact with the patient. Of course, if the physician believes the nurse has a better rapport with the patient and family based on their continual contact at the bedside, then he or she may delegate responsibility for delineating the patients preferences to the nurse.

Thus, the taxonomy of the decision context allows decision-making to be delegated in a controlled fashion. The fact that different team members have different areas of expertise is gracefully handled at the same time by this "divide and conquer" approach. Once the various elements of the decision context have been defined, decision analysis provides a methodology for logical synthesis into recommendations and insight.

Decisions about adjusting FIO_2 for a post-operative patient dependent on a ventilator illustrate how the decision analysis approach can be used. We start with the task of encoding respiratory medicine domain knowledge, a task that is assigned to the pulmonary specialist physician. We ask the physician to represent his or her knowledge so the bedside physician and the nurse can easily use it to create influence diagrams for specific patients and decisions. He or she can do this by creating *decision-framing templates* that express common organizing principles of life-support decisions and by creating *knowledge maps* that articulate medical facts and details [16].

For example, Figure 5.9 presents a decision-framing template for life-support decisions. We represent life-support therapy generically with a decision node, a rectangle labeled "Life-Support R_x." We indicate that

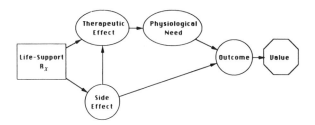

Figure 5.9. A decision-framing template expresses the common organizing principles underlying life-support decisions.

life-support therapy has a therapeutic effect and a side effect with chance nodes—ovals labeled "Therapeutic Effect" and "Side Effect"—that are linked to the decision by conditioning arcs from the decision node. The side effect may modulate the therapeutic effect. Consequently, there is an arrow from "Side Effect' to "Therapeutic Effect." The therapeutic effect is directed toward satisfying a fundamental patient physiological need. We represent this with an arrow from "Therapeutic Effect" to "Physiological Need." The patient outcome depends both on how well the patient's physiological need is satisfied and on how great a side effect is generated to accomplish that. This is indicated by the arrows from "Physiological Need" and "Side Effect" into "Outcome." The patient preferences over the outcomes are represented by the value node and the arrow from "Outcome" to "Value."

The value of this template is that it provides a ready-made structure for building an influence diagram for any life-support therapy—whether it is for oxygen therapy, fluid, inotropes, positive end-expiratory pressure, intra-aortic counterpulsation, or transfusion. Of course, for each specific therapy, the diagram will need to be further developed with the appropriate details for therapeutic effect, side effect, physiological need, outcome and value. The critical care specialist can provide significant guidance for this development and greatly enhance its efficiency by articulating the relevant medical facts and details in the form of knowledge maps.

For example, the immediate therapeutic effect of oxygen therapy is that increasing the inspired fraction of oxygen increases the alveolar partial pressure of oxygen. This effect is described by the alveolar gas equation [17]. Figure 5.10 is a knowledge map of the alveolar gas equation:

$$PAO_2 = PIO_2 - PACO_2 [FIO_2 + (1 - FIO_2)/R],$$

where

$$PIO_2 = 713 \times FIO_2.$$

PAO_2 is partial pressure of alveolar oxygen; PIO_2, the partial pres-

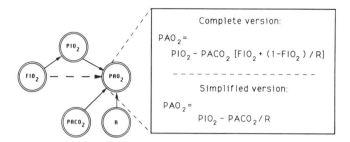

Figure 5.10. A knowledge map graphically represents the alveolar gas equation. Note that the simplified version that is commonly used clinically differs from the complete version, because it removes the conditioning arc from FIO_2 to PAO_2. See text for abbreviations.

sure of inspired oxygen; $PACO_2$, the partial pressure of alveolar carbon dioxide; FIO_2, the fractional inspired concentration of oxygen; and R, the respiratory quotient.

We graphically indicate that the fractional inspired oxygen concentration directly affects the partial pressure of inspired oxygen. The partial pressure of inspired oxygen, together with the partial pressure of alveolar carbon dioxide and the respiratory quotient, determine the partial pressure of alveolar oxygen. Note the arrow from "FIO_2" to "PAO_2." This direct influence of fractional inspired oxygen on the partial pressure of alveolar oxygen is deleted in the commonly used approximate form of the alveolar gas equation [3]. This gives the equation:

$$PAO_2 = PIO_2 - PACO_2/R$$

In a similar fashion, the critical care specialist will be responsible for encoding his or her knowledge about side effects of oxygen therapy and about the underlying physiological needs that oxygen therapy must satisfy. Sample knowledge maps for these elements are shown in Figure 5.11 and Figure 5.12. We note that the critical care specialist creates the knowledge maps and templates without the time pressure of meeting immediate clinical needs. Such decision engineering requires undistracted reflection. As we shall see, the work done by the critical care specialist

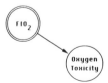

Figure 5.11. A knowledge map can represent the key side effect of FIO_2.

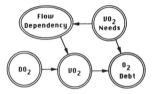

Figure 5.12. A knowledge map can represent the physiological relationships related to the need for oxidative metabolism. VO$_2$, oxygen consumption; DO$_2$, oxygen delivery.

represents an "off-line" investment that expedites the "on-line" in-fluence diagram-building tasks of the bedside physician and nurse.

The bedside physician frames the FIO$_2$ adjustment decision by using the knowledge maps to expand the decision-framing template. Using oxygen therapy as an example, the physician might build a decision framework as illustrated in Figure 5.13. This structurally complete in-fluence diagram characterizes what is relevant to decisions about adjust-ing the FIO$_2$ on a specific patient for an interval of time. The diagram explicitly identifies survival as the value node. This may not be appro-priate for all cases; here, the bedside physician is simply identifying the appropriate value function for the specific patient situation. Likewise, the remainder of the diagram is not meant to be universal—it simply repre-sents the physician's synthesis of the various knowledge elements into a

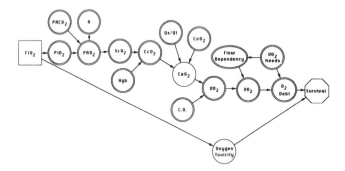

Figure 5.13. The bedside physician frames the FIO$_2$ adjustment decision by using the knowledge maps created by the critial care specialist to expand the decision-framing templete. PIO$_2$, partial pressure inspired oxygen; PACO$_2$, partial pres-sure alveolar carbon dioxide; R, respiratory quotient; PAO$_2$, partial pressure alveolar oxygen; ScO$_2$, oxygen saturation pulmonary capillary blood; Hgb, hemoglobin concentration; CcO$_2$, oxygen content pulmonary capillary blood; Qs/Qt, pulmonary right-to-left shunt; CvO$_2$, oxygen content venous blood; CaO$_2$, oxygen content arterial blood; C.O., cardiac output; DO$_2$, oxygen delivery; VO$_2$ oxygen consumption.

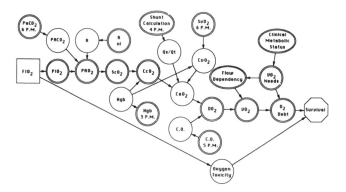

Figure 5.14. The nurse details the FIO_2 adjustment at 6 p.m. by linking currently available values for patient data intò the physician framework. $PaCO_2$, partial pressure arterial carbon dioxide; SvO_2, oxygen saturation mixed-venous blood; R nl, normal respiratory quotient.

partial decision model appropriate to the particular patient situation for an interval of time.

The physician provides this decision framework to the nurse as guidance. Then, based on the changing patient circumstances as represented by the continually collected data, the nurse parametrically completes the influence diagram by assessing the values for the "border" nodes. For example, at 6P.M., the nurse can enter into the model assessments for the measure partial pressure of arterial carbon dioxide (P_aO_2), which can serve as an approximation for the partial pressure of alveolar carbon dioxide ($PACO_2$). Likewise, he or she can enter values for the measured hemoglobin. The result is presented in Figure 5.14.

Once the nurse has entered the value that describe the patient's circumstances, a complete influence diagram is obtained. It is important to recognize that this diagram not only captures the decision structurally, but because of the mathematical relationships encoded in its constituent knowledge maps and the data provided by the nurse, it also captures the specific details of the decision at hand. Some of these assessments are shown in Figure 5.15. With appropriate algorithms, the fully assessed influence diagram can be evaluated to show how the value node depends on the different possible values of the decision variable. In technical terms, the influence diagram of Figure 5.15 is transformed to the *minimal influence diagram* in Figure 5.16. The multiple assessments underlying the full influence diagram are reduced to the single assessment shown in Figure 5.16 that summarizes the essence of the decision—the relationship between the value node and the decision node. The graph in Figure 5.17 shows this relationship between FIO_2 and probability of survival in detail for our hypothetical patient given the data available at 6 P.M.

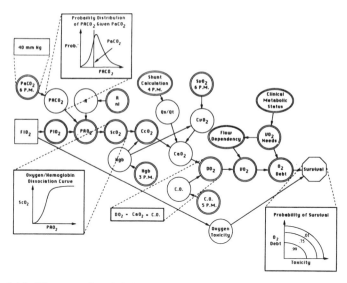

Figure 5.15. The completed influence diagram is mathematically well defined, both structurally and parametrically.

The nurse viewing this graph at 6P.M. notes that an FIO_2 of 95% provides the highest probability of survival—0.75. The graph also shows that probability of survival is very sensitive to the FIO_2—the probability of survival markedly diminishes for FIO_2 less than 90%.

Three hours later, however, the nurse may have new measurements for hemoglobin and partial pressure of the arterial carbon dioxide. Updating the decision framework provides a new influence diagram appropriate for the patient's circumstances at 9P.M., as presented in Figure

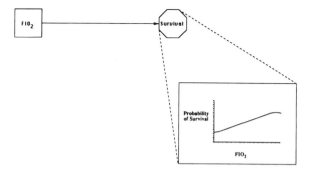

Figure 5.16. Using appropriate algorithms, we can reduce the comprehensive influence diagram into a simpler diagram that captures the essence of the FIO_2 decision. The assessment of probability of survival conditioned on FIO_2 is shown in more detail in Figure 5.18.

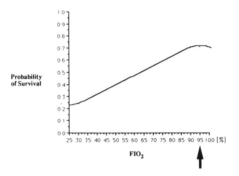

Figure 5.17. The graph of FIO_2 versus probability of survival shows that the optimal FIO_2 given the date at 6 P.M. is 95%.

5.18. This influence diagram can be evaluated to generate the graph shown in Figure 5.19.

This graph shows that at 9 P.M. the highest probability for survival is obtained with an FIO_2 of 60%. However, more important than the recommendation to decrease the FIO_2, from 95% to 60% are the *insights* the graph provides. Comparing this graph with the earlier graph shows that the patient has improved—his probability of survival is uniformly higher. Furthermore, survival is no longer sensitive to the value of FIO_2. In addition, other insights can be derived from the decision model. For example, the nurse can use the influence diagram to explore the sensitivity of survival to other variables, such as cardiac output. This would generate the graph shown in Figure 5.20.

This graph shows that probability of survival is quite sensitive to cardiac output. While the patient presently has a cardiac output (indicated by the arrow) consistent with the highest probability of survival, any

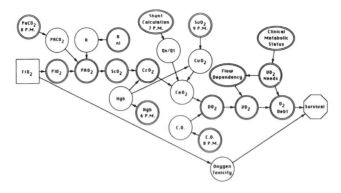

Figure 5.18. The nurse updates the influence diagram at 9 P.M. with the recent values for patient data.

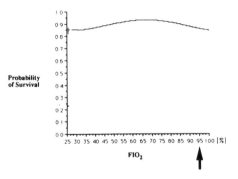

Figure 5.19. The new information leads to an updated decision model at 9P.M., which is evaluated to generate a new graph of FIO_2 versus probability of survival.

change would lead to a significant decrease. Prompted by this discovery, the nurse calls, the physician to point out the sensitivity of patient survival to cardiac output. The physician now reassesses the patient and expands the patient's life support to include fluid administration that will ensure that the cardiac output is maintained at the desired level. He creates a new decision framework to guide the nurse, as presented in Figure 5.21.

This oxygen therapy example shows how the decision analysis approach can be applied in critical care. The critical care specialist, the bedside physician, and the bedside nurse each contribute their special expertise to build an influence diagram that captures what can be done, what is known, and what is desired. This influence diagram can then be evaluated both to generate a recommendation and to provide insight.

This approach goes considerably beyond existing critical care decision practice. For example, rather than calling the physician when the cardiac output is already low and the patient is in trouble, the nurse calls much

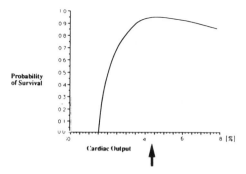

Figure 5.20. A graph of the sensitivity of survival to cardiac output suggests that cardiac output is a sensitive variable.

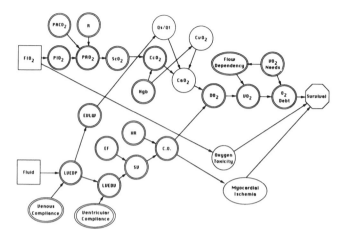

Figure 5.21. To buffer the sensitive variable, cardiac output, the physician re-frames the problem to include fluid therapy that can maintain cardiac output at the desired level. LVEDP, left ventricular end-diastolic pressure; LVEDV, left ventricular end-diastolic volume; SV, stroke volume; EF, ejection fraction; HR, heart rate; EVLW, pulmonary extra-vascular lung water. See also Figure 5.14.

earlier (while there is still time to act) to inform the physician that cardiac output is an important variable to control and that additional therapy should be included to keep this output in the desired range. The contrast with standing orders is also dramatic. The influence diagram provides the equivalent of on-demand standing orders that are quickly reformulated in response to changing circumstances, that are consistent with the physicians overall strategy for patient care, and that are less brittle or ephemeral. Furthermore, the decision analysis approach provides the tools to appraise the decision recommendation within its appropriate con-text. Clinicians not only receive recommendations, but also insight. They not only know what to do, but why.

Orchestra: **An Intelligent Decision System for Critical Care**

The critical care team members will need a significant amount of assis-tance to be able to encode decision templates and knowledge maps, to create decision frameworks, and to complete, evaluate, and interpret influence diagrams. Figure 5.22 shows a top-level architecture for a com-puter system that will help each member of the critical care team con-tribute the appropriate elements to the decision context.

The critical care specialist uses a decision-engineering workbench to encode the decision templates and knowledge maps. (We use the term "decision engineering" to refer to the task of analyzing a class of

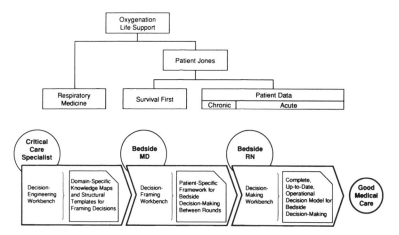

Figure 5.22. Using a sequence of computer-based decision work-benches, the critical care team members collaboratively formulate the decision model.

decisions—e.g., critical care decisions—in decision analytic terms.) These templates convert the decision-engineering workbench into a decision-framing workbench, which serves as the software tool for the bedside physician. He then uses this program to create the patient-specific decision framework that serves to guide the nurse's decision-making between rounds. And this patient-specific decision framework converts the decision-framing workbench into a decision-making workbench. This is the tool the nurse uses to add to the decision framework the data elements that describe the patient's evolving circumstances. All this results in a completed influence diagram that can be evaluated on the decision-making workbench to generate a recommendation. This diagram can be "mined" using the decision-making workbench to generate the insights that will lead to good medical care.

Using this approach, we are now building a pilot system, called *Orchestra*, for ventilator management. Its elements are illustrated in Figure 5.23. The system runs on the Apple Macintosh II personal computer. The system constituents are a user interface, a data acquisition and storage system, a decision-engineering workbench, and a ventilator management knowledge base. The decision-engineering workbench, called MacAnalyst[TM1], is now complete, and it provides tools for formulating (using a graphical interface), evaluating, and appraising influence diagrams (Figure 5.24). It also provides tools for the entry of decision-framing templates and knowledge maps. The data acquisition system, also completed, is called Respirator Workstation. It provides a programming en-

---

[TM]MacAnalyst is a trademark of IDS Partners.

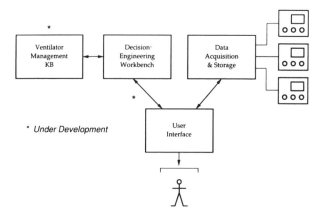

Figure 5.23. A pilot system for ventilator management, *Orchestra* has four major components. The major components exist at the prototype level, and efforts are focused on knowledge engineering and integration.

vironment, called WISP, that allows for the interactive creation and execution of software drivers for medical instrumentation that supports the RS232 protocol. The Respirator Workstation thus allows flexible data acquisition from a wide variety of medical instrumentation. Drivers have now been written for the Puritan-Bennett 7200a microprocessor ventilator, for the Ohmeda 3700 pulse oximeter, and for the Bard urine-output measuring device. Drivers will be written for the Siemens 1281 physio-

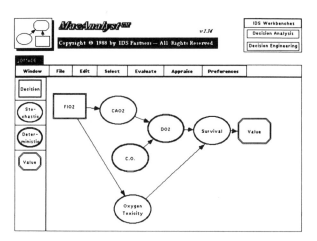

Figure 5.24. The decision-engineering workbench in *Orchestra*, called Mac-Analyst, provides tools for formulating, evaluating, and appraising influence diagrams.

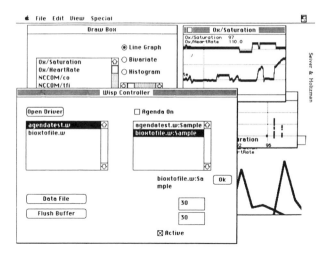

Figure 5.25. *Orchestra's* user interface provides easy control of the data acquisition system and allows display of the data in multiple formats. (Reprinted by permission of IDS Partners.)

logical monitor and for the Oximetrics mixed-venous oximeter when interface boards for those instruments are released by their manufacturers. The *Orchestra* user interface allows graphic display of the data, entry of noninstrument data by the clinician, and easy control of the data acquisition functions (Figure 5.25). A link to the decision-engineering workbench is now under development. This will allow the nurse to incorporate the acquired data into the decision framework easily. Also under development is the ventilator knowledge base, which, running on the decision-engineering workbench, forms an expert system that in response to inputs from the critical care team effects the sequential transformation of the decision-engineering workbench first to a decision-framing workbench and then to a decision-making workbench.

Summary

We feel that decision analysis can address all major ICU decision defects through a consistent, comprehensive, and efficient decision-making methodology. In addition, intelligent decision systems can make professionl-level decision analysis available at the bedside by greatly reducing its cost and by increasing its speed. *Orchestra* illustrates how intelligent decision systems technology supports the application of the decision analysis approach to critical care. This new clinical decision-making approach has great potential for improved critical care decision-making.

References

1. Brimm JE. Computers in critical care. Crit Care Nurs Q 1987, March 53–63.
2. Gardner RM. Computerized management of intensive care patients. MD Comput 1986; 3:36–51.
3. Bone RC. Monitoring respiratory function in the patient with adult respiratory distress syndrome. Semin Resp Med 1981; 3:45–55.
4. Shoemaker WC. Relation of oxygen transport patterns to the pathophysiology and therapy of shock states. Intensive Care Med 1987; 13:230–43.
5. Knaus WA, Draper EA, Wagner DP. An evaluation of outcome from intensive care in major medical centers. An Intern Med 1986; 104:410–18.
6. Civetta JM, Hudson-Civetta J. Cost-effective use of the intensive care unit. In Eiseman B, Stahlgren L. (ed): Cost-Effective Surgical Care 1987.
7. Howard RA. Decision analysis: applied decision theory. In: Hertz DB, Melese J (eds): Proceeding of the Fourth International Conference on Operations Research. New York: Wiley-Interscience, 1986; 55–71.
8. Laplace PS. A Philosophical essay on probabilities. 6th ed. New York: Dover, 1951.
9. Bernoulli D. Specimen theoriae novea de mensora sortis. Papers of the Imperial Academy of Sciences in Petersburg 1738; 5:175–92.
10. Pauker SG, Kassirer JP. Decision analysis. New Engl J Med 1987; 316:250–8.
11. Howard RA, Matheson JE. Influence diagrams. In: Howard RA, Matheson JE (eds): Readings on the Principles and Applications of Decision Analysis, Vol. II Menlo Park, CA: Strategic Decisions Group, 1984:719–62.
12. Olmsted S. On representing and solving decision problems. PH.D. dissertation. Stanford, Calif.: Engineering-Economic Systems Department, Stanford University, 1983.
13. Shachter RD. Evaluating influence diagrams. Operations Res 1986; 34:871–82.
14. Holtzman S. Intelligent decision systems. Reading, MA. Addison-Wesley, 1989; pp. 90–107.
15. Howard RA. Knowledge maps. Management Science 1989; 35(8):903–922.
16. Comroe JH, Forster RE, DuBois AB, Briscoe WA, Carlsen E. The Lung. 2nd edition. Chicago: Year Bood Medical Publishers, 1962:339–41.

II
Decision Support Data Links

Chapter 6
Standardized Acquisition of Bedside Data: The IEEE P1073 Medical Information Bus

M. Michael Shabot

Introduction

Imagine the following scenario: your team has just completed the implementation of a successful computerized Patient Data Management System (PDMS) in your busy intensive care unit. A new instrument, an electronic urimeter which continuously measures urine output and core body temperature (Bard Urotrack Plus, C.R. Bard Company, Murray Hill, NJ), is introduced into your ICU. The device is interesting because it has an RS-232 data output port which reports all device measurements every second. Furthermore, the data output port appears to be as straightforward as possible, because it is the "simplex" (send only) implementation of RS-232 and used only two wires, "data out" and "ground." It seems both easy and attractive to interface this device to the PDMS in order to capture and display urine output and core body temperature automatically.

The scenario above occurred at Cedars-Sinai Medical Center, but the reality of the implementation was much more complex than originally envisioned. As frequently occurs, the RS-232 ports on the PDMS computer (Hewlett-Packard 78709 PDMS, Hewlett-Packard Co., Waltham, MA) were configured differently from the urimeter's RS-232 output ports. A protocol conversion device was required to resolve the incompatibility. In addition, one computer port had to be fanned out to 20 bedside urimeters using two multichannel controllers. Extensive PDMS software had to be written to switch the controller ports and acquire urimeter data. Eventually the interface required the purchase of several thousand dollars' worth of hardware and months of software development [1].

The results were gratifying, however. Since our ICU delivers 5,600 patient-days of ICU care per year, we conservatively estimated that the

Adapted from an article in the *Int J Clin Monit Comput* 6:197–204, 1989. Reprinted with permission of Kluwer Academic Publishers.

interface could eliminate up to 134,400 manual urine output measurements (at a savings of 20 sec per measurement), 33,600 rectal temperature measurements (saving 2.5 min per measurement), and 134,400 instances of manual results charting (saving at least 10 sec per instance). Potential nurse time savings were calculated at over 2,500 h per year, or 27 min per patient day [1].

A few months later, the Medical Center installed bedside pulse oximeters (Ohmeda Biox 3700, Ohmeda Co., Boulder, CO). This device also has an RS-232 data output port and again it seemed desirable automatically to capture real time saturation values and alarms for the PDMS. However, the configuration of the RS-232 on the pulse oximeter was different from the urimeter *and* the PDMS computer. As a result, all new software and a separate RS-232 data communications network had to be created for the pulse oximeter. Only the general schema for polling bedside devices and storing results into the PDMS database could be transferred from the urimeter experience.

The utility of interfacing multiple bedside devices to a data management system cannot be denied. Figure 6.1 shows a Cedars-Sinai PDMS real-time status display screen which combines inputs from the bedside urimeter, oximeter, and physiologic monitor. To this point virtually all the pioneering efforts in medical data management have involved the construction of bedside data links [2–4]. However, it remains impractical for most medical centers to develop this hardware and software [5].

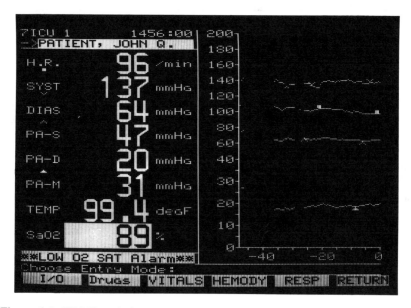

Figure 6.1. PDMS real time status display of vital signs, bladder temperature, and transcutaneous O_2 saturation.

Problem Statement

A concise statement of the problem is that *the absence of interface standards for bedside medical devices has precluded the connection of most bedside devices to patient monitoring computer systems and alarm networks.* In addition, the absence of standards has markedly limited the success of comprehensive clinical computer systems, because most bedside data can not be captured automatically. Although virtually all new medical devices have a data output port, these ports adhere to different versions of various hardware and software standards. It is uneconomical for hospitals and medical computer system vendors to provide different interfaces to the myriad of bedside devices currently available.

Pilot Standards Efforts

A pilot Medical Information Bus has been developed by Gardner, Hawley and colleagues at the LDS Hospital in Salt Lake City, Utah [6–8]. Infusion pumps, ventilators, pulse oximeters, and other bedside instruments now transmit data to host computers in the ICU. Although the precise design of the LDS MIB differs from the IEEE P1073 Draft Standard, valuable lessons have been learned and problems solved with the LDS experience. For instance, the importance of implementing a "filter" function to control device reporting was an LDS insight, because without such a filter, minor variations in physiologic measurements were found to flood the network with trivial data. The IEEE P1073 Medical Device Data Language (described below) now specifies a variety of filter functions.

The IEEE P1073 Medical Information Bus Committee

In 1982, a small group of individuals met in the board room of Phoenix Baptist Hospital, Phoenix, Arizona, to form a Medical Information Bus Committee. The objective of the committee was to develop a hardware and software communications standard for medical devices which would permit "plug and play" connection of bedside devices to data monitoring and management systems. The MIB Committee met every few months and rapidly enlarged its membership to include interested vendors and users from various health care organizations across the United States.

In 1984, the committee affiliated with the Engineering in Medicine and Biology Society (EMBS) of the Institute for Electrical And Electronics Engineers (IEEE). The MIB Committee applied for and received recognition as an official Standards Committee of the IEEE under the auspices of the EMBS, and was officially renamed the IEEE P1073 Medical Information Bus Committee. Under IEEE guidance, international vendors and users joined the committee. The EMBS and IEEE affiliations will allow formal balloting and approval processes so that the 1073 Standard can be promulgated as an official IEEE and American National Standards Institute (ANSI) Standard. Currently over 150 individuals and vendors subscribe to MIB Committee publications, and about 50 members meet four times a year to create and revise the standard in preparation for formal balloting.

Use of Existing Standards

Although there are no existing standards for *medical* device communications, there are many other viable hardware and software standards available. The MIB Committee made a commitment to use existing standards whenever possible in order to speed and simplify development of the MIB. In particular, the International Standards Organization-Open Systems Interconnection (ISO-OSI) seven-layer data communications reference model was incorporated into the MIB (Fig. 6.2). As communication technologies continue to evolve, it will be possible to replace one layer of the MIB protocol without affecting any other layer. Selected existing standards are used for portions of bedside (intra-room) communications, inter-room communications, and the Medical Device Data Language.

User Requirements

One of the first actions of the MIB Committee was to create a User Requirements (UR) Subcommittee. The members of this subcommittee are nurses, physicians, and administrators who actually use or are responsible for medical devices and systems. Their task was to define the *clinical* requirements for the MIB without regard to the engineering, hardware, or software required to meet those needs. The resulting clinical requirements indicated that standard local area networks such as RS-232 or Ethernet would be inadequate to meet the demands of the bedside medical environment.

The UR Subcommittee discovered that medical devices are quite different from ordinary computer peripherals like printers and terminals. One major difference is that medical devices are closely associated with a *bedside*, because each bedside is associated with a particular patient. This binding of patient, device, and bedside is critical to associating data with the proper patient. A second unique characteristic of medical devices is that they are frequently moved from patient to patient. While certain equipment may be fixed at bedsides (i.e., physiologic monitors), other devices like intravenous infusion pumps, ventilators, and pulse oximeters

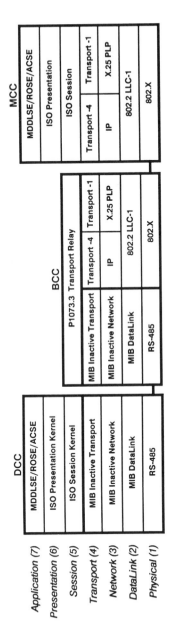

Figure 6.2. ISO-OSI seven layer model of the MIB. *DCC to BCC. 1073.1* **Layer 7**—MDDLSE/ROSE/ACSE—The kernel subset of Medical Device Data Language Service Elements, ISO 9072 Remote Operation Service Elements and ISO 8649/8650 Application Control Service Elements. **Layer 6**—MIB Presentation—The kernel subset of ISO 8822/8823 Presentation layer services. **Layer 5**—MIB Session—The kernel subset of ISO 8326 Session layer services. *10.73.2* **Layer 4**—MIB Inactive Transport (MIT)—service primitive and parameters appear identical to ISO Transport service primitives and parameters, but most parameters are defaulted in the MIT protocol. **Layer 3**—MIB Inactive Network (MIN)—A functionally inactive layer, with a control header specified for use in future revisions. **Layer 2**—MIB DataLink—A specified subset of High level Data Link Control (HDLC), using Two Way Alternate Normal Response Mode (TWA-NRM), with the Bedside Communications Controller node (BCC) as the primary station and the Device Communications Controller nodes (DCC) as the secondary stations. **Layer 1**—RS-485—Data transfer uses EIA RS-485 at a signaling rate of 375kb using Non-Return to Zero (NRZI) encoding. BCC provides 12V DC+/–3V current limited to 250mA of power to DCC. A unique MIB 6-pin connector and a shielded cable with two twisted wire pairs is specified. *BCC to MCC Host:* (standard LAN protocols) **Layer 4**—Transport Protocol 1—basic error recovery protocol. Transport protocol 4—error detection and recovery protocol. **Layer 3**—Internet Protocol. CCITT X.25 Public Link Protocol. **Layer 2**—IEEE 802.2 Logical Link Control. **Layer 1**—IEEE 802.X Carrier Sense Multiple Access with Collision Detection (Ethernet), Token Ring, Token Passing Bus or other LAN.

are switched from patient to patient as required. Furthermore, when a patient is transported for a test, many battery-backed-up devices are unplugged to travel with the patient and are plugged back in when the patient returns to his/her bed. The UR Subcommittee told the engineers that it was essential for safety reasons that devices *automatically* report their location at a particular bedside as soon as they were plugged in. It was neither adequate nor practical to make the nurse or other user remember to *tell* the computer system at which bedside a particular device was located. For similar safety reasons, the UR Subcommittee required that each MIB device continuously display a positive visual indicator of meaningful communication with the host computer.

In addition, the UR Subcommittee specified that devices automatically identify themselves as to type and capability when plugged in, rather than require a nurse to *tell* the computer what kind of device was connected, and when. The User Requirements Subcommittee suggested that similar parameters from similar devices, such as transcutaneous oxygen saturation from pulse oximeters, be communicated in a generic rather than a vendor-specific fashion. Thus, a variety of intravenous pumps, oximeters, and other devices could be connected to the network with commonly measured parameters such as IV flow rate or O_2 saturation displayed by a host computer system in a standard, vendor-independent manner. In fact, the UR Subcommittee guided the MIB effort to produce a true vendor-independent design which will allow for maximum freedom in selecting medical devices. As long as instruments adhere to the MIB Standard, plugging them in to an MIB network will require no user programming or configuration at all [9].

Finally, the UR Subcommittee helped solve a particularly thorny problem concerning the unique identification of similar devices at a bedside. The most common example is a patient with three IV pumps, each of which is running a different fluid or drug. The nurse needs to identify each pump in an unambiguous fashion to the host computer in order to specify the fluid being delivered. The UR Subcommittee helped specify that each device likely to be duplicated at bedside must contain a two-digit display which the host computer can set uniquely upon initial connection. Thus, Pump 1 could be identified as a distinct entity from an otherwise identical Pump 2. In summary, the UR Subcommittee presented the MIB engineers with a stringent set of requirements that dictated new and unique solutions to unique network problems.

Data Link

The Data Link Subcommittee developed the hardware and data link control standards required to implement the network. A simple "bus" was deemed impractical, because such a bus would not easily allow automatic

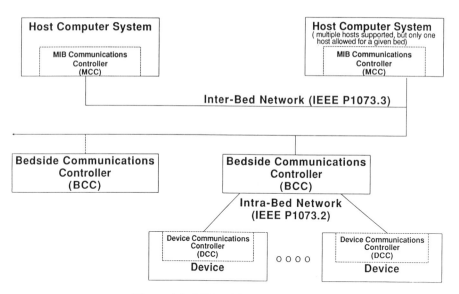

Figure 6.3. MIB arhitecture diagram.

association of a given device to a particular patient's bedside. Eventually an architecture was evolved which utilizes a bus topology between bedsides and a star topology at each bedside (Fig. 6.3) [10]. The network is controlled by a Master Communications Controller (MCC) which communicates to dedicated Bedside Communications Controller (BCC) over a standard IEEE 802.X network such as Ethernet. Each bedside controller can handle up to 16 individual data ports per bedside. If more data ports are required at the bedside, additional BCCs can be installed, each configured to the same bed location.

Each device will contain a Device Communications Controller (DCC) which handles communications to the BCC. RS-485 running at 375 Kbaud (thousand bits per second) and High level Data Link Control (HDLC) have been selected as the communication method between DCC and BCC.

While the MIB Standard will completely specify the DCC, BCC, and MCC nodes, these are logical rather than physical entities. It is recognized that a "smart" bedside device (such as a personal computer) might function as a BCC, MCC, and host system all in one. Another likely configuration will be a bedside physiologic monitor which contains "MIB Standard" data ports for connection of auxiliary devices. Auxiliary data from IV pumps, ventilators, and gas monitoring devices could be transmitted centrally over the vendor's standard monitoring network. *The key MIB connection is the one between the device and the bedside data port.* As long as that connection conforms to MIB hardware and software standards, the actual configurations of the BCC, MCC, and host are immaterial.

Physical Interface

The Physical Subcommittee specified the connectors and cables which connect MIB-compatible devices to the data ports on the wall. Many suggestions from the User Requirements Subcommittee were taken into consideration and the choice of the connector turned out to be a difficult decision for the committee. Eventually selected was a safe, durable, miniature connector which is keyed to prevent similar computer connectors from being inserted into MIB ports.

Applications Interface

The Applications Interface Committee worked diligently to create a new computer language called Medical Device Data Language (MDDL). The purpose of MDDL is to provide a simple and well-designed method of data communication between medical devices and host systems. In keeping with the policy of using existing standards when at all possible, the MIB Committee adopted ISO 9072 Remote Operation Service Elements (ROSE) as the structural framework for MDDL. ROSE's flexibility allowed the MIB Committee to define its own types of data operations so that medical transactions could occur on an efficient and timely basis. A comprehensive parameter list was developed so that similar parameters from like devices would be described, transmitted, and displayed in a common manner. However, the MDDL also allows the identification of devices down to the manufacturer, revision and serial number level so that unique identification of a particular device is possible for inventory control or remote biomedical testing.

Communications between a host system and bedside devices are fully bidirectional on the MIB. Closed loop applications are entirely possible, depending on the capabilities of particular devices and host systems. In addition, devices will be able to query the status of other devices, not directly but rather through the host, with appropriate host system software.

Current Status of the Standard

The MIB P1073 Standard has been divided into three sections for draft development and balloting. Section P1073.1 describes the application interface and the MDDL language. Section P1073.2 describes the connection of devices to bedsides. Section P1073.3 describes the connection of bedsides to a host computer system. Section P1073.2 is scheduled for submission for EMBS balloting in 1989. The other sections are scheduled for balloting in 1990. If the review and balloting processes proceed smoothly, parts of the Medical Information Bus could become an IEEE Standard as early as 1990. Following that, it will be submitted to the American National Standards Institute (ANSI) and other standards organizations for further national and international recognition.

The Future

The absence of standards for medical device communications has stymied the acceptance and success of automated clinical data management systems. Even devices with simple RS-232 data output ports require special interfacing hardware and software. Due to the number and variety of medical devices available, each with their own peculiar data output configuration, it has been impractical to interface with most of them. Limited by manual data entry, most computerized patient data management systems have failed to deliver the productivity gains their users expected.

The forthcoming IEEE P1073 Medical Information Bus (MIB) Standard promises to correct this situation with a single powerful bedside device interface method. The MIB will provide specifications for all hardware and software necessary for medical data communications. The MIB handles the need for automatic recognition of new devices placed at a bedside, automatic reconfiguration of the network, binding of a device to a particular patient's bedside, and many other issues unique to the medical data communications environment. The MIB is expected to undergo formal IEEE balloting in 1990 and promises to open a new era in data management for clinical patient care.

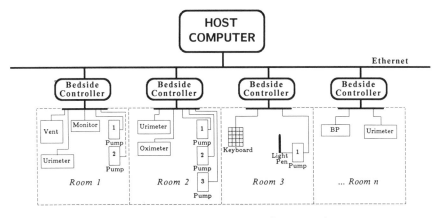

Figure 6.4. MIB device connection example.

By the mid 1990s it should be possible for medical device manufacturers and computer vendors to produce systems which integrate virtually all electronic data at a patient's bedside (Figure 6.4). Medical device vendors can produce devices with a standard, inexpensive interface and be confident that their instruments will be compatible with data monitoring and management networks. Computer system vendors can develop new monitoring and documentation systems with the assurance that vital bedside data can be automatically acquired. The major limitation of current systems with be erased and it is expected that the use of comprehensive clinical computer systems will rapidly expand. The clinical benefits of the MIB in the operating room, ICU, and floor care areas are readily apparent. The patient will benefit because computerized telemetry, monitoring, and data management will occur in a manner which is much more practical that current methodologies. More than just a new data network, the Medical Information Bus is the path to a whole new era in medical data management.

1993 Footnote: At the time of publication of this book, the MIB standard has still not been finalized by the IEEE, but progress in writing the standard and in obtaining the concensus needed for approval continues.

Further Information About the MIB

Individuals wishing additional information about the MIB Standard and MIB Committee are encouraged to write to the secretariat:

IEEE Standards Department
445 Hoes Lane
P.O. Box 1331
Piscataway, NJ 08855-1331
(908) 562-3810
(908) 562-1571 FAX

References

1. Shabot MM, Lobue M, Leyerle BJ. An automatic PDMS interface for the Urotrack Plus 220 urimeter. Int J Clin Monit Comput 1988; 5:125–31.
2. Shubin H, Weil MH. Efficient monitoring with a digital computer of cardiovascular function id seriously ill patients. Ann Intern Med 1966; 65:453–60.
3. Osborn JJ, Beaumont JO, Raison JC, et al. Measurements and monitoring of acutely ill patients by digital computer. Surgery 1968; 64:1057–70.
4. Sheppard LC, Kouchoukos NT, Kirklin JW. The digital computer in surgical intensive care automation. Computer 1973; 6:29–34.
5. Shabot MM. Software for computers and calculators in critical care medicine. Software in Healthcare 1985; 3:26–39.

6. Gardner RM, Hawley WL. Standardizing communications & networks in the ICU. Patient monitoring and data management conference. AAMI Technology Analysis and Review. 1985; TAR No. 1–85:59–63.
7. Gardner RM. Computerized management of intensive care patients. MD Comput 1986; 3:36–51.
8. Hawley WL, Tariq H, Gardner RM. Clinical implementation of an automated medical information bus in an intensive care unit. SCAMC 1988; 12:621–24.
9. Nolan-Avila L, Paganelli B, Norden-Paul R. The medical information bus: An automated way of capturing patient data at the bedside. Comput Nurs May/June 1988; pp 115–121.
10. Schwartz M. Telecommunication networks: Protocols, modeling and analysis. Reading, MA: Addison-Wesley, 1987.

Chapter 7
Real-Time Data Acquisition: Recommendations for the Medical Information Bus

Reed M. Gardner, William L. Hawley, Thomas D. East, Thomas A. Oniki, and Hsueh-Fen W. Young

Introduction

Communication is one of the most important tasks performed by health care professionals. Data underlie every medical decision, and except for the personal observations made by and acted upon by physicians at the bedside, should be communicated. Often, the data are communicated through several people and via electronic strips, hand-written notes, computer displays, and computer printouts before getting to the medical decision-maker. Each step in the process, especially if it involves people and hand-written records, can result in delays and errors.

For patients in intensive care units (ICUs) and those undergoing anesthesia and surgery, this need is especially urgent [1]. Information in the medical record should be easily retrievable and reviewable in a temporal relationship with other associated data. Records having these characteristics would facilitate the routine processing of data required for medical decisions. The HELP system uses an integrated database and has decision-making capability [2,3]. Traditional manually recorded medical records lack these attributes. In the modern ICU it is not unusual for a patient to be connected to several computerized monitoring devices (see Fig. 7.1) [2].

With the on-line bedside monitoring situation, historically each supplier of monitoring equipment wanted to "do it all." Each vendor wanted to provide *every* monitoring device for *every* bedside. Unfortunately, none of the vendors are large enough, flexible enough, or innovative enough to invent *all* the new monitoring devices. As a result. there is a

Adapted with permission from A modification of real time data acquisition: Experience with the Medical Information Bus (MIB) by Gardner RM, Hawley WL, East TD, Oniki TA, Hsueh-Fen Young W, SCAMC 1991; 15:813–7.

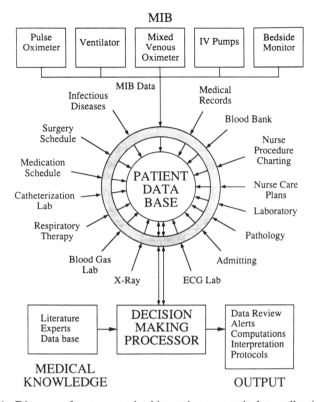

Figure 7.1. Diagram of a computerizcd intensive care unit data collection system.

veritable "Tower of Babel" situation with data flowing from bedside devices. Bedside monitoring devices today are being designed with microprocessors as the principal tool to solve the complex measurement tasks. For example, microprocessor-based, small, portable, infrared sensor based devices are now "shined" onto the eardrum for quick, noninvasive, and accurate measurement of patient temperature. Thus, the challenge is to acquire, store, report, and use this data for diagnostic and therapeutic decision-making. To facilitate automatic data acquisition from the multitude of physiological devices located at the bedside, we have integrated data flowing from these devices using the Medical Information Bus (MIB). Devices such as bedside monitors, infusion pumps, pulse oximeters, venous oximeters, and ventilators have been interfaced to the MIB. The MIB is being standardized by the Institute of Electrical and Electronic Engineers (IEEE) with their MIB standards committee IEEE P1073 established in 1984 [4].

This report discusses some of the practical issues faced in developing an optimum "real-time" data acquisition from bedside monitoring devices. Our report is based on 5 years' experience at collecting data from several devices and integrating the data collection into medical and nursing clinical practice.

Methods

To assist the IEEE P1073 MIB committee in developing appropriate standards and solve some of its internal data acquisition problems, in 1985 we built a prototype MIB. Since that time, interfaces have been built and tested for the following devices: 1) infusion pumps; 2) pulse oximeters; 3) mixed venous oximeters; 4) ECG and blood pressure monitors, including noninvasive blood pressure "Dinamap"-type devices; 5) ventilators; 6) gastric pH monitors; 7) urimeters; and 8) blood gas machines. In the process of testing these devices several common issues continued to appear: A) the *complex electrical interfacing issues*, B) the *people issues* of integrating the MIB data flow into clinical practice, and C) the *data selection issues*, since most devices produced much more data than was being charted manually or than was desired and these signals currently contain considerable "noise."

Since there is much in common for all devices interfaced, this report will summarize some of the findings for all devices interfaced. Also presented are specific issues for each device to illustrate the nature of the problems that must be solved.

Results

Complex Electrical Interfacing Issues

Shabot stated the problem most clearly in his 1989 article [4] "The absence of interface standards for bedside medical devices has precluded the connection of most bedside devices to patient monitoring computer systems and alarm networks." Even though most bedside instruments provide "data" interfaces they come in a variety of forms, e.g., RS-232, TTL-Level serial bit streams, 20 ma current loop, 4 bit BCD with synchronization pulses, full or half-duplex, just to name a few. Although some devices do not have any software or hardware capability to check for transmission errors, others have their own proprietary data checking protocols. As a result of this circumstance, and in cooperation with IVAC corporation, we developed a microprocessor-based Device Communications Controller (DCC) designed to allow interfacing of most bedside devices [5,6].

Figure 7.2 is a block diagram of the prototype MIB system we constructed. The system was built such that each DCC could plug into "standard" connectors on a wall connector box in the patient's room. Each pa-

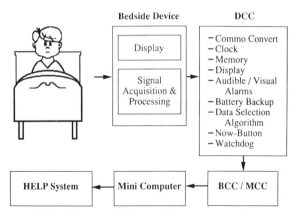

Figure 7.2. MIB block diagram, DCC, Device Communications Controller; BCC, Bedside Communications Controller; MCC, Master Communications Controller.

tient room will likely have a variable number and mixture of devices. For example, we have had patients with 12 infusion pumps connected as well as a bedside monitor, a ventilator, pulse oximeter, and a mixed venous oximeter connected.

People Issues Involved in Integrating the MIB into Clinical Practice

Experience gained during the implementation of the prototype MIB system pointed out the need to have flexible software in the DCC. We found, as others have, that systems were most easily integrated into "clinical" applications that required minimal changes in the user's environment [7]. If the MIB data gathering scheme does not allow a user to correct or change a procedural mistake simply, the user will revert to manual methods. After our experience with implementing the MIB for infusion pumps, pulse oximeters, ECG and blood pressure monitors, and ventilators [8], we have become much more aware of the need to integrate the functionality of MIB into nursing and clinical care practices. With infusion pumps we are now using the MIB routinely with excellent nurse acceptance. For example, many nurses put "keep open" IVs on the MIB because it is an easier and more consistent way to chart. Bedside ECG and blood pressure monitors automatically collect data every 15 min in our ICUs and every 5 min in surgical suites with excellent physician and nurse acceptance [9]. A rigid system is least likely to be embraced by the users independent of its sophistication or perceived benefit.

Even if all the other obstacles can be overcome, there are still subtle concerns about *data ownership* in an integrated computerized medical record, *timeliness* of data entry, and selection of *accurate* or *representative* data.

Data ownership. It is common practice for several health professionals to record the same data and not share it effectively. For example, at our institution, ventilator data (e.g., FiO_2) are entered into the medical record by nurses, respiratory therapists, blood gas technicians, and physicians. This would be acceptable if they "shared" their data and stored them in a common place. Unfortunately the data are neither shared nor consistent. This inconsistency does not usually cause a problem for the "manual" record, but it can clearly cause a problem for the care of the patient. If a physician needs to know what the FiO_2 data on a patient is, he may ask three caretakers and get three different answers! In fact, we have documented that problem with our computerized ICU medical record. We found that the FiO_2 data recorded in the computer record at the time a blood gas sample was drawn were correct only about 50% of the time!

Timely data recording. Manual records do not require timely data recording. What is "timely" recording? To the engineer or computer scientist it is data recording as it occurs. To the nurse or therapist it may mean recording data by the "end of the shift." Since most computerized systems allow data review by professionals from locations outside the unit, data entry must be timely. Timely "external" review of patient data is "foreign" to nurses and therapists, who typically have only dealt with manual charting. They expect to provide verbal reports to physicians as they come into the unit for rounds or discuss the patient status via telephone. Thus, we have had to make a fundamental "cultural" and philosophical change to improve the timely recording of data by nurses and therapists. These health care professionals must realize that they must enter data in a timely fashion, much as personnel in the laboratory or radiology must do.

Entry of accurate and representative results. It is expected that human observers take all the important factors into consideration when they record observations at the bedside. For example, is the patient stable, is the physiological parameter stable and representative for the time period? Unfortunately, our observations made from MIB data collection experiments in which we have compared nurse or therapist manual data entry with on-line logging have shown more data logging errors than expected.

Figure 7.3 shows examples of these errors. Figure 7.3 A shows there was about a 3 hr (180 min) time interval when a patient was on a ventilator with 55% oxygen while the therapists record showed 40%. Even when the therapist made a data entry in the middle of the time interval they still logged 40%. Figure 7.3B shows that a nurse charted a 77% oxygen saturation from a pulse oximeter at 18:00 when the median saturation for the hour before was 82%. This data entry error was likely a "timeliness" error. The nurse most likely measured the saturation at 18:20 and to fit the patient care order for making the observation at 18:00 decided that it was "close enough." Figure 7.3C shows that the patient's median saturation had been 94% and yet for an interval of less than 2 min the satura-

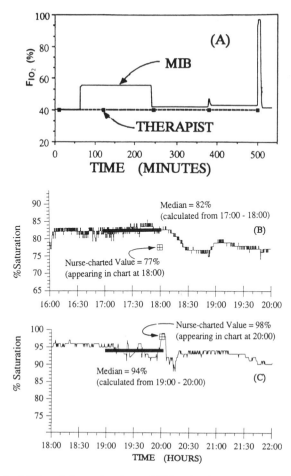

Figure 7.3. A: MIB and therapist charted FiO$_2$. B, C: MIB and nurse charted O$_2$ Saturations. B has a timeliness error and C an atypical data error.

tion was 98%—the nurse chose to chart the 98% data—*not* a representative or typical saturation for the time interval.

For effective computerized decision-support systems, data must be entered promptly and correctly. It is no longer adequate to have the "chart" correct only at the time of shift change.

Data Selection Issues

Bedside monitoring devices such as heart rate meters, blood pressure monitors, pulse oximeters, ventilators, etc., generate a flood of data. Up to 1.5 Mbytes per patient per day are produced every day if just heart rate data are recorded! Obviously this amount of data could quickly overwhelm storage and display capabilities of any clinical computer system.

Thus, a better way must be developed to preserve a "reasonable" data storage and display strategy. Recently Gravenstein has suggested physiologically based methods for establishing data collection rates [10]. It appears that recording most physiological parameters every minute is acceptable. Other parameters such as temperature can be recorded at longer intervals. If one decided to record data at 1, 5, or 15 min intervals, what should be recorded? Maximum value, minimum value, an average, a mathematical "median" or some other time-weighted function? Answers to these questions are not yet known for certain. Development of a "consensus" by physicians, ethicists, nurses, therapists, and medical informatics professionals with input from legal representatives will be necessary. During this process the need for data recording will come under close scrutiny, and it is likely that there will be a better understanding of the clinical importance of each of the measured parameters.

Figure 7.4 illustrates the problem of data selection for a patient on a ventilator. Plotted along the x-axis is the time of day in hours. Along the y-axis is the tidal volume (TV) delivered by the ventilator in liters. Tidal volume is but one of 33 parameters available from the modern ventilator every 10 sec! Figure 7.4A shows ventilator data recorded at 10 sec intervals. Figure 7.4B is illustrative of a "moving average" filtering mechanism used to reduce the amount of data stored and presented. Figure 7.4C shows the same data recorded by a respiratory therapist at roughly 2 hr intervals.

Early experience with collecting data from our prototype MIB devices has shown that data collection and selection techniques have shown major flaws. These flaws occur with both the human data recorder and the simpler computerized data selection technologies already applied. We have found it necessary to permit easy selection and collection of episodic data such as may occur when thermodilution cardiac output and wedge pressures are measured. Other similar occasions occur when a patient is in a particular position or stable condition. In these episodic situations a single button push allows the collection of these data easily and simply.

Based on our experience with selecting data from devices we have found the following: Infusion pumps—Flow rates charted when a new rate has been stable for 2 min and at 1 ml volume increments are adequate. Pulse oximeters—arterial oxygen saturation and heart rate can be determined reliably and nearly free of artifacts. Recording this data at 30 sec intervals and storing median values every 15 min has resulted in an acceptable record. A competing strategy might be to record beat-to-beat information. Such a strategy would result in a large amounts of artifact. Using the manual recording alternative of logging data every few hours also seems inappropriate. Ventilators—with these devices one must record not only the delivered volumes. oxygen concentrations, and rates, but also those set on the ventilator. The number of parameters we have chosen to store is large (20 with one ventilator as noted below) and the required interval of recording is about 3 min.

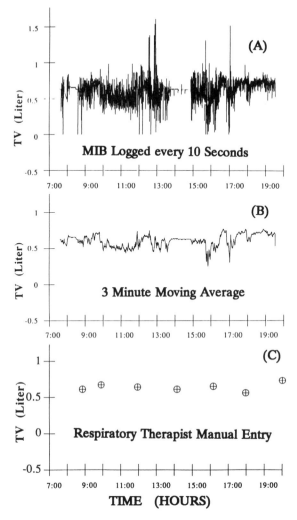

Figure 7.4. A: Tidal volume (in liters) logged every 10 sec for a 12 hr period. B: Tidal volume data obtained by using a 3 min moving average filter to get more "representative" data for the same time period. C: Tidal volume recorded by a respiratory therapisl for the same 12 hr period.

Recommendations

Monitoring manufacturers have *not* been careful to eliminate artifact and often transmit invalid data. A first and major effort must be undertaken by the manufacturers to eliminate known artifacts. In many cases, simple signal processing would dramatically reduce the false results presented as output [9].

Based on more than five years of experience in the clinical setting with data selection schemes, we make the following recommendations for data recording. These data selection strategies are not meant to replace the alarm functions built in bedside devices, but only to help in the data recording process. The data selection recommendations made below have only been tested in our ICUs and *must* receive the scrutiny of many other clinical and manufacturing institutions. We are certain that modifications will be made to these recommendations. However. we feel that presenting our recommendations as a target will elicit a movement to optimize these strategies.

1. DEVICE—Heart Rate, ECG
   First priority heart rate signal. Collect data every 30 sec and store a moving median every 15 min. If a 5 min median has a greater than 5 beat per minute heart rate change, store that value.

2. DEVICE—Heart Rate, Direct Arterial Blood Pressure
   Second priority heart rate signal. Collect data every 30 sec and store a moving median every 15 min. If a 5 min median has a greater than 5 beat per minute heart rate change, store that value.

3. DEVICE—Heart Rate, Pulse Oximeter
   Third priority heart rate signal. Collect data every 30 sec and store a moving median every 15 min. If a 5 min median has a greater than 5 beat per minute heart rate change, store that value.

4. DEVICE—Blood Pressure, Arterial Blood Pressure
   Be certain that data selection algorithms for direct arterial blood pressure are built into the bedside monitor [9]. Collect systolic/diastolic and mean blood pressure every 30 sec and store a moving median every 15 min. If a 5 min median has a greater than 10mmHg pressure change, store that value. If automated noninvasive blood pressure is measured it will be the second priority signal and finally manually (auscultatory) measured blood pressure will be the third priority blood pressure signal source.

5. DEVICE—Oxygen Saturation, Pulse Oximeter
   Collect data every 30 sec and store a moving median every hour. If the 10 min media has a greater than 4% saturation change in either direction, store that value.

6. DEVICE—Oxygen Saturation, Mixed Venous
   Collect data every 30 sec and store a moving median every hour. If the 10 min media has a greater than 4% saturation change in either direction, stored that value.

7. DEVICE—Mechanical Ventilator
   General: Collect data every 10 sec and make the data selections based on the rules noted elow. Also, any time a therapist, nurse or physician activates a data collection button.
   Settings: Store every ventilator *setting* that lasts for more than 3 min. Ventilator settings recommended for collection are indicated below:

1. Ventilation Mode
2. Respiratory Rate (IMV Rate)
3. Tidal Volume
4. Inspiratory Flow
5. Oxygen %
6. Trigger Sensitivity
7. PEEP
8. Plateau Time or Percentage
9. I/E Ratio
10. Pressure Support or Control Level
11. Flow-by Support Level
12. Flow-by Sensitivity

Measured parameters: Calculate a 3 min moving median from the 10 sec data collected. Store a moving median for each 1 hr time interval. In addition, store measured parameters where there is a change greater than the thresholds noted below that lasts for more than 3 mins.

Ventilator *measured* parameters recommended for collection are indicated below:

1. Peak Airway Pressure > 10 cm H_2O Change
2. Mean Airway Pressure > 5 cm H_2O Change
3. Spontaneous Tidal Volume > 100 ml Change
4. Corrected Expired TV > 50ml Change
5. Spontaneous Rate > 5 beat per minute Change
6. Machine Assisted Rate > 2 beat per minute Change
7. Plateau Pressure > Every Change
8. Measured I/E Ratio > 25% Change

8. DEVICE—IV Pump
   Record volume infused to the nearest milliliter and record changes in-flow rate once it has remained stable for at least 2 mins.

It is not uncommon for a patient to be attached to three or four devices that derive heart rate. We have only indicated a priority for selecting the signal from which heart rate should be determined. In the future, there should be strategies developed to combine data from these multiple signals to establish representative heart rates.

Conclusions

The basic premise that the MIB can be used as an automated data collection and communications system has been proven in the clinical setting. However, MIB standards must be developed and accepted; artifacts present in the raw physiological signals must be reduced; consensus must be reached on what data to collect, how often to collect the data, how to select the data, and data ownership; and sociological medical-legal issues must still be addressed.

Physicians, nurses, medical informatics professionals, and manufacturers should unite and push forward and complete the MIB standard. Once a first standard is produced, there will be the impetus for the industry to move forward.

As stated earlier, monitor vendors must take a more careful look into their methods of artifact rejection and transmission of nonrepresentative data. Eventually the MIB and data selection methodology should be built into every monitor.

The recommendations presented above are given as a starting point. These recommendations should be carefully tested and validated and, where needed, better recommendations proposed and tested.

Data ownership and sociological issues will continue to be a problem, but must also be addressed. There is an emotional issue of losing something with automation. We have all been taught to write with a pencil on paper and are reluctant to have that "security blanket" taken away from us. If one is charting data, one must write it down: we surmise that this process will cause the observer (nurse, physician, therapist) to think about or process the data [11]. Despite what most people believe about their accuracy as data loggers, we have clear evidence that human observers do not always record data accurately nor in a timely fashion.

Finally the medical-legal factors must also be considered. We feel that the factors that can be raised here are best solved by an open discussion and the development of a consensus of the data needs for optimum patient care.

The people factors and data selection strategies are likely to be more difficult to accomplish than the device engineering interface and computerized acquisition factors. For optimum care of our patients, we must make the major cultural and philosophical changes needed to achieve a consistent, timely, and accurate real-time computerized medical record.

Acknowledgments

This work was supported in part by a grant from Marquette Electronics (Milwaukee, W1).

References

1. Dick RS, Steen EB, (eds). The computer-based patient record: an essential technology for health care. Insitute of Medicine. National Academy of Sciences Press 1991.
2. Gardner RM, Bradshaw KE, Hollingsworth KW. Computerizing the inten-

sive care unit: Current status and future directions. J Cardiovasc Nurs 1989; 4:68–78.

3. Kuperman GJ, Maack BB, Bauer K, Gardner RM. The impact of the HELP computer system on the LDS hospital paper medical record. Top Health Rec Management 1991; 12:1–19.

4. Shabot MM. Standardized acquisition of bedside data: The IEEE P1073 Medical Information Bus. Int J Clin Monit Comput 1989; 6:197–204.

5. Hawley WL, Tariq H, Gardner RM. Clinical implementation of an automated Medical Information Bus in an intensive care unit. SCAMC 1988; 12:621–4.

6. Tariq H, Gardner RM, Hawley WL. Implementation of Medical Information Bus (MIB) at LDS hospital. Proc Ann Int Conf IEEE Engin Med Biol Soc 1988; 10:1799–800.

7. Weaver RR. Assessment and diffusion of computer decision support systems. Int J Technol Assess Health Care 1991; 7:42–50.

8. East TD, Yang W, Tariq H, Gardner RM. The IEEE Medical Information Bus for respiratory care. Crit Car Med 1989; 17:580.

9. Gardner RM, Monis SM, Oehler P. Monitoring direct blood pressure: Algorithm enhancements. IEEE Comput Cardiot 1986; 13:607–10.

10. Gravenstein JS, deVries A Jr, Beneken JEW. Sampling intervals for clinical monitoring variables during anesthesia. J Clin Monit 1989; 5:17–21.

11. Gardner RM. Patient-monitoring systems. In: Shortliffe EH, Perreault LE (eds): Medical Informatics: Computer Applications in Health Care. Reading, MA: Addison-Wesley, 1900:366–99.

Chapter 8
A Common Reference Model for Healthcare Data Exchange: P1157 MEDIX System Architecture

David V. Ostler, John J. Harrington, and Gisle Hannemyr

Introduction

The IEEE Engineering in Medicine and Biology Society has been sponsoring the P1157 working group's development of a standard for exchange of data between Hospital Information Systems (HIS). This work to date has focused on the following objectives:

1. Support both inter- and intramedical center communications, among patient care settings and ancillary services.
2. Do not assume a particular decomposition of the health care system into subsystems.
3. Structure the standard in a flexible manner so that multiple subsets of features are allowed.
4. Provide a framework allowing the migration of applicable health care standards into a common reference model.
5. Define a standard set of interface transactions which allow health care information systems to exchange data.
6. Specify standard representations of transaction data items, while allowing for domain-specific variations.
7. Ensure data integrity, consistency, security, reliability, and ownership.
8. Ensure compatibility of multiple vendor systems at the application interface through the use of ISO/OSI Application Service Element standard protocols.
9. Ensure that successive protocol versions are compatible.

* Reprinted with permission of IEEE from SCAMC 1990; 14:235–238.

Reference Model

It is not possible to give a precise definition of what constitutes an automated health care information system. The P1157 working group has taken the view that an automated health care system provides a computational model of the underlying health care environment (Fig. 8.1). In defining a model for data exchange between automated health care systems, a common context must be defined so that each message received has a unique meaning. This can be viewed as a mapping between the health care environment and a conceptual schema. This schema is then mapped into a specific hardware and software realization or computational model.

The conceptual schema cannot be based on ancillary departments or functions within a hospital since the health care environment does not have a single decomposition of the services performed. For example, a hospital may have a single department providing laboratory results, but a group of practicing physicians may receive these services from a variety of providers. To provide a common schema across all health care systems, the building blocks of common context need to be at the level of patients, physicians, and services provided.

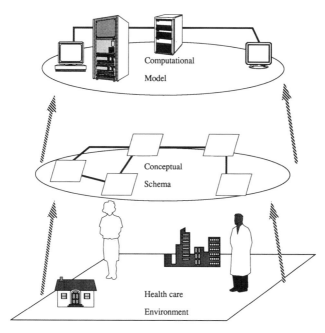

Figure 8.1. Models of the health care environment.

Object Model

The working group has selected an object-oriented paradigm to describe the reference model. Each P1157 object represents a real world or conceptual entity which is relevant to the domain of health care. An object has attributes and actions. Attributes are measurable properties of the object, or refer to another objects. The state of an object is expressed by the value of its measurable properties, and the action it performs at that instance. The state of a system is the accumulation of the states of all the objects in the system.

Object orientation in general is based upon a direct modeling of application domain entities (both concrete and abstract) and concepts. Direct modeling uses objects to model entities and object classes to model concepts. Direct modeling is supported by the notion of objects that have characteristics similar to the entities: Objects are identifiable units, with clear boundaries to their environment and a definite set of operations that can be performed. Objects exist over time and are carriers of state information (represented by local data items), and objects are the primary source of actions (i.e., they act on their own and my respond to messages sent to them).

In addition the usual classification of application domain entities into concepts (or categories of objects) is supported by classes of objects, and specializations of general concepts is directly supported by subclasses of objects.

When object-orientation is used in system development, the functional specification of the system is made in the context of the object model of the system. The functionality of the system is represented by action sequences of the identified objects, or by functions associated with the objects.

The object model of the application domain (without functions added) is more stable than the functionality of the system; even though the required functionality of a system may change according to new requirements, the system will still handle the same set of entities and concepts. The same argument is also valid in the definition of a reference model for the structure of health care data. The set of health care concepts is more stable than the functionality of the applications.

A reference model is also the conceptual schema that not only defines the characteristics of the system for use of the customers and suppliers of applications, but also for users of the applications, e.g., health personnel. A reference model should not only be understood by the suppliers of applications, but also by health personnel using the applications.

A traditional data model will give a static structure to either all parts of the health care system (and that will not be possible to obtain agreement on), or it will give a static structure on only that part for which agreement may be obtained. The last alternative may be so small that it is not interesting and that much of the work in health care will belong to the part which is not part of the model.

Using object-orientation makes it possible to make a model (and use a method for arriving at it and for maintaining it) that caters to special cases.

As an example, the notion of a patient is common to all parts of a health care system.

Information about a patient is used in many different situations, and not all information is needed in all situations. One alternative is to agree on the maximum set of attributes characterizing a patient and then make different extracts of this for special purposes. Agreement on the maximum set of attributes may cause problems. Another alternative is to agree on a common and smaller set of attributes of a general class of patients and then provide for the definition of as many different special classes of patient as there are different needs. The approach assumes that special classes will have the attributes of the general class, and that they will in addition have attributes that are needed for the special cases. It will be easier to obtain a common agreement on this smaller set of attributes, and as the model provides the means for tailoring it to different needs it will be acceptable also to those especially concerned with their special definition of a patient.

Inheritance

The class/subclass mechanism makes it possible to specify only once the common properties associated with a general class of objects. Objects of subclasses get the properties defined in the general (super) class (by "simple inheritance"); in addition they get the properties defined for the subclasses. Many health care objects will share characteristics. The use of subclassing will reflect this.

As a simple example consider the concept of patient, modeling the fact that health care is concerned with real patients. In order to communicate about patients, data objects representing these patients have to be generated and communicated. There is, however, also a need for communication about persons in general. The properties of persons will be properties that are also valid for patient, but patients will have additional properties. In addition there may be other specializations of the general-class Person, e.g., Physician. This will in an object-oriented language be reflected by three classes: Person, Patient, and Physician (Fig. 8.2). The class Patient is specified as a subclass of person, implying that Patient objects will get the properties Name and Address of class Person.

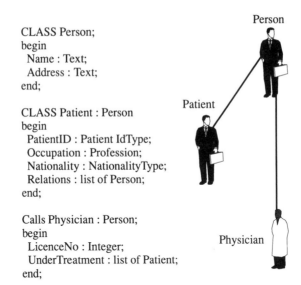

```
CLASS Person;
begin
  Name : Text;
  Address : Text;
end;

CLASS Patient : Person
begin
  PatientID : Patient IdType;
  Occupation : Profession;
  Nationality : NationalityType;
  Relations : list of Person;
end;

Calls Physician : Person;
begin
  LicenceNo : Integer;
  UnderTreatment : list of Patient;
end;
```

Figure 8.2. An example of the use of objects to model health care concepts.

Polymorphism

Once a class has been established as part of the standard MEDIX architecture, it cannot be redefined. Polymorphism circumvents this restriction.

Polymorphism allows an object that is a member of a particular class to be regarded as and to act like one or more of its superclasses. Essentially, this means that the standard may be extended by letting objects with extended capabilities be defined as subclasses of established classes without breaking systems based on the already established (super)classes.

Encapsulation

Encapsulation is a mechanism that ensures the integrity an object, It requires that all communication with an object be accomplished by sending "messages" to the object. It means that internal operation of an object is not accessible unless the object recognizes and accepts a "message" that are defined to change or expose the state of some of its attributes or actions.

Medical Client/Agent Server Model

To implement the object-based reference model described, each MEDIX system on the network provides an agent process that maintains and interface to some set of MEDIX object (Fig. 8.3). A MEDIX system that

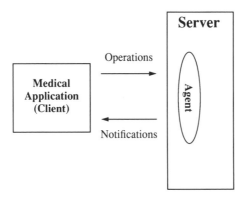

Figure 8.3. Medical client/agent/server model.

requires information about a set of objects that it does not maintain connects to a server that is maintaining these objects. The set of objects supported by an individual system depends upon the specific part of the health care environment supported.

The use of an object-oriented reference model does not require that all HIS systems convert to object-oriented databases, or for that matter, to object-oriented programing. The Reference Model assumes that a Medical Application that uses MEDIX will be a client of the available information on the network. Each MEDIX system that supports a set of objects is a server for that information. A MEDIX server provides an agent that transforms the object operations into non-object based operations that the system supports (i.e., SQL queries, reports, etc.)

An Example

If a network contained three systems, the first a general ADT (Admit, Discharge, Transfer) system, the second an Laboratory Information System, and the third a Clinical Information, System for the ICU (Figure 8.4)—(i.e., Structured query language (SQL) queries. . . .)

The ADT system would maintain a set of objects describing a patient's billing, demographics, and admit diagnoses.

The Laboratory Information System would maintain objects relative to specimens drawn with references to patient objects.

The Clinical Information System could maintain connections for access to both of these sets of objects or instantiate copies of these objects and maintain a distributed set of these objects within it's own database.

When a new patient is admitted into the ADT system the patient object is created and registered within the network. The ICU system with recognize the new object and duplicate the object in its database. The patient would then move to the ICU and have specimens drawn for labora-

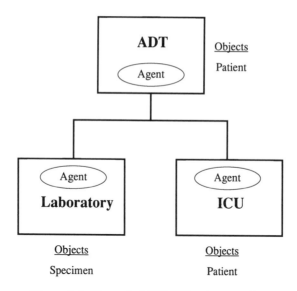

Figure 8.4. Example MEDIX implementation.

tory tests. These specimens are created in the laboratory system and as updates to these specimens create results. Upon request the ICU looks for specimen data and finds it registered under the lab system, requests the information, and receives a response to the query.

The common view of the network is one of availability of objects. The agent in each of these systems could translate the object actions into the appropriate database or functions on each system. When the ICU system creates the specimen object the laboratory agent would translate that action into creating a new specimen and test record. When the results are entered into the laboratory system, the agent would create an event report to be sent to the ICU.

P1157 Architecture

The P1157 architecture is based on the previously described reference model with a set of common service elements to support application interaction with the underlying objects and a set of functional specifications which refine the common service elements and data model to meet the needs of particular application functions.

The P1157 working group is developing a family of standards. The Architecture and Document Structure are described in an overview standard. The overview describes two branches to the document structure for these standards.

The first branch contains a methods document that describes a standard format and method for defining Medical Object Sets. The remaining documents in this branch define sets of Medical Objects for various medical functional areas.

The second branch contains a methods document that describes a standard format and method for defining communication profiles to be used to support communications between systems relative to the instantiation of sets of Medical Objects.

This architecture and document structure allow a common Reference Model to be used with multiple automated health care applications and object sets. Today's focus may be on the ADT functions and laboratory results data exchange, but future standards can address pharmacy objects, blood bank objects, financial support object, materials management objects, etc.

Specific MeDical Objects (SMDO)

A Specific Medical Object document is created for each new capability added to the MEDIX family of standards. For example, a basic set of objects will be defined for the functionality defined by ADT. The document will also defined the basic set of operations performed on these objects.

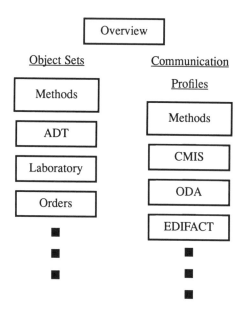

Figure 8.5. P1157 Document structure.

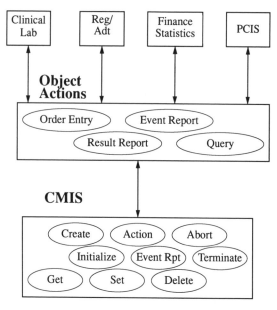

Figure 8.6. MEDIX reference model.

Communication Profiles

Communication Profiles define specific mappings, of OSI environment Application Services to the operations required to support any SMDO. For example SMDOs are defined for the Clinical Lab, ADT, Pharmacy, tc. (Fig. 8.6).The SMDO includes the definition of the set of object actions to perform the basic operations that each SMDO requires (i.e., order entry, or result report.) The Methods of Data Format and Associations (MDFA) maps these object action onto a set of Application Service Elements. The example in Figure 8.5 uses CMIS [2]. Since CMIS is already used to support object operation exchanges, the object operations do not require any further mapping.

Another example is the use of the Office Document Architecture (ODA) [3]. ODA defines a standard for exchanging documents. Since much of health care is delivered in a non-automated environment, the definition of an exchange using document formats would be appropriate. The MDFA for ODA would map the object actions onto specific documents types and allow the information to be created as a human readable document if necessary.

Conclusions

This architecture and Reference Model will allow the MEDIX standard to continue to grow as the needs of the health care environment change. In addition, the specific lack of required decomposition will allow this standard to be appropriate for the various healthcare environments that exist worldwide.

Presently, the working group has progressed drafts for the overview document and several object sets. Work is also underway to define the first communication profile documents.

References

1. Wallace RH, Stockenberg JH, Charette RN. A Unified Methodology for Developing System. New York: Intertext Publications, Inc., McGraw-Hill, 1987.
2. ISO DIS 9595, Common Management Information Service (CMIS) Definition.
3. ISO DIS 8613, Text and Office Systems—Office Document Architecture and Interchange Format.

III
Clinical Alerting Tools

Chapter 9
Development of a Computerized Laboratory Alerting System

Karen E. Bradshaw, Reed M. Gardner, and T. Allan Pryor

Introduction

The role of the clinical laboratory is primarily to provide physicians with patient data for use in clinical decision-making. Studies have shown that laboratory test results are the data most frequently used by physicians in decision-making [1,2]. For such decision-making to be effective, the clinical laboratory must provide accurate laboratory test results in a timely fashion, and physicians must identify and utilize important test results in making appropriate patient care decisions. Factors which make it difficult to achieve these goals are 1) problems in data communication, 2) unavailability of the attending physician, 3) information overload, and 4) human imperfectibility 3].

Over the past two decades, the number of laboratory tests performed by clinical laboratories has steadily increased, with laboratories in large hospitals performing several million tests per year [4]. This increase has been due in part to advances in technology which allow batteries of tests to be run simultaneously at low cost, and in part to increased physician utilization of laboratory tests to aid in screening and early diagnosis of patients [5]. As the number of tests performed by clinical laboratories has grown, so have the problems of data communication, information overload, and human error, both for the clinical laboratory and for the physician.

Man is limited in his ability both to process large amounts of information (due to sensory overload) [6,7] and to recognize important events which occur randomly and infrequently [8] Even physicians who have been trained, educated and have the best intentions do err, especially when called upon to deal with large amounts of patient data [9–13].

Adapted from an article published in *Comput Biomed Res* 22:575–587, 1989. Reprinted with permission of Academic Press, Inc.

How, then, can the computer help in providing physicians with important patient information generated by the clinical laboratory, and in ensuring the correct interpretation of that information by physicians? It has been suggested that computers are most helpful when they concentrate on areas in which physicians are known to be imperfect [14], and that they are most readily accepted when they are accessible, easy to use, and are perceived as enhancing the patient-management capabilities of physicians [15,16].

To date, laboratory information systems have been designed mainly to handle clerical, financial, and managerial functions, including data acquisition, presentation, and storage [17]. Some efforts have also been made to develop computerized decision aids to help in the interpretation of laboratory test results [18–21]. However, little has been done to develop decision aids in the hospital setting which would automatically alert clinicians to laboratory information that needs their immediate attention. Such alerting systems would be most effective if they were integrated into a total hospital information system containing most or all of a patient's data available from such diverse sources as laboratory, pharmacy, radiology, and patient history [22,23].

This paper describes the development of a new decision aid using the HELP medical information system at LDS Hospital [24,25]. The decision aid, called the Computerized Laboratory Alerting System (CLAS), monitors and alerts for the presence of life-threatening conditions in hospitalized patients, so that appropriate treatment can be more rapidly instituted. CLAS was designed to aid the clinical laboratory in the timely communication of important laboratory test results, to deal with the problems of physician absence, information overload, and human imperfectability, and to enhance the patient management capabilities of the physician in a way that is convenient and easy to use.

Methods

Background

LDS Hospital is a private 520-bed tertiary care facility which is part of the intermountain Health Care (IHC) hospital system. It is a teaching hospital associated with the University of Utah College of Medicine and has more than 300 private physicians on staff. The computer facilities at the hospital include 10 Tandem TXP central processing units, 18 minicomputers, and over 600 terminals and printers distributed throughout the hospital. At least four terminals and one printer are located in each nursing division. Intensive care units (total of 60 beds) and the 48-bed 8 West nursing division are equipped with a terminal at each bedside, and there are plans to place terminals at each bedside throughout the hospital in the near future [26].

The hospital's computer facilities are used to provide a hospital-wide

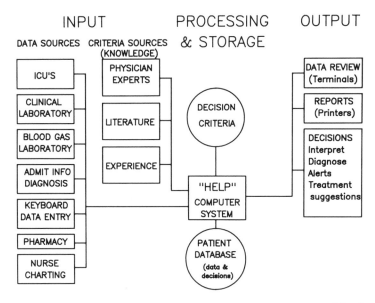

Figure 9.1. The HELP System. Data from many sources are stored in the computerized patient database. The data are then available for review or for use in reports or computerized decision-making. The HELP knowledge base consists of decision criteria developed from expert opinion, the literature, and experience.

comprehensive medical information system called HELP [24]. The HELP system has flexible medical decision-making capabilities and is able to evaluate data within specific time constraints. Medical knowledge is encoded into decision modules or frames which can then be evaluated by the HELP system. Frames can be automatically evaluated without human intervention (data-driven) whenever a data item is stored in the computerized patient database. A diagram of the HELP system is shown in Figure 9.1.

The laboratory information system used by the central laboratory at LDS Hospital is fully integrated into the HELP system, so that as soon as laboratory tests are completed and verified, the results are transmitted to HELP and stored in the HELP computerized patient database. Laboratory test results are then available for use in evaluating computerized decision logic (frames), or for review at any terminal, both inside and outside the hospital.

Design of the CLAS System

The purpose of CLAS was to monitor and alert for life-threatening conditions in hospital patients. To achieve this purpose, it was necessary to develop a knowledge base defining the life-threatening conditions and an efficient method for transmitting alerts to the clinicians responsible for the

```
Title: Metabolic Acidosis (13:1:5)

Message:    |-<13 3 1 5 4˜Metabolic Acidosis--CO2
            is (Val^CO2;##), BUN is (Val^BUN;##)-
            |

Author: Karen Bradshaw

Type: Diagnosis

Destination: Patient File, Nearest Terminal

Variable Declarations:
     CO2 which is |-13 1 1 1 4˜CO2--SMA-7-|;
     BUN which is |-13 1 1 1 5˜BUN--SMA-7-|;

Logic:     Val^CO2 = CO2;
           Val^BUN = BUN;
           If CO2 < 15 and BUN > 50
           or CO2 < 18 and BUN < 50
           or CO2 < 18 and Not Exist BUN
           then conclude true;
              end;

Evoke: If CO2 < 18;
```

Figure 9.2. Frame for the metabolic acidosis alert contained in the CLAS medical knowledge base. Frames in the knowledge base are data driven. This means that frames are automatically activated when pertinent laboratory data are stored in the HELP patient database.

patient's medical care. CLAS's medical knowledge base was developed in conjunction with physicians at LDS Hospital; it included alert criteria for hyponatremia, hypernatremia, falling sodium, hypokalemia, hyperkalemia, falling potassium, metabolic acidosis, hypoglycemia, hyperglycemia, and falling hematocrit [27]. Once the alert criteria were developed, they were incorporated into decision modules called frames. These frames were "data-driven," so that they were activated whenever pertinent laboratory data was stored in the computerized patient database. The frame for the metabolic acidosis alert is shown in Figure 9.2.

It was decided that the best alert feedback mechanism would be one which functioned automatically, without the need for a human messenger, and one which notified appropriate health care personnel in a timely fashion (within minutes). This would allow CLAS to function effectively 24 hr a day, 7 days a week. The architecture of the CLAS alert feedback mechanism is shown in Figure 9.3.

When laboratory tests are ordered for a patient, laboratory personnel perform the tests and enter the results into the laboratory computer system. Results are then transmitted to the HELP system, stored in the patient database, and evaluated by the data driver component of the HELP

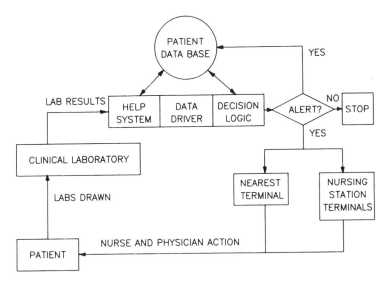

Figure 9.3. Architecture of the Computerized Laboratory Alerting System (CLAS). Patient laboratory test values are evaluated by data driven decision logic to determine if a life-threatening condition is present. Resultant alerts are transmitted to the computer terminals on the nursing division where the patient is located. Alerts are reviewed by nurses and physicians and appropriate action is taken to treat the patient.

system to determine if alert decision logic should be invoked. Alert decision logic modules are invoked for sodium, potassium, carbon dioxide (pCO_2), glucose, and hematocrit laboratory values which fall within specified ranges or rates of change. The alert decision modules further evaluate laboratory values in conjunction with other patient data (e.g., past laboratory values or medications) contained in the computerized patient database. If a life-threatening condition is detected, an alert is generated. The alert is stored in the patient database and is transmitted and displayed on computer terminals in the nursing division where the patient is located. The alert is transmitted to all the terminals at the central nursing station (usually four terminals), as well as to the terminal closest to the patient (bedside terminal or satellite terminal located closest to the patient's room). A nurse or physician can then review the alert on the computer terminal and use the alert information to help determine appropriate patient care.

The clinical staff were originally notified of the existence of an alert by having the patient's room number displayed in the lower left-hand corner of the terminal screen. This method of alert notification was chosen because of practical limitations on where and how a message could be displayed on a computer terminal while it was in use, and because of concerns about alarming a patient's family or friends if a message containing the word "alert" appeared on the terminal at the patient's bedside. When a nurse or physician observed their patient's room number on the terminal, they selected the Lab Alert menu option on the terminal screen, specified the patient's room number, and the alert message was displayed on the screen. Once an alert was reviewed in this manner, the room number was cleared from the left-hand corner of the terminal screen. The CLAS alert review program also allowed medical personnel to review (via terminal or printed report) all alerts on an individual patient or all alerts on the patients of a specific nursing division.

User Education and Initial Evaluation

Once the alert feedback mechanism of CLAS was operational, efforts were made to educate the clinical staff about CLAS and to teach them how to use the system. These efforts included presentations to computer user groups, demonstrations to head nurses, written instruction sheets for individual users, memos to hospital staff, and a contest for the nursing division which achieved the best response (most alerts reviewed) to CLAS. These educational efforts were conducted over a two-month period. At the end of the educational period, overall response to the CLAS was evaluated in terms of the number of alerts which were reviewed (acknowledged) on the computer terminal, and the length of time between alert posting (indication of an alert on the terminal) and alert acknowledgment. Acknowledgment of an alert consisted of review of an alert by a health care provider by displaying the full alert message on the terminal. In the initial evaluation of response to the CLAS, it was found that, though a large percentage of alerts were being acknowledged, the time between alert posting (on the terminal) and alert acknowledgment was often unacceptably long (several hours). Occasionally alerts for "life-threatening" conditions would not be acknowledged for several days. The average time before alert acknowledgment and the number of alerts acknowledged for each nursing division within the hospital are shown In Table 9.1 for the two weeks following the two-month educational period.

Modification of the CLAS System

Because of the long acknowledgment time, two different methods were explored for improving the CLAS alert feedback system in the hope that alert response time could be shortened. First, a flashing yellow light was designed and installed on the West 8 nursing division. The alert feedback mechanism was modified so that a special code was transmitted along with the alert to terminals on the nursing division where the patient was located. The special code activated the flashing light so that health care personnel knew immediately when there was a new alert. After the alert

Table 9.1. Average Number of Alerts Acknowledged and Average Acknowledgment Time After Educational Period April 6, 1987 to April 19, 1987

Nursing unit	Date	No. Acknowledged/ No. generated	%	Average time to acknowledge (hr)
Med/Surg ICU	4-6-87 to 4-12-87	5/11	45	27.4
Med/Surg ICU	4-13-87 to 4-19-87	0/8	0	NA
Shock/Trauma ICU	4-6-87 to 4-12-87	4/15	27	39.0
Shock/trauma ICU	4-13-87 to 4-19-87	15/20	75	33.6
Coronary Care Unit	4-6-87 to 4-12-87	6/6	100	15.4
Coronary Care Unit	4-13-87 to 4-19-87	3/6	50	35.6
Thoracic ICU	4-6-87 to 4-12-87	0/8	0	NA
Thoracic ICU	4-13-87 to 4-19-87	0/3	0	NA
West 3	4-6-87 to 4-12-87	3/3	100	16.1
West 3	4-13-87 to 4-19-87	8/13	61	15.1
West 4	4-6-87 to 4-12-87	1/4	25	14.9
West 4	4-13-87 to 4-19-87	0/3	0	NA
West 6 South	4-6-87 to 4-12-87	3/5	60	13.2
West 6 South	4-13-87 to 4-19-87	3/3	100	39.0
West 6 North	4-6-87 to 4-12-87	0/7	0	NA
West 6 North	4-13-87 to 4-19-87	0/5	0	NA
West 7	4-6-87 to 4-12-87	7/8	87	43.2
West 7	4-13-87 to 4-19-87	8/10	80	33.6
West 8	4-6-87 to 4-12-87	7/14	50	49.4
West 8	4-13-87 to 4-19-87	1/10	10	5.1
East 8	4-6-87 to 4-12-87	6/12	50	58.2
East 8	4-13-87 to 4-19-87	2/4	50	38.7
North 4	4-6-87 to 4-12-87	0/6	0	NA
North 4	4-13-87 to 4-19-87	4/5	80	23.3
North 6	4-6-87 to 4-12-87	1/1	100	21.1
North 6	4-13-87 to 4-19-87	0/0	NA	NA

was acknowledged, another code was transmitted which turned the light off. The flashing light was installed on one nursing division as a trial, and was found to reduce dramatically the time between alert posting and review (0.1 hr after vs. 28.0 hr before). Because the flashing light was successful in shortening alert acknowledgment time, plans were made to install flashing lights on all nursing divisions within the hospital. However, the unavailability of parts needed for constructing the lights caused a two-month delay in the light construction. In the meantime, a second method for reducing alert response time was developed. The second method of reducing alert response time involved making modifications to the laboratory review component of the HELP system so that the terminal first displayed any unacknowledged alerts on a patient (along with appropriate laboratory data) whenever any of the patient's laboratory test results were reviewed.

Data Collection and Final Evaluation

At the time CLAS was implemented, a special computer file was set up to capture pertinent information for each alert generated, including patient number, type of alert, time of alert, time of acknowledgment, hours till acknowledged, and patient room. The information captured on each alert allowed tracking of user response to CLAS, and aided in determining the success of modifications (flashing light, etc.) which were made. Six months after CLAS implementation, the computer file was further modified to capture information on CLAS users by type (nurse, physician, ward clerk, or other). Data captured in the special computer file were downloaded to a personal computer, edited using WordPerfect, and analyzed using Lotus 123.

Results

Table 9.1 shows the percentage of alerts which were reviewed and acknowledged on each nursing division for a two-week period after CLAS had been implemented for two months. The average time between alert posting (on the terminal) and alert acknowledgment for this period ranged from a low of 3.1 hr to a high of 72.7 hr. After installation of the flashing light on the West 8 nursing division, data were again collected and analyzed to see if the flashing light had any effect. The results of the analysis are shown in Table 9.2.

For the "pre"-flashing light period, from March 24, 1987 to May 3, 1987, the 686 alerts generated hospital-wide had an average acknowledgment time of 38.7 hr. For the West 8 nursing division, 70 alerts were generated, and the average acknowledgment time was 28.0 hr. After the

Table 9.2. Results of Efforts to Improve CLAS Feedback and Acknowledgment System—Flashing Light Prelight—3/24/87 to 5/3/87; Postlight—5/28/87 to 8/10/87)

Location	Pre/post	Average hr till acknowledged	Alerts acknowledged (%)
Entire hospital	Pre	38.7 ± 31.8	41.4
West 8	Pre	28.0 ± 28.1	28.6
West 8	Post	$.1 \pm 0.2$	100.0

flashing light was installed on the West 8 nursing division, the average West 8 acknowledgment time dropped to 0.1 hr or about 6 min (103 alerts). Before the flashing light was installed on West 8, 28.6% of the alerts generated were acknowledged. After the light was installed, the percentage of alerts acknowledged on West 8 rose to 100%.

A similar analysis of average acknowledgment time and number of alerts acknowledged was performed on data collected for two weeks before (July 28 to August 11, 1987) and after (August 14 to August 28, 198.7) the integration of alert review and acknowledgment with the HELP laboratory review program. The data from the analysis are summarized in Table 9.3. during the "pre" period (118 alerts generated), the average alert acknowledgment time for the hospital, excluding the West 8 nursing division, was 64.6 hr, with 71.2% of the alerts acknowledged. Data collected during the "post" period (149 alerts generated) showed that the average acknowledgment time for the hospital, not including West 8, had fallen to 3.6 hr, with 94.6% of the alerts acknowledged. The distribution of alert acknowledgment times for the first 220 min after alert posting during the "post" period is shown in Fgure 9.4. After alert/laboratory review integration, 29% of the alerts were reviewed within 20 min of posting, 47% were reviewed within 1 hr of posting, and 78% of the alerts were reviewed in the first 220 min after posting.

Data on users of the CLAS system were collected for $2\frac{1}{2}$ months after CLAS implementation. Each time an alert was acknowledged, the user was asked to indicate whether they were a ward clerk, nurse, M.D., or "other" hospital personnel. The data gathered on users of the CLAS system are shown graphically in Figure 9.5. The percentage of users in each user group did not vary greatly between the general nursing floors and the ICUs. The largest difference was for ward clerks, who acknowledged alerts 15.9% of the time on the floor and 7.5% of the time in the ICUs. Physicians acknowledged alerts 32.0% of the time in the ICUs, and

Table 9.3. Results of Efforts to Improve CLAS Feedback and Acknowledgment System—Alert/Lab Review Integration (Pre-Integration—7/28/87 to 8/11/87; Post-Integration—8/14/87 to 8/28/87)

Location	Pre/post	Average hr till acknowledged	Alerts acknowledged (%)
Hospital except West 8	Pre	64.6 ± 67.1	71.2
Hospital except West 8	Post	3.6 ± 6.5	94.6

BRADSHAW, GARDNER, AND PRYOR

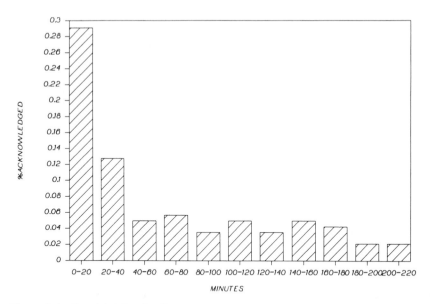

Figure 9.4. Graph of the distribution of alert acknowledgment times following integration of alert acknowledgment and laboratory review (8/14/87 to 8128187). During this period, 149 alerts were generated (not including alerts for patients on the West 8 nursing division), and 78% of these alerts were acknowledged within 220 min of posting (on the terminal).

25.9% of the time on the floors. Nurses acknowledged alerts 53.8% of the time in the ICUs and 51.9% of the time on the floors. "Other" personnel acknowledged alerts 7.7% of the time in the ICUs and 6.3% of the time on the floors.

Discussion

For physician decision-making to be effective, the clinical laboratory must provide accurate laboratory test results in a timely fashion, and physicians must identify and utilize important test results in making appropriate patient care decisions. The CLAS decision-aid was designed to help accomplish both of these goals. In its original implementation, however, few of CLAS's alerts were actually reviewed by the clinical staff, and those that were often so delayed as to be of little value. CLAS was initially unsuccessful in meeting its design goals because it required clinicians to develop new habits (checking the computer terminal for alerts, accessing a special

COMPUTERIZED LABORATORY ALERTING SYSTEM

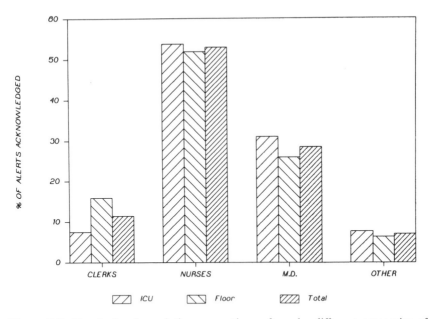

Figure 9.5. Graph showing relative proportions of use by different categories of hospital staff for the floor, ICU, and hospital as a whole.

alert review menu option), and because the alert acknowledgment process required several steps and was time consuming (3–4 min).

For CLAS to be truly effective in relaying important laboratory results to physicians in a timely manner, the alert feedback and acknowledgment system had to be modified to more nearly meet the needs and habits of the users. The two methods used to improve alert acknowledgment were successful to different extents and for different reasons.

The flashing light on the West 8 nursing division caused an immediate and marked improvement in the speed and completeness of alert acknowledgment because it made the presence of an alert obvious and because the light was bright enough and obnoxious enough to make people want to respond. On the other hand, incorporation of alert acknowledgment within the laboratory result review component of HELP was effective because it was logical (as alerts were based on patient laboratory test results) and because it used a mode of access to patient information which was both familiar to and frequently used by nurses and physicians. Although both methods greatly reduced the alert acknowledgment time (28.0 hr before vs 0.1 hr after the flashing light and 64.6 hr before vs 3.6 hr after integration) and increased the number of alerts reviewed (28.6%

before vs. 100% after the flashing light and 71.2% before vs. 94.6% after integration), average acknowledgment time using alert/laboratory integration was still several hours, with only 29% of the alerts reviewed within 20 min.

Since CLAS was designed to warn of life-threatening conditions, a 3–4 hr average response time was unacceptable. On the other hand, our experience showed that constant use of the flashing light was not desirable, as it was distracting and somewhat irritating to hospital staff. For these reasons, we elected to combine the two methods, so that alerts could still be acknowledged at the time of laboratory data review, and so that the flashing light was activated whenever alerts were not reviewed and acknowledged within 20 min of posting on the terminal. The combination of alert/laboratory review integration and flashing light then became an effective and accepted method for alert feedback and acknowledgment.

During the development of CLAS, physicians were asked their opinion of the best method of alert feedback. They responded that the alerts should first be relayed to nurses who could then evaluate them and use their judgment as to whether to notify the physician. Data collected on CLAS users showed that the most frequent users of the system were in fact nurses (nurses acknowledged 53.0% of all alerts). An unexpected result was that a large portion (28.5%) of the alerts were acknowledged by physicians. This result reflects a high degree of physician involvement in review of laboratory data using the computer terminal. As more physicians make use of a recently available option to review laboratory data on terminals in the physician's home or office, the percentage of physicians acknowledging alerts may increase.

Now that CLAS has been tested and modified so that it effectively meets design goals and is accepted by clinicians, further evaluation can be carried out to determine CLAS's effect on the patient care process and on patient outcome. Such evaluation will allow us to judge whether the CLAS system truly improves the quality of the patient care process, and whether its associated costs are justified. If CLAS does have a positive impact on patient care, the system can then be expanded to meet additional data communication and decision-making needs within the hospital.

Summary

Using the capabilities of the HELP medical information system at LDS Hospital, researchers developed a Computerized Laboratory Alerting System (CLAS). CLAS monitors and alerts for the presence of life-threatening conditions in hospitalized patients which are indicated by laboratory test results. Alerts are posted on computer terminals in the hospital's nursing divisions, where they are reviewed and acknowledged by hospital staff so that appropriate treatment can be rapidly instituted. CLAS was evaluated to determine its effectiveness in relaying alerts to the clinical staff, and improvements were made to develop an effective user interface. Initial average alert response times on nursing divisions ranged from 5.1 to 58.2 hr. The average alert response time dropped to 3.6 hr when alert review was integrated with laboratory result review, and to 0.1 hr after installation of a flashing light to notify hospital staff of the presence of new alerts.

References

1. McDonald CJ, Wheeler LA, Glazener T, and Blevins L. A data base approach to laboratory computerization. *Am J Clin pathol* 1985; 83:707.
2. Bradshaw KE, Gardner RM, Clemmer TP, Orme JF, Thomas F, and West BJ. Physician decision-making—Evaluation of data used in a computerized ICU. *Int J Clin Monit Comput* 1984; 1:81.
3. McDonald CJ, Wilson GA, and McCabe GP. Physician response to computer reminders. JAMA 1980; 244:1579.
4. Miller RE, Steinbach Gl,and Dayhoff RE. A hierarchical computer network: An alternative approach to clinical laboratory computerization in a large hospital. Proceedings of the Fourth Annual Symposium on Computer Applications in Medical Care. Washington, DC: IEEE Computer Society Press, 1980; p. 105.
5. Schneiderman MD, DeSalvo L, Baylor S, and Wolf PL. The "abnormal" screening laboratory results. *Arch Int Med* 1972; 129:88.
6. McDonald CJ. Protocol-based computer reminders, the quality of care and the nonperfectability of man. *N Engl J Med* 1976; 195:1351.
7. Drinkwater BL. Performance of civil aviation pilots under conditions of sensory input overload. *Aerosp Med* 1967; 38:164.
8. Alluist EA. Attention and vigilance as mechanisms of response. In EA Bilodeau (ed): Acquisition of Skill. New York: Academic Press, 1966; p 201.
9. Wheeler LA, Brecher G, and Sheiner LB. Clinical laboratory use in the evaluation of anemia. *JAMA* 1977; 238:2709.
10. Olsen DM, Kane RL, and Proctor PH. A controlled trial of multiphasic screening. *N Engl J Med* 1976; 294:925.
11. Byrd RB, Horn BR, Solomon DA, Griggs GA, and Wilder NJ. Treatment of tuberculosis by the pulmonary physician. *Ann Inter Med* 1977; 86:799.
12. Dixon RH, Laszio J. Utilization of clinical chemistry services by medical staff: An analysis. *Arch Intern Med* 1974; 134:1064.
13. Shapiro S, Slone D, Lewis GP, Jick H. Fatal drug reactions among medical inpatients. *JAMA* 1971;216:467.
14. Friedman RH. The use of computers to assist physicians in patient management. *Adv Intern Med* 1986; 31:71.
15. Teach RL, Shortliffe EH. An analysis of physician attitudes regarding computer-based clinical consultation systems. *Comput Biomed Res* 1981; 14:542.
16. Siegel C, Alexander MJ. Acceptance and impact of the computer in clinical decisions. *Hosp Community Psychiatr* 1984; 35:773.

17. Enlander D (ed). Computers in Laboratory Medicine. New York: Academic Press, 1975.
18. Speicher CE, Smith JW, Jr. Interpretive reporting in clinical pathology. JAMA 1980; 243:1556.
19. Evans RS, Gardner RM, Bush AR, Burke JP, Jacobsen JA, Larsen RA, Meier FA, Warner HR. Development of a computerized infections disease monitor (CIDM). *Comput Biomed Res* 1985; 18:103.
20. Myers JD. The computer as a diagnostic consultant with emphasis on the use of laboratory data. *Clin Chem* 1986; 32:1714.
21. Spackman KA, Connelly DP. Knowledge-based systems in laboratory medicine and pathology. *Arch Pathol Lab Med* 1987; 111:116.
22. Lindberg D. "The Growth of Medical Information Systems in the United States. Lexington, MA: Lexington Books, 1979.
23. Shortliffe EH. Computer programs to support clinical decision making. JAMA 1987; 258:61.
24. Pryor TA, Gardner RM, Clayton PD, Warner HR. The HELP system. *J Med Systems* 1983; 7:87.
25. Pryor TA. The HELP medical record system. *MD comput* 1988; 5:22.
26. Johnson DS, Burkes M, Sittig D, Hinson D, Pryor TA. Evaluation of the Effects of Computerized Nurse Charting. Proceedings of the Eleventh Annual Symposium on Computer Applications in Medical Care. Washington, DC: IEEE Computer Society Press, 1987; p 363.
27. Bradshaw KE. Computerized alerting system warns of life-threatening events. Proceedings of the 10th Annual Symposium of Computer Applications in Medical Care. Washington, DC: IEEE Computer Society Press, 1986; p 403.

Chapter 10
Inferencing Strategies for Automated Alerts on Critically Abnormal Laboratory and Blood Gas Data
M. Michael Shabot, Mark LoBue, Beverley J. Leyerle, and Stuart B. Dubin

Introduction

A relatively insignificant amount of human thought is required to recognize critically abnormal events. After a few weeks of training on the ward, most medical students can recognize seriously abnormal results of common laboratory tests and take some definitive action, such as calling a supervising physician. The "gestalt" by which laboratory results are appreciated as clinically dangerous is complex and challenging to duplicate in a modern digital computer.

In 1984 we implemented a comprehensive ICU patient data management system (HP 78709A PDMS, Hewlett-Packard Co., Waltham, MA) [1]. The PDMS has network connections for automatic acquisition of all laboratory and blood gas data required for a patient's ICU flow sheet. In 1988 we decided to implement a decision support system which would evaluate all incoming laboratory data for critically abnormal results. If found, a critical value message is posted on the affected patient's bedside terminal and the central station terminal. Implementation of the decision support package occurred in phases, corresponding to our understanding of the inferencing strategies required to detect critical laboratory values. Although three major strategies are presented here, refinement of critical event detection algorithms remains a continuing process.

Methods

Data Management Network

The Cedars-Sinai Surgical Intensive Care Unit PDMS is networked to two major data-producing computers as well as 60 physiologic monitors

Adapted from an article published in the Proceedings of the Thirteenth Annual Symposium on Computer Applications in Medical Care, Washington, DC, November 5–8, 1989. Reprinted with permission of IEEE.

and other instruments at 20 beds [2]. The networked data-producing computers include a Laboratory Information System which operates within a cluster on a VAX 8530 computer running Sunquest Flexilab software. The second network connection is to a Blood Gas Information System which operates on a DEC 11/23 computer running Forth software. In both systems, laboratory data records are automatically transmitted to the PDMS as soon as the data is stored. In 1984 we wrote an additional PDMS software module which notifies the ICU staff that laboratory data has been received by placing a specific message such as "**Chem I Lab Data Ready**" on the appropriate patient's bedside terminal and the central station terminal [3]. In addition to laboratory data, all objective flowsheet data is maintained by the PDMS. Connections to bedside instruments provide for the automated acquisition of hemodynamic, respiratory, and intake and output data. Flowsheet calculations and other information are provided directly by the PDMS.

Inferencing Module

A new software module called "ALERTS" was written for the PDMS to provide inferencing capabilities. All laboratory records received by the laboratory interface module are sent to the ALERTS processor and the standard PDMS data storage processors (Figure 10.1). Within the ALERTS processor, all incoming data passes through a central decision node to determine if it is an ALERT key. If not, the ALERTS process is aborted. If the parameter is an ALERT key, it is subjected to various inferencing strategies as described below. If necessary for the inferencing

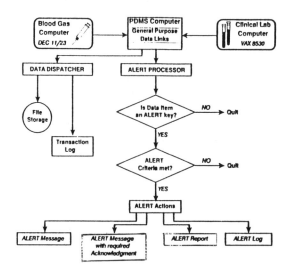

Figure 10.1. Inferencing system.

algorithm, the ALERTS processor can recall prior values or related laboratory data from the patient's PDMS data base.

If an ALERT condition is detected, a more urgent laboratory data message such as "*K + **Chem I *ALERT***" is posted to the appropriate terminals [4]. All laboratory "Ready" and "ALERT" messages have pre-configured life spans of 60 min for clinical laboratory data and 30 min for blood gas data. All ALERTS are also logged in a flat ASCII file which is periodically transferred to a personal computer over a serial data link. In the PC the ALERT log Is imported into a dBASE IV data base for further analysis [5].

Overall Inferencing Strategy

The Cedars-Sinai laboratory data inferencing module operates on four levels. It is similar to previous rule-based strategies [6]. At each inferencing level, progressively more complex sets of conditions are applied to the data in order to detect ALERT conditions. The first-order decision which must be made is to determine which laboratory data qualify as ALERT keys. In critically ill SICU patients, a significant percentage of laboratory data is abnormal but need not generate undue alarm in the health care team. Certain laboratory parameters do not qualify as ALERT keys regardless of the degree of abnormality. An example is serum bilirubin, which in adults does not require an emergency response even if the level is very high. A serum bilirubin of 20 mg/dl may well require a medical response, but not an ALERT response. (Note that if the patient is a neonate, the same bilirubin level might represent an ALERT condition, with immediate treatment indicated to prevent kernicterus.) For the Cedars-

Table 10.1. ALERT parameters.

Serum Chemistries	*Drug levels*
Sodium	Phenytoin
Potassium	Theophylline
Chloride	Phenobarbital
Bicarbonate	Quinidine
Calcium	Lidocaine
Hematology	Procainamide
Hemoglobin	NAPA
Hematocrit	Digoxin
White Blood Count	Thiocyanate
Partial Thromboplastin Time	Gentamicin
Prothrombin Time % Activity	Tobramycin
Arterial blood gas	*Cardiac Enzymes*
pH	Creatinine kinase (CK)
PO_2	CK-MB
PCO_2	

Table 10.2. Inferencing Strategy Levels

Types of Alerts
High and low limits
Calculation-adjusted limits
Trend alerts

Sinai SICU. 26 variables have been selected as appropriate for ALERT responses (Table 10.1).

Once parameters have been identified as ALERT keys, they are subjected to the three levels of inferencing strategy in Table 10.2.

Strategy I: Critical Value ALERTS

Certain laboratory results indicate life-threatening situations if they reach a critically high or low level, usually well beyond the "normal" range. A common example is serum potassium, which is associated with serious or fatal cardiac arrhythmias at levels below 3.0 mmol/L and above 6.5 mmol/L. Examples of parameters and their associated critical value limits are given in Table 10.3.

Strategy II: Calculation-Adjusted Critical Value ALERTS

Some laboratory parameters represent appropriate ALERT keys if other criteria are met. A common example is serum calcium, which is associated with tetany for levels below 7 mg/dl. However, total serum calcium as measured by the laboratory is directly affected by both serum albumin concentration and pH. Most ICU patients with seemingly critical hypocalcemia are merely hypoalbuminemic and in no danger. The reason is that

Table 10.3. Critical Value Limits

	Low	High
Na+	120	160
K+	3.0	6.5
Cl−	80	156
HCO_3	10	40
Hgb	7	18
Hct	21	60
WBC	2	35

IF exist Serum Albumin (within 48 hours)
  Ca++ = Ca++ + 0.8 X (4.0 - Albumin)
ENDIF

IF exist arterial pH (within 2 hours)

$$\text{Ca++} = \text{Ca++} \times \left[\frac{0.55 + (7.40 - \text{pH})/4}{0.55}\right]$$

ENDIF

IF Ca++ < 7.0 or > 12.0 then ALERT

Figure 10.2. Calculation-adjusted calcium limits.

calcium is normally 55% bound to albumin, and only the unbound or ionized calcium is physiologically active. Albumin binding is also affected by blood pH. Therefore the measured serum calcium must be subjected to a calculation adjustment before passing it through high/low critical value filters (Figure 10.2).

Whenever related laboratory values are used in calculation-adjusted limits, one must specify a time "window" for which the related values are medically valid. Because serum albumin changes very slowly (in the absence of albumin infusions), we recognize it as valid for 48 hr. Arterial pH may change very rapidly, so for adjustment purposes we use it for only 2 hr. Another important calculation-adjusted parameter is the percentage of creatinine kinase (CK), which is due to the myocardial fraction, CK-MB. CK is a muscle enzyme and the CK-MB component is found chiefly in heart, although a small percentage is present in many other tissues, including skeletal muscle. CK-MB is very useful in diagnosing cardiac muscle damage due to myocardial infarction or, as is commonly seen

IF CK-MB >4.0 then ALERT
IF exist CK .and. CK-MB then
  IF 300< CK >1000 then
    IF (CK X CK-MB/100) >15 then ALERT
  ENDIF
  IF 1000< CK >2000 then
    IF (CK X CK-MB/100) >35 then ALERT
  ENDIF
  IF CK > 2000
    IF (CK X CK-MB/100) > 100 then ALERT
  ENDIF
ENDIF

(Where total CK is in IU/L and CK-MB is reported as percent of total CK)

Figure 10.3. Calculation-adjusted CK-MB limits.

in trauma, myocardial contusion. The challenge is to separate patients whose laboratory results are suggestive of myocardial infarction or myocardial contusion from those whose elevations in CK might simply reflect skeletal muscle damage, a task that cannot be performed completely, even in principle. However, since the latter group generally has very high total CK values (typically > 2,000 IU/L, a level not commonly seen in disease of cardiac origin), we have constructed a useful decision support strategy (Fig. 10.3).

Strategy III: Trend ALERTS

The most complex inferencing schemes involve detection of critically adverse laboratory data trends. Human recognition of critical trends probably involves multifactorial parallel processing with analog weighting and is difficult to duplicate in a rule-based digital computer. We found that computer recognition of critical trends required a strategy which encompassed four important criteria:

- Amount of change
- Rate of change
- Time span between samples
- Proximity of current value to a critical value limit

Thus far we have implemented critical trend ALERTS for hemoglobin, hematocrit, and serum sodium. The schema for hemoglobin is shown in Figure 10.4.

If a basic critical value limit is exceeded (hemoglobin <7 g/dl or >18 g/dl), a limit ALERT is declared and no tests for critical trends are performed. If the current hemoglobin passes the limit filters, the PDMS recalls the most recent previous hemoglobin. If a hemoglobin result is found within the preceding 36 hr, a subtraction is performed to determine the amount of change. This test is performed to determine whether a sig-

IF Hgb < 7 .or. Hgb > 18 then do $\boxed{\text{LIMIT\_ALERT}}$
  ELSE IF exist Prior_Hgb (within 36 hours) then
    IF (Prior_Hgb - Hgb) > 1.5 then

$$\text{IF Hgb} \geq 10 \text{ .and.} \left[\frac{(\text{Prior\_Hgb} - \text{Hgb}) / \text{Hours}}{\text{Prior\_Hgb}}\right] \times 100 > 1.0$$

$$.\text{or. Hgb} < 10 \text{ .and.} \left[\frac{(\text{Prior\_Hgb} - \text{Hgb}) / \text{Hours}}{\text{Prior\_Hgb}}\right] \times 100 > 0.66$$

      then do $\boxed{\text{TREND\_ALERT}}$
      ENDIF
    ENDIF
  ENDIF
ENDIF

Figure 10.4. Hemoglobin trend ALERT algorithim.

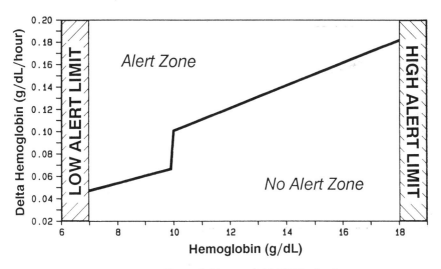

Figure 10.5. Hemoglobin trend ALERT criteria.

nificant change has occurred, in order to avoid declaring false ALERTS due to minor measurement variations. For hemoglobin we consider a decrease by more than 1.5 to be significant. If a significant decrease has occurred, we then determine the rate of change and test it against a pre-configured limit. Note that the equations are structured so that the rate limit becomes more sensitive in inverse proportion to the hemoglobin level. That is, as the hemoglobin level declines, progressively smaller rate changes are required to trigger a trend ALERT. Finally as the hemoglobin declines below 10 g/dl and approaches the low critical value limit, we introduce a step change to make the ALERT trigger even more sensitive. In so doing we are attempting to emulate the process by which clinicians consider progressively lower values to be increasingly worrisome. The trend ALERT criteria for hemoglobin are graphically illustrated in Figure 10.5.

We are considering more subtle trend alert analyses for future implementation. For example, a rising indirect bilirubin level, although perhaps not reflecting an immediate medical concern, might indicate the early phase of a delayed hemolytic transfusion reaction. This early period is often missed in clinical management, and thus a trend ALERT applied in this case might lead to immediate action in obtaining the appropriate antigen-free blood for subsequent transfusion.

Clinical Results

Over a ten week period a total of 386 ALERTS were detected on 330 specimens. There were 55 specimens with multiple ALERTS. Alerts occurred in the following proportions:

52%—blood gas
27%—hematology
14%—chemistry
6%—cardiac enzyme
1%—drug levels

On a clinical basis the ALERTS module was considered to be a major enhancement to the functionality of the ICU computer system.

Summary

Automating the recognition of critically abnormal laboratory and blood gas results is a non-trivial task. Human judgment is remarkably multi-factorial with regard to evaluation of incoming data and appreciation of seriously abnormal events. We have implemented a decision support module for a comprehensive ICU patient data management system which examines all incoming laboratory and blood gas data for critical events. Three inferencing strategies were required to make computerized laboratory alerts both sensitive and specific. The most straightforward strategy simply subjects certain lab tests to critical value high/low band pass filters. Intermediately complex laboratory tests are passed through a calculation algorithm in which related laboratory results are analyzed and corrections applied before application of critical value filters. By far the most complex inferencing schemes involve detection of critically adverse laboratory data trends. We found that recognition of critical trends required a strategy which encompassed the amount of a parameter's change, the rate of change, the time span between samples and proximity of the current value to a critical value limit. The choice, application, and results of these strategies are discussed in this paper.

Conclusions

Bedside ALERTS for critically abnormal laboratory data are both possible and desirable. For laboratory results and ALERTS to be clinically useful, data must be transmitted from the Laboratory Information System to the ICU computer automatically and without delay. The recognition of critical laboratory ALERTS is a complex process which is difficult to duplicate in a digital computer. Nonetheless, application of appropriate limits, calculations, and trend detection algorithms can yield an ALERTS subsystem which materially enhances the value of common laboratory data.

References

1. Leyerle B, Nolan-Avila L, Shabot MM, et al. Implementation of the comprehensive computerized ICU data management system. *Proceedings of the Ninth Annual Symposium on Computer Applications in Medical Care (SCAMC)*, MJ Ackerman (ed), New York, NY: IEEE Computer Society Press, 1985; pp 386–387.
2. Leyerle BJ, LoBue M, Shabot MM. The PDMS as a focal point for distributed patient data. *Int J Clin Monit Comput* 1988; 5:155–161.
3. Avila L, Lobue M, Shabot MM. Electronic Event Messaging in a Patient Data Management System. *Proceedings of the Sixth Annual Conference on Computing in Critical Care*, Los Angeles, California, January 29–31, 1986; pp 61–62.
4. Shabot MM, LoBue M, Leyerle BJ, Dubin S. PDMS clinical alerts. *Proceedings of the Ninth Annual Conference on Computing in Critical Care*, Dallas, Texas, February 28–March 2, 1989, p 39.
5. LoBue M, Leyerle B, Shabot MM. Data base and statistical techniques for PDMS data. *Proceedings of the Eighth Annual Conference in Computers in Critical Care*, Hershey, Pennsylvania, February 12–13, 1988; p 47.
6. Gardner RM. Computerized laboratory alerting system (CLAS). In Kuperman GJ, Gardner RM (eds): *The HELP System—A Snapshot in Time*. Department of Physics, LDS Hospital, Salt Lake City, Utah, 1985; pp 105–111.

Chapter 11
Decision Support Alerts for Clinical Laboratory and Blood Gas Data

M. Michael Shabot, Mark LoBue,
Beverley J. Leyerle, and Stuart B. Dubin

Introduction

The process by which clinicians recognize potentially dangerous laboratory data is difficult to computerize. Normal value limits are useful reference points, but although a significant percentage of ICU laboratory results are abnormal, most should generate no undue alarm. Critical value limits such as $K^+ < 3.0$ mmol/L or hemoglobin < 7.0 g/dl are more relevant to critical care areas and are relatively easy to program into a data management computer system. However, simple limits are inadequate for more complex laboratory results, which must be correlated with other data to insure that true critical values are present. For example, hypocalcemia is a relatively common finding in surgical ICU patients in whom bowel disorders, abdominal surgery, stress, and sepsis may rapidly produce a hypoalbuminemic state. Because calcium is bound to albumin, in such a setting the hypocalcemia may be more apparent than real. Critical value limits will also fail to identify subtle but dangerous trends such as falling hemoglobin or hematocrit until the blood loss is quite severe and a critical value threshold is exceeded.

We have designed and implemented a computerized ICU decision support alert system which analyzes all incoming laboratory and blood gas data for critically abnormal values and trends. Calculation-adjusted critical values are also detected. Over an eight-month prospective trial this system was tested to determine the number and type of critical laboratory data events and their association with ICU outcome measures.

Adapted from an article published in *Int J Clin Monit Comput* 7:27–31, 1990. Reprinted with permission of Kluwer Academic Publishers.

Methods

The ALERTS system runs on a computerized patient data management system (HP 78709A PDMS, Hewlett-Packard Co., Waltham, MA) which serves 20 Surgical ICU beds. This system maintains electronic flowcharts which contain all the objective hemodynamic, respiratory, laboratory, intake/output, and other clinical data required for direct patient care [1]. This system also provides the official medicolegal record in the form of laser-printed flowsheet reports. The PDMS is networked to a Clinical Laboratory Information System (Sunquest Flexilab software on VAX 8530 hardware) and a blood gas computer system (Forth software on DEC 11/84 hardware) [2]. Laboratory data is transmitted to the PDMS over an RS-232 data link which utilizes a cyclic redundancy check (CRC) to ensure the integrity of all transmitted data.

Inferencing Strategies

The ALERTS subsystem operates on the PDMS as an automatic decision support computer program which is triggered by the receipt of fresh laboratory data (Fig. 11.1). Our inferencing strategies for lab data ALERTS have been described in detail elsewhere [3]. In brief, three

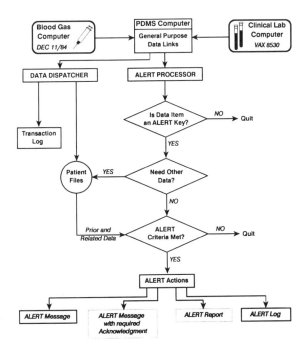

Figure 11.1. ALERT detection system.

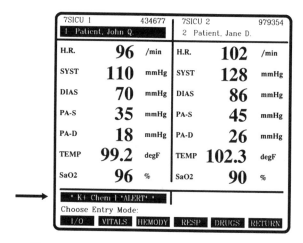

Figure 11.2. Bedside terminal ALERT message.

types of ALERTS are detected: 1) high and low critical values 2) calculation-adjusted critical values, and 3) critical trends. The logic for the high and low critical values is based on simple rules and is similar to a system previously described by Gardner [4]. More complex calculation-adjusted ALERTS are provided for serum calcium and myocardial enzymes. Serum calcium (Ca^{++}) is corrected for albumin and/or pH (if available within appropriate time windows) before application of critical value tests, as follows:

Table 11.1. ALERT Parameters

Serum chemistries	Drug levels
Sodium	Phenytoin
Potassium	Theophylline
Chloride	Phenobarbital
Bicarbonate	Quinidine
Calcium	Lidocaine
	Procainamide
Hematology	NAPA
Hemoglobin	Digoxin
Hematocrit	Thiocyanate
White blood count	Gentamicin
Partial thromboplastin time	Tobramycin
Prothrombin time, % activity	
Arterial blood gas	Cardiac enzymes
pH	Creatinine Kinase (CK)
PO_2	CK-MB
PCO_2	

$Ca^{++}_{(corrected)} =$

$(Ca^{++}_{(measured)} + (0.8\,(4.0\text{-albumin}))) \times (0.55 + (7.4\text{-pH})/4)/0.55$

[for abumin within 48 hours and arterial pH within 2 hours]

Our inferencing strategy for myocardial enzyme ALERTS is somewhat more complex. The Creatinine Kinase × Creatinine Kinase-Myocardial Band% (CK × CK-MB%) product is compared to progressive critical value limits for different ranges of total CK in order to alert reliably for myocardial damage in the face of skeletal muscle trauma [3].

The most complex alerts involve recognition of adverse trends in hemoglobin, hematocrit, and serum sodium values, independent of critical limits. Our trend ALERT algorithms compare the current laboratory value to the most recent previous result with respect to amount of change, rate of change. time span, and proximity of the current value to a critical value limit. The equations are structured so that the trend ALERT trigger becomes progressively more sensitive as the current value falls [3].

When an ALERT condition is detected, a specific ALERT message is displayed at the bottom of the patient's bedside PDMS terminal (Fig. 11.2). The ALERTS program was written in Fortran 77 and all ALERT parameters are listed in Table 11.1.

Data Collection

Over an eight-month period (January 1, 1989-August 31, 1989) all laboratory data transmissions were evaluated by the ALERTS subsystem. When an ALERT was detected, the lab data record was stored in a separate PDMS data file at the time it was dispatched to SICU terminals and the electronic flowsheet. Demographic, severity of illness, and length of stay data were maintained or calculated by the PDMS and stored separately [5,6]. These data sets were eventually transferred to a personal computer and stored in a relational database (dBASE IV, Ashton-Tate, Torrance, CA) for subsequent analysis. Mortality data was obtained from the hospital's mainframe computer and was merged into the severity database.

Results

Over the eight-month test period a total of 1,515 ALERTS were detected among approximately 115,000 individual lab results transmitted to the PDMS. Multiple ALERTS occurred in 134 specimens. During the test period 4,058 days of care SICU were delivered to 1,474 patients. The overall distribution of ALERTS is given in Table 11.2.

Blood gas data generated just over one-half of all ALERTS (Table 11.3). Four hundred forty-six blood gas ALERTS were due to critically high pH or low CO_2 levels. However, many of these results occurred in

Table 11.2. ALERTS Detected

	No. of ALERTS	%
Blood gas	758	50.04
Hematology	233	15.38
Hemoglobin trend	167	11.03
Chemistry	139	9.17
Cardiac enzymes	104	6.86
Hematocrit trend	69	4.55
Coagulation	33	2.18
Drug levels	12	0.79
Total	1,515	100.0

Table 11.3. Arterial Blood Gas ALERTS

	No. of ALERTS	Mean	Standard deviation
Low pH	165	7.17	0.08
High pH	188	7.60	0.04
Low PO_2	87	37.8 torr	10.1
Low PCO_2	258	21.3 torr	2.7
High PCO_2	60	74.4 torr	15.3
	758		
Total	758		

Table 11.4. Hematology ALERTS

	No. of ALERTS	Mean	Standard deviation
Low hematocrit	74	18.6%	1.74
Low hemoglobin	68	6.2 g/dL	0.52
High hematocrit	1	61.8%	0.0
High hemoglobin	3	18.9 g/dL	0.85
Low WBC	16	$1.1 \frac{\times 1,000}{\mu}$	0.74
High WBC	71	$47.8 \frac{\times 1,000}{\mu}$	13.2
Total	233		

Table 11.5. Trend ALERTS

	No. of ALERTS	Mean	Standard deviation
Fall in hemoglobin	167	2.5 g/dl	1.06
Fall in hematocrit	69	5.6%	1.70
Total	236		

Table 11.6. Calculation-Adjusted ALERTS

	No. of ALERTS	Mean	Standard deviation
Low Calcium	22	6.44 mg/dl	0.38
High Calcium	8	13.20 mg/dl	0.74
High CK-KB%	79	6.51 %	3.23
CK-MB% for critical CK × CK-MB% product	25	2.28 %	0.78
Total	134		

Table 11.7. Chemistry ALERTS

	No. of ALERTS	Mean	Standard deviation
Low potassium	51	2.74 mmol/L	0.17
High potassium	22	7.01 mmol/L	0.39
Low sodium	6	117.0 mmol/L	1.53
High sodium	10	167.7 mmol/L	3.03
Low bicarbonate	5	5.8 mmol/L	2.60
High bicarbonate	15	50.9 mmol/L	14.52
Total	109		

head trauma patients who were receiving hyperventilation therapy to reduce intracranial pressure. Hematology ALERTS were the next most common (Table 11.4), and usually represented very serious conditions requiring immediate therapy. Hemoglobin and hematocrit trend ALERTS (Table 11.5) also represented serious clinical problems. We noted some false hematocrit ALERTS due to discrepancies between the results of centrifuge spun and automated Coulter counter measurement methods.

A significant number of calculation-adjusted calcium and CK-MB ALERTS are noted in Table 11.6. Not shown in the table are 35 specimens with raw measured calciums of less than 7 mg/dl for which an ALERT notification was *withheld* because the calculation-adjustment

Table 11.8. Coagulation & Drug Level ALERTS

	No. of ALERTS	Mean	Standard deviation
Low PT % Activity	1	7.30%	0.0
High PTT	32	131.3 sec	20.0
High digoxin	9	4.4 ng/ml	1.36
High theophylline	2	20.5 μcg/ml	0.25
High lidocaine	1	6.0 μcg/ml	0.00
Total	45		

raised the calcium over the threshold for the critical low limit. Routine chemistry, coagulation, and drug level ALERTS are shown in Tables 11.7 and 11.8.

ICU length of stay and mortality were correlated with ALERT occurrences for 507 consecutive SICU patients over a three-month period (January 1, 1989–March 31, 1989). For 126 patients receiving one or more ALERT message, the SICU length of stay averaged 6.62 days, the SICU mortality rate was 9.52%, and the overall hospital mortality rate was 15.87%. In contrast, 381 patients with no ALERT messages had an average ICU stay of just 1.57 days and corresponding SICU and hospital mortality rates of 0% and 1.31%, respectively.

Conclusions

A comprehensive ICU PDMS which is networked to a Laboratory Information System can detect critically abnormal laboratory results and instantaneously transmit a bedside video ALERT to the ICU staff. We detected ALERTS in 1.32% of all results transmitted to a busy general surgical ICU. Rule-based calculation adjustments can be used to optimize true positive ALERTS and minimize false positives. Access to prior laboratory data allows clinically adverse trends to be detected. Access to clinical flowsheet data will permit further optimization of the results presented above, which is not feasible with raw lab data alone. Since the PDMS electronic flowsheet contains complete respiratory therapy, neurologic monitoring and Glasgow coma score data. we plan to adjust dynamically the thresholds for low CO_2 and high pH ALERTS on patients receiving therapeutic hyperventilation.

Our severity data shows that the occurrence of critically abnormal laboratory results is associated with prolonged ICU stays and high ICU and hospital mortality rates. Immediate detection of laboratory data ALERTS and automated notification of the ICU staff may allow for earlier treatment of these high risk patients.

References

1. Leyerle BJ, Nolan-Avita L, Shabot MM et al. Implementation of a comprehensive computerized ICU data management system. *SCAMC* 1985; 9:386–7.
2. Leyerle BJ, LoBue M, Shabot MM. The PDMS as a focal point for distributed patient data. *Int J Clin Monit Comput* 1988; 5:155–61.
3. Shabot MM, LoBue M, Leyerle BJ, Dubin SB. Inferencing strategies for automated ALERTS on critically abnormal laboratory and blood gas data. *SCAMC* 1989; 13:54–57.
4. Gardner RM. Computerized laboratory alerting system (CLAS). In Kuperman GJ, Gardner RM (eds): *The HELP System*. A Snapshot in Time. LDS Hospital: Salt Lake City, 1985; 105–11.
5. Shabot MM, Leyerle BJ, LoBue M. Automatic extraction of intensity-intervention scores from a computerized surgical intensive care unit flowsheet. *Amer J Surg* 1987; 154:72–8.
6. Leyerle BJ, LoBue M, Shabot MM. Computerized data bases: Medical data management beyond the bedside. *Int J Clin Mon Comput* 1990; 7:83–89.

Chapter 12
Assessing the Effectiveness of a Computerized Pharmacy System
Reed M. Gardner, Russell K. Hulse, and Keith G. Larsen

Introduction

As medical knowledge has expanded and the acuity of hospitalized patients has increased, physicians have had an ever-increasing amount of patient data to evaluate and assess. One result from this expansion of knowledge has been the application of computers for classification and analysis. The computerized pharmacy alerting system at LDS Hospital [1] has gained wide physician acceptance and is now financially subsidized by the hospital administration.

Investigators have pointed out the value and conceptual worth of computerized pharmacy systems [2–9], such as the MENTOR system [2], the Boston Collaborative Drug Surveillance Program [6],and outpatient pharmacy systems [8,9]. Educational methods have been shown to improve prescribing behavior, but may not be long-lasting [4]. The work presented here resulted from quantitative and qualitative assessment procedures and illustrates the benefits of a computerized pharmacy system.

Materials and Methods

The LDS Hospital in Salt Lake City, Utah, is a 520-bed facility with a clinical computer system (HELP) that gathers data from many services within the hospital [10,11]. The result is a rich clinical patient database. Data in the system is obtained from automated equipment in clinical laboratories and intensive care units, as well as from pharmacy, surgery, multiphasic screening areas, admitting, and medical records areas [10,11].

Adapted from an article published in the Proceedings of the Fourteenth Annual Symposium on Computer Applications in Medican Care, Washington, DC, November 4–7, 1990. Reprinted with permission of IEEE.

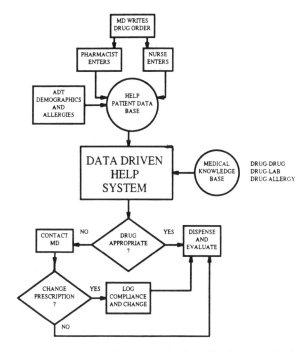

Figure 12.1. Flow diagram of computerized medication monitoring system.

Figure 12.1 is a flow chart of the pharmacy module of the HELP system in operation since 1975. Medication orders are entered by hand into the patient chart, then are entered into the HELP computer system by a pharmacist or a nurse [10,11]. The integrated database and decision-making capabilities of the HELP system made it possible to evaluate the medication orders for Drug-Drug, Drug-Laboratory, and Drug-Allergy interactions. If the drug is appropriate, the pharmacist dispenses the medication. If the computer indicates that the medication is not appropriate, a pharmacist contacts the prescribing physician.

Assessment of the effectiveness of the system is based on five evaluations: 1) the number and type of alerts, 2) physician compliance with pharmacy alerts, 3) physician attitudes toward the pharmacy system, 4) the type of patient data used to make decisions, and 5) benefit/cost estimation of the alerting system. The procedure for each of the five assessments is presented below.

Number and Type of Alerts

Statistics on the number and type of each generated alert have been kept since the system's inception in 1975. In 1979 the alerts were subdivided into two categories: informational and action-oriented. "Informational" alerts were important to the care of the patient, but did not require immediate therapy change. "Action oriented" alerts required prompt physician interaction to change therapy. With each "action-oriented" alert, a clinical pharmacist contacted the responsible physician for a detailed assessment of the medication order.

Physician Compliance Rates

The attending pharmacist was responsible for assessing physician compliance with the alert. Assessment of physician compliance rates was based on data derived from the physician compliance log shown in Figure 12.1.

Physician Attitudes

Evaluation of physician attitudes toward the HELP system was based on a questionnaire sent to 360 staff members in the spring of 1989 112]. Several questions about the value of the pharmacy system and its effect on their practice were asked.

Data Sources Required for Pharmacy Alerts

Alerts were categorized according to the sources of data required to trigger them. Drug-Drug alerts compared new medication orders to data in the patient's medication profile. Drug-Allergy alerts required not only drug information, but also knowledge about the patient's allergies to medications. Drug-Laboratory alerts required knowledge about medications plus data from the clinical laboratory.

Benefit/Cost Analysis

A charge of $0.35 per monitored patient day was instituted to cover the cost of the computer resource, and developmental costs for the program were funded by a grant from the Public Health Service. As a result, the denominator of the benefit/cost ratio was readily determined.

Evaluating the benefit of the alerting scheme was much more difficult [13]. Two clinical pharmacists from LDS Hospital and three clinical pharmacists from the University of Utah College of Pharmacy assessed the value of each alert using a modified Delphi approach [14,15]. The pharmacists were provided a list of current hospital costs and were asked to estimate probable complications resulting from each adverse drug reaction addressed in the alerting system. Each was then asked to assess the value of the alert to the patient in terms of dollar costs. They were asked to make this judgment in response to the question, "If this adverse drug reaction occurred in the patient, what would it cost to treat the adverse reaction?" No further instructions were given and each expert was asked to make an independent judgment of dollar value.

The benefit was calculated by using the dollar value of each alert. The dollar value was determined from an average of the five pharmacists' responses multiplied by actual incidence rate of the alerts for a two-year period. We noted that some alerts that were judged to be life-threatening and had very high benefits as judged by the clinical pharmacists never occurred during the year. As a result, the effect of having these alerts was assumed to have no value. However, had they occurred, the computer system would have provided a lifesaving alert!

Results

Number and Type of Alerts

During 1989, LDS Hospital admitted 20,470 patients who stayed for a total of 114,108 days (average length of stay, 5.58 days). Approximately 1.3 million doses of medications were given. Figure 12.2 plots the alerting experience at LDS Hospital from the inception of the computerized medication monitoring system in 1975 through 1989. In 1979, the logging of total alerts and "action-oriented" alerts was begun. Note that, except for the years 1988 and 1989, the number of alerts has grown almost continuously. In 1981 alerts decreased as the HELP system was transferred from the old hardware platform to the Tandem hardware. The downturns noted in 1988 and 1989 were due to changes in the software operating sys-

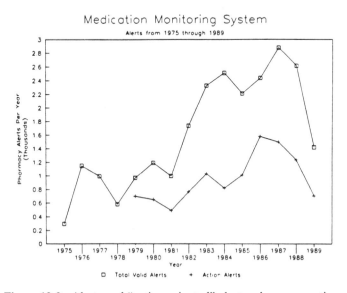

Figure 12.2. Alerts and "action oriented" alert—change over time.

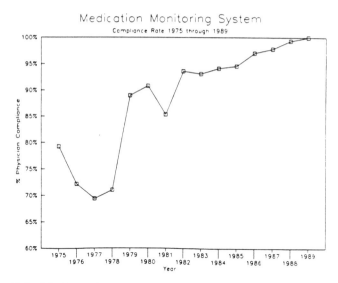

Figure 12.3. "Action-oriented" alert compliance plot from 1979 through 1989.

tems that reduced the effectiveness of some of the data driven capability of the HELP system. The situation causing the problem has now been corrected.

Physician Compliance Rates

Figure 12.3 plots the physician compliance rate to the pharmacy alerting system. The compliance rate in 1975, the first year of operation, was about 80% and dropped to about 70% in 1977. In 1979, the alert categories were changed so compliance assessments were made only from "action-oriented" alerts. As a result, in 1979 the compliance rate jumped to about 90%. Since 1979, except for the year 1981 when we changed the HELP system to a new hardware platform, there has been a continual improvement in rate of physician compliance to alerts. In 1989 there were 703 "action-oriented" alerts and all 703 resulted in physician compliance!

Physician Attitudes

Two hundred forty-six of the 360 physician questionnaires mailed in the spring of 1989 were returned (65% return rate). The questionnaires provided a rich source of assessment data on a variety of subjects. The questions and responses regarding the pharmacy system are noted below.

When physicians were asked to rank existing computer features they ranked "Alerts that warn of potentially dangerous situations such as life-threatening laboratory abnormalities or drug interactions" at the top with a score of 4.63 (out of a possible high of 5). "Medication monitoring and

Table 12.1. Physician Ranking of Computer Features

	1st	2nd	3rd	Score	Sum First 3 Choices
1. Lab Results	132	27	10	1,848	169
2. Vital Signs	11	36	35	1,264	82
3. Pharmacy Alerts	20	40	19	1,262	79

generation of pharmacy alerts at the time an order is placed" was given a score of 4.34. When physicians were asked to rank what future computer features were needed, they placed "Direct physician access to the pharmacy knowledge base for prescription advice" with a score of 4.26, second only to expansion of laboratory alerting [16].

Physicians were also asked to rank the ten features of the LDS Hospital computer system that most contributed to their professional practice. Table 12.1 shows that the pharmacy alerts ranked third.

Data Sources Required for Pharmacy Alerts

Figure 12.4 shows the percentage of time each data source resulted in a pharmacy alert. Drug-Laboratory alerting had the largest percentage of alerts (55.5% of the time) while Drug-Drug interaction capability produced 36.3% of the alerts.

Benefit/Cost Analysis

Benefit/cost analysis was based on the assessments by five clinical pharmacists. Results of this analysis presented in Table 12.2. Benefit for

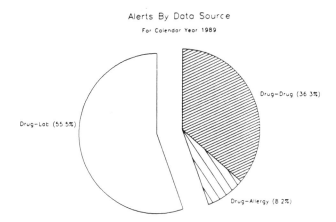

Figure 12.4. Pie chart of percentage of each alert type.

Table 12.2. Experience with 24 Most Beneficial Alerts—2 Years Activity That Accounts for Approximately 90% of the Benefit

Rank by $ Value	Alert	# Compliance	$ Benefit Average 5 Experts	Total $ Benefit
1	Aminoglycoside monitoring	256	360	92,160
2	K+ when hyperkalemic	85	380	32,300
3	Digitalis & hypokalemia	90	341	30,690
4	K+ spare diuretic—hyper K	43	590	25,370
5	Codeine allergy	139	170	23,630
6	Penicillin allergy	65	202	13,130
7	K+, renal failure	44	286	12,584
8	Gentamicin, renal status	19	651	12,369
9	Aspirin allergy	67	170	11,390
10	Meperidine allergy	53	170	9,010
11	TNC antacids	178	49	8,722
12	Lomotil excess	35	235	6,023
13	Chloramphenicol	19	317	5,040
14	K+ with K+ diuretic	14	360	4,396
15	Coumarin	28	157	3,680
16	Sulfonamide allergy	20	189	2,478
17	KCl—hypo K+ & hypoCl-	21	118	2,210
18	Morphine allergy	13	170	2,072
19	Low Na+ diet	14	148	1,700
20	Coumarin, thyroid	17	100	1,210
21	Cholestyramine	22	55	750
22	NaF—Ca	30	25	416
23	Amp—allopurinol	13	32	391
24	Laxative & anti-laxative	17	23	
	TOTAL for all 86 Alerts Types	1,459		$339,752

each type of alert was determined by averaging the dollar value estimates from the five clinical pharmacists. There were wide variations between the estimates of the clinical pharmacists because of their uncertainty about severity of the reaction. For example, with penicillin allergy it was necessary to evaluate two separate questions: 1) What was the incidence of reaction for those who "claimed" to have penicillin allergy? and 2) What was the severity of the reaction when a person with positively known penicillin allergy was given penicillin? Some patients think they are allergic to penicillin, because they get a skin reaction from ampicillin Thus the incidence of true penicillin allergies from the population who think they have penicillin allergies may be only about 50%. On the other hand, for a patient known to have a penicillin allergy one could use a worst-case analysis and assume that every patient given penicillin would

Table 12.3. Computerized Alerting Experience and Benefit to Cost Analysis

Patients monitored	53,006
Patients days monitored	246,5421
Drugs orders monitored	312,518
Number of alerts	2,110
% Patients with alerts	3.98%
% Drug orders with alerts	0.68%
Cost per patient day for system	$0.35
Cost for 2 years service	$86,282
Estimated Benefit (see Table 12.2)	$339,751
Benefit/cost ratio	3.94

have anaphylactic shock and could die. There is a continuum of reactions ranging from no reaction or a mild reaction to a severe reaction or death.

Table 12.3 summarizes the benefits and the benefit/cost ratio for the computerized alerting system. During the two-year experience, over 53,000 patients were monitored for more than 246,000 patient days. Less than 4% of the patients had medication alerts and less than 0.7% of the drugs ordered resulted in an alert. Charges of $0.35 per day resulted in the charge for service of just over $86,000 for the two-year period. Table 12.3 also shows the benefit to the patient was more than $339,000, or a benefit/cost ratio of 3.94. Features that were felt to be of value but were not considered as benefits in this analysis included 1) administrative support such as billing, dispensing, and printing of medication labels; 2) pharmacy data review and reporting capabilities used by nurses and physicians; 3) pharmacy support of other computerized decision support capabilities, such as the computerized microbiology system operating on the HELP system [17–19]; 4) the printing of patient profiles; 5) reduced malpractice risks for physicians and the hospital; and 6) availability of the database for research.

Discussion

It was demonstrated that a computerized pharmacy system could be used in a clinical setting to the benefit of patients. Physicians appreciated and responded appropriately to the medication alerts. In addition there was a continuing growth in the number of alert conditions. The alerts could have resulted in a learning effect that would reduce the number of alerts over time. If there was a learning effect, it was small. Tierney and associates have shown a similar lack of learning effect with a computerized ordering system [20]. Physicians were very responsive to the alerts and appreciated the "safety net" effect of the computerized system. In 1989,

100% of the "action-oriented" alerts were responded to appropriately. A questionnaire determined that our physicians appreciated the alerts and wanted even more computerized capability. It become apparent through examination of the patient data used to generate the alerts that an integrated database with at least a link to the laboratory data was crucial. There seemed to be a salutary benefit-to-cost ratio. However, better methods need to be developed to prove the actual benefit of such a system.

Tierney, Shortliffe, and McDonald have pointed out the need for computer systems that aid physicians in their decision making [20–22]. The pharmacy alerting system described and assessed here is an important step in using computers to improve the care process. The use of such systems may improve the care process much as surgeons have found that there is "high cost for low frequency events" [23]. A computerized system is clearly the best "safety net" yet developed for such improvements.

Summary

Quantitative and qualitative assessments were conducted to determine the value of a computerized pharmacy system in operation since 1975. Patient prescriptions were processed and critiqued for contraindications. It was found that the number of medication monitoring alerts increased over the 15-year period. Physicians have increasingly complied with the changes recommended by the computer system and want to expand the computer capability. Integration of patient data from multiple sources, especially clinical laboratory, was essential to making the medication monitoring system effective. A benefit/cost analysis showed that there was about a 4:1 benefit-to-cost ratio for the system.

Acknowledgments

This work was supported in Part by Public Health Service grants HS-02463 and HS-01053.

References

1. Hulse RK, Clark SJ, Jackson JC, Warner HR, Gardner RM. Computerized medicantion monitoring system. Am J Hosp Pharm 1976; 33:1061–1064.
2. Speedie SM, Skarupa S, Oderda L, et al. MENTOR: Continuously Monitoring Drug Therapy with an Expert System, MEDINFO 1986; pp 237–239.
3. Knapp DA, Speedie MK, Yaeger DM. Drug prescribing and its relation to length of hospital stay. Inquiry 1980; 17:254–259.
4. Soumerai SB, Avorn J. Predictors of physician prescribing change in an educational experiment to improve medication use. Med Care 1987; 25:210–221.

5. Morrell J, Podlone M, Cohen SN. Receptivity of physicians in a teaching hospital to a computerized drug interaction monitoring and reporting system. Med Care 1977; 15:68–78.

6. Cohen MR. A compilation of abstracts and index of articles published by the boston collaborative drug surveillance program. Hosp Pharm 1977; 12:455–492.

7. Steel K, Gertman PM, Crescenzi C, Anderson J Iatrogenic illness on a general medical service at a university hospital. N Engl J Med 1981; 304:638–642.

8. Kirking DM, Thomas JW, Ascione FJ, Boyd EL. Detecting and preventing adverse durg interactions: The potential contribution of computers in pharmacies. Soc Sci Med 1986; 22:1–8.

9. Rascati KL, Carole LK, Foley PT, Williams RB. Multidimensional work sampling to evaluate the effects of computerization in an outpatient pharmacy. Am J Hosp Pharm 1987; 44:2060–2076.

10. Pryor TA, Gardner RM, Clayton PD, Warner HR. The HELP System. J Med Systems 1983; 7:87–102.

11. Pryor TA. The HELP Medical Record System. MD Computing 1988; 5:22–33.

12. Lundsgaarde HP, Gardner RM, Menlove RL. Using attitudinal questionnaires to achieve benefits optimization. SCAMC 1989; 13:703–708.

13. Weinstein MC, Stason WB. Foundations of cost-effective analysis for health and medical practices, N Engl J Med 1977; 296:176–726.

14. Linstone HA. The Delphi Method Techniques and Applications, Murray Turoff Editors. Reading, MA: Addison-Wesley, 1975.

15. Sackman H. Delphi Critique. Lexington, MA: Lexington Book, DC. Health and Company, 1975.

16. Bradshaw KE, Gardner RM, Pryor TA. Development of a computerized-laboratory alerting system. Comp Biomed Res 1989; 22:575–587.

17. Evans RS, Larsen RA, Burke JP, Gardner RM, Meier FA, Jacobson JA, Conti MT, Jacobson JA, Hulse RK. Computer surveillance of hospital-acquired infections and antibiotic use. JAMA 1986; 256:1007–1011.

18. Larsen RA, Evans RS, Burke JP, Pestotnik SL, Gardner RM, Classen DC. Improved perioperative antibiotic use and reduced surgical wound infections through use of computer decision analysis. Infect Control Hosp Epidemiol 1989; 10:316–320.

19. Pestotnik SL, Evans RS, Burke JP, Gardner RM, Classen DC. Therapeutic antibiotic monitoring: surveillance using a computerized expert system. Am J Med 1990; 88:43–48.

20. Tierney WM, Miler ME, McDonald CJ. The effect on ordering of informing physicians of the charges for outpatient diagnostic tests. N Engl J Med 1990; 322:1499–1504.

21. Shortliffe EH. Computer programs to support clinical decision-making. JAMA 1987; 258:61–66.

22. McDonald CJ, Tierney WM. Computer-Stored medical records: Their future role in medical practice. JAMA 1988; 259:3433–3440.

23. Couch NP, Tilney NL, Rayner AA, Moore FD. The high cost of low-frequency events—The anatomy and economics of surgical mishaps. N Eng J Med 1981; 304:634–637.

IV
Clinical Systems and
Decision-Making

Chapter 13
Clinician Decisions and Computers
George A. Diamond, Brad H. Pollock, and Jeffrey W. Work

In his masterful sociologic dissection of the medical profession, Eliot Freidson [1] identifies five attributes that characterize the behavior of the typical practicing clinician:

He believes in what he is doing. He believes that he is doing good rather than harm. He has faith in the efficacy of his treatments, and believes that what he does makes the difference between success and failure. When things go right, he takes the credit.

He prefers action to inaction. Successful action is preferred to unsuccessful action, but action with little chance of success is preferred over no action at all.

He is pragmatic. He is prone to seeing apparent cause/effect relationships (even in the absence of any theoretical foundation), and is inclined to "tinker" with conventional methods—to bend the rules—if he isn't getting the results that he expects.

He is highly subjective. He depends more on his own first-hand experience and "gut feelings" than on abstract principles or "book knowledge."

He emphasizes uncertainty in his defense. He is prone to justify this pragmatic reliance on personal experience by citing the Lawlessness of Chance instead of the Laws of Science. When things go wrong, it's not his fault.

In Freidson's view, the clinician's behavior stems from the pressures engendered by the nature of the work. The clinician deals with individuals rather than groups, and therefore cannot rely on epidemiologic concepts or probabilities derived from population statistics. He or she is often forced to make critical decisions in the face of overwhelming uncertainty. In emergencies, there isn't even time to think. In response to these pressures, the clinician has developed a set of shortcuts—rules of

Adapted from an article published in the *J Am Cell Cardiol* 9:1385–1396, 1987. Reprinted with permission of the American College of Cardiology.

thumb—and those of us who use them well are said to possess "good clinical judgment." (According to S.I. Hayakawa [2], the word *judgment* "is *sense* applied to the making of decisions, especially correct decisions, and thus it depends to some degree upon the exercise of discernment or discrimination." *Decision*, on the other hand, refers to "a choice among alternatives . . . [and imparts] a note of acting with dispatch and, perhaps, of using an ability to improvise as one goes along without stopping constantly for a new search after methods or motives." Thus, although judgment requires decision, decision does not require judgment. Our use of the word *belief* implies neither sense nor action.) Indeed, these short-cuts work very well most of the time. but for just this reason we tend to overlook the times when they mislead us. This is when computer decision aids may be helpful.

Why Do We Need Computer Decision Aids?

Words Distort Meaning

Many medical beliefs are expressed imprecisely [3]. What do physicians actually mean—and what do they communicate—when they employ vague words such as *often* and *sometimes* as substitutes for precise numeric statements? When 205 individuals were asked what numeric probability they thought was intended by a variety of semiquantitative words, the range of estimates was striking [4–7]. The word *often*, for example, was thought to communicate a probability ranging from a low of only 0.2 to a high of 0.9. Given the wide numeric range associated with these words, we should not be surprised that all meaning is sometimes totally lost. We'll never know, for instance, what geologist David Johnston was trying to tell us about Mount Saint Helens in early 1980 when he announced, "there's probably pretty good evidence that an eruption may be likely." He died in the subsequent eruption [8].

Rhetoric Distorts Logic

According to Thomas [9], "The great thing about human language is that it prevents us from sticking to the matter al hand." So powerfully can language direct our actions, in fact, that both patients and physicians can be led to apparently irrational decisions just by the way we phrase a problem [10–12]. Suppose you are told that 600 people are going to die this year in your coronary care unit. There are two new treatments available (thrombolysis and angioplasty, for those who require concrete examples). If you give everybody treatment A only 400 people will die. If you give everybody treatment B there is one chance in three that nobody will die and two chances in three that all 600 people will die. Which of these two treatments do you prefer? Although there's really no mathematical difference between the two expected outcomes, 72% of 152 people confronted with this decision preferred the latter treatment [12]. When decision problems are framed in terms of mortality, we tend to be willing to take risks in the hope that fewer will die. This is called *risk-seeking* behavior.

Suppose instead that two other treatments are available. If you give everybody treatment C, 200 people will be saved. If you give everybody treatment D, there is one chance in three that all 600 people will be saved and two chances in three that nobody will be saved. Which of these two treatments do you prefer? Although these outcomes are identical to the preceding outcomes, 78% of 155 people now preferred the former treatment [12]. When the same decision problem is framed in terms of survival, we tend to avoid risks in the hope that more will be saved. Such behavior is called *risk aversion*.

Words that communicate survival and mortality can be especially compelling. For example. McNeil et al. [11] were able to get experienced physicians, graduate students with formal training in statistics, and hospitalized patients with a variety of unrelated diseases to prefer treatment presented in terms of *improved survival* to one presented in terms of *reduced mortality*, even though the data they were given favored the latter.

Irrational perceptions of risk have been cited as another source of biased decision making. For example, we tend to inflate the apparent risk of situations that we perceive to be *infrequent, unfamiliar, and uncontrollable* [13]. Thus, under the right circumstances, physicians and patients are both more fearful of sudden cardiac death and airplane crashes than of automobile accidents or a fatal fall in the bath. Actuarial statistics—and insurance company premiums—clearly show, however, that the latter two are much more likely.

Preconception Distorts Belief

Physicians tend to hold a systematic preconception toward an assumption of illness—the patient is guilty until proved innocent, so to speak. The classic example of this bias comes from a 1934 survey on physician referrals for tonsillectomy by the American Child Health Association [14]. Of 1,000 children, 611 had already had their tonsils removed. When the remaining 389 children were examined by a new group of physicians, 174 (45%) were thought to be in need of tonsillectomy. This left 215 children with apparently normal tonsils, but when they were again examined by a second group of physicians, 99 (46%) were thought to be in need of tonsillectomy. This left 116 children with apparently normal tonsils, but when they were again examined by a third group of physicians, 51 (44%) were thought to be in need of tonsillectomy. Thus like the teacher who "grades on a curve" and gives a certain proportion of the class failing grades no matter what the overall quality of the class, these physicians were incline to remove a certain proportion of tonsils regardless of the signs and symptoms observed. So much for second opinions.

Overconfidence Distorts Accuracy

Despite such cognitive limitations, people tend to be overconfident about the accuracy of their beliefs when faced with decision problem of anything more than trivial difficulty. For example, one group of investigators [15] gave their subjects a 20-min lecture explaining the concepts of odds and probability some detail. The subjects were then asked to state which of two conditions (such as diabetes and suicide) they thought occurred more often, and to express how sure they were in stating the odds that they were correct. When the stated odds were low (<5:1) their beliefs were well calibrated because the actual error rate was close to that expected from those odds (>17%). However, when the stated odds were high (≥5:1) their error rates were much higher than expected from the stated odds. For example, in 157 instances in which the subjects thought the odds were 1.000,000:1 against being wrong—a predicted error rate of only 0.0001%—they were actually wrong 10% of the time!

In a study conducted at the Université Laval in Quebec (LeClere and Bordage, personal communication). medical students and physicians with various levels of clinical experience were given a portion of text to read from Harrison's *Principles of Internal Medicine*. Immediately thereafter, they were asked to state a percentage that represented their *comprehension* of the text and a second percentage that represented the amount of material they thought they would *recall* at a later time. They were then tested formally for comprehension and recall. All subjects were overconfident, regardless of their level of training. Measured comprehension averaged 33% compared with a stated value of 90%, whereas measured recall averaged 25% compared with a stated value of 80%.

These errors are not caused solely by a lack of knowledge [16]. The same investigators [17] evaluated the origin of diagnostic errors by presenting a series of 20 case histories that had been previously misdiagnosed by other physicians to a new group of 59 physicians at various levels of training. The subjects were first asked to make a diagnosis on the basis of the available clinical information, and were then given a true-false test to determine if they possessed the factual knowledge needed to correctly diagnose these cases. Almost half of the cases (45%) were misdiagnosed, and because most of the errors (57%) were made by individuals who possessed adequate factual knowledge, they were attributable more to faulty reasoning than to inadequate knowledge. It is nevertheless said that everyone complains of their memory, but no one of their judgment.

When Are Computer Decision Aids Most Effective?

The Blois Rubric

When the clinician first encounters a patient, he must prepared to consider any of an infinite number of possibilities. As the problem becomes

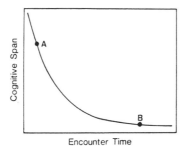

Figure 13.1. The Blois rubric: clinical judgment and computers. (Adapted from [18].)

better defined, however, he needs to focus his attention on only a few alternatives. Blois [18] illustrates this process using a diagram similar to that in Figure 13.1. One can think of the horizontal axis on this diagram as representing some function of clinical encounter time, and the vertical axis as the cognitive span required to solve the problem. Thus, point A is an early stage in the clinical encounter (for example, just after eliciting the patient's chief complaint) when a broad (if superficial) knowledge base is needed, and point B is a later stage (for example, after completing the history and physical examination) when only a small (but detailed) knowledge base is needed. Blois contends that carbon brains (MIT's Marvin Minsky irreverently refers to them as "meat machines") are designed to function best at point A, whereas silicon brains function best at point B. Thus. it should be more difficult to construct computer decision aids to handle Blois type A problems compared with Blois type B problems. Moreover. type A programs should be expected to function less successfully than type B programs.

The Thomas-Weisbrod Rubric

Thomas [19] characterizes the technology of medicine on three qualitatively different levels. The first level, which he calls "nontechnology," is directed at those untreatable conditions for which medicine can offer only supportive therapy (for example, hospice care). The second level, which he calls "halfway technology" (but which most of us tend to think of as conventional high technology), is directed it the treatable consequences of an incurable disease (for example, cardiac transplantation and renal dialysis). The third level, which he calls *real* high technology to distinguish it from *conventional* high technology, is directed exclusively at prevention and cure (for example, immunization and antibiotics).

Whereas Thomas [19] sees these levels of technology as "so unlike each other as to seem altogether different undertakings," Weisbrod [20] bases his conceptual model of health expenditure on the view that they lie

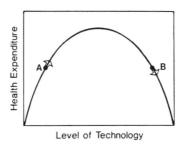

Figure 13.2. The Weisbrod rubic: medical technology and health expenditure. (Adapter from Weisbrod [20].)

along a continuum. According to this model, halfway technology is more expensive than both nontechnology and high technology. Thus, an advance in technology (through introduction of a computer decision aid, for example) can either increase or decrease health expenditures, depending on one's current position along this so called Weisbrod curve (Fig. 13.2). According to this model, a computer decision aid directed at a Weisbrod type A problem (located to the left of the curve's peak) will not be cost-effective unless it represents a major technologic leap. In contrast, a computer decision aid directed at a Weisbrod type B problem (located to the right of the peak) will be cost-effective even if it represents only a marginal advance. (The Weisbrod curve is reminiscent in some ways of the better known Laffer curve—the theoretical basis for supply-side economics. Unfortunately, the real world is more complex than would appear from the Laffer curve [21] and the same might be said with respect to the Weisbrod curve.)

How Do Computer Decision Aids Organize Medical Knowledge?

Computer decision aids do more than just store and retrieve information; they encode *knowledge* (information in context). The characteristics of eight such systems [22–29] are shown in Table 13.1.

Structure

The most common approaches to encoding knowledge are based on *algorithms* (arithmetic computation) or *heuristics* (symbolic rules). The distinction between the two is best described by analogy with a split-brain model [30], whereby algorithms are analogous to the analytic, ratiocinative functions of the left hemisphere, whereas heuristics are analogous to

Table 13.1. Characteristics of Representative Computer Decision Aids [22–29]

Aid	Domain	Hardware	Structure	Function
MYCIN	Infectious disease	Main	Heuristic	Consultant
Acid-base electrolyte	Internal medicine	Mini	Algorithm	Management
Internist-1	Internal medicine	Main	Heuristic	Consultant
ATTENDING	Anesthesiology	Main	Heuristic	Critiquing
Digitalis advisor	Cardiology	Main	Algorithm/heuristic	Management
CADENZA	Cardiology	Micro	Algorithm/heuristic	Consultant
HT-ATTENDING	Cardiology	Micro	Heuristic	Critiquing
Predictive instrument	Cardiology	Calc	Algorithm	Management

[1]Calc, calculator; Main, = mainframe; Micro, = microcomputer.

the synthetic, intuitive functions of the right hemisphere. As for the brain, this analogy suggests that optimal performance will be achieved by using a combination of both approaches.

Algorithms

One of the most popular multivariate algorithms is based on *Bayes's theorem*, whereby a posttest outcome measure (for example, disease probability) is calculated from the pretest measure and some index of the observation with respect to the outcome (for example, sensitivity and specificity). The resultant posttest probability then serves as the pretest probability for the next test [31]. There are three problems with this approach: 1) reliable estimates of pretest probability are often not available; 2) sensitivities and specificities are sometimes highly biased [32–34]; and 3) it is usually assumed without adequate justification that all observations are conditionally independent [35–38]. In the face of these limitations, the empiric performance of the method is best summarized by the quip that a good Bayesian does better than a non-Bayesian, while a bad Bayesian gets clobbered.

Discriminant Analysis

This analysis employs an algorithm that maximizes a mathematic function derived from some set of continuous variables that discriminate between two or more mutually exclusive outcomes [38]. Despite its strong theoretical foundations, however, this algorithm has important practical limitations. First, unlike probabilities, discriminant scores are abstract constructs with no natural clinical interpretation. Second, the model requires 1) that input variables derive from a multivariate normal distribution; 2) that interaction terms are included to account for conditional nonindependence; and 3) that the degree of dependence among input variables is the same for each outcome group. At least one of these assumptions is usually violated in the process of clinical application.

Logistic Regression

This algorithm is more robust than discriminant analysis because no distributional assumptions for the input variables are required and, as with Bayesian analysis, because the output measure is directly interpretable as a probability [38]. Unlike the others, however, this algorithm is capable of discriminating only between two groups and, as with discriminant

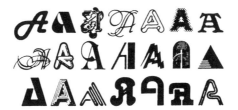

Figure 13.3. Heuristics: what is the essence of *A*-ness?

analysis, interaction terms must be included if the input variables are not independent.[1]

Heuristics. Rules of thumb are much more appealing than algorithms largely because they are not mathematical and because they seem to approximate more closely the way people make decisions ("always kick on fourth down" or "never vote for the incumbent"). But such simplicity is often deceptive [40]. Although few of us have any difficulty identifying each representation in Figure 13.3 as a stylized variation on the letter *A*, it is not easy to come up with a simple rule that defines what we might call the "essence of *A*-ness"—a rule that correctly characterizes all *A*'s without ever incorrectly characterizing any other letters such as *H*'s and *V*'s. Fortunately, medical classification tasks are much less difficult than pattern recognition tasks such as this. Here is a simple, reasonably good medical heuristic:

IF the patient has posttussive rales. *AND* the patient has no fever, *THEN* the patient probably has heart failure.

---

[1] The common belief that logistic and discriminant regression do not require the unpalalable independence assumption [39] is not necessarily correct. Two variables (such as age and gender) are *conditionally independent* if knowledge about the probability (p) of one of them provides no information about the other $p(age) = p(age|gender)$ and $p(age) = p(gender) = p(age$ and gender$)$. But two variables that are conditionally independent with respect to each other need not be conditionally independent with respect to a third variable. Neither age nor gender, for example, are conditionally independent with respect to the presence of coronary artery disease (CAD): $p(CAD|age) <\neq> p(CAD|age$ and gender$)$; and $p(CAD|age) \cdot p(CAD|gender) <\neq> p(CAD|age$ and gender$)$. The exponent of a logistic equation that predicts coronary artery disease using variables defined to be independent only in the first sense takes the form: $C = C_{age} \cdot age + C_{gender} \cdot gender$. However, the resultant logistic equation does not account for independence defined in the second sense (*interaction*). To do so, one needs to compute a revised exponent that includes at least the additional first order interaction term: $K = K_{age} \cdot age + K_{gender} \cdot gender + K_{age \cdot gender} \cdot age \cdot gender$. Ignoring the interaction terms is equivalent to assuming that age and gender (although conditionally independent with respect to each other) are also conditionally independent with respect to disease status. This is materially equivalent to assuming conditional independence with respect to serial Bayesian analysis.

Heuristic rules like this are the basis of knowledge representation in a number of so-called "expert systems" [41] Such programs are readily updated with new knowledge and can be made to explain the "reasoning" behind their conclusions. On the other hand, heuristics provide less satisfactory ways to express confidence [42] than do computational algorithms (in which uncertainty is readily quantified as a standard deviation, for example).

Function

Consultative systems. Computer decision aids can perform a diversity of functions. Consultative systems accept patient information as input and provide specific diagnostic or therapeutic advice as output. For example, the individual patient's medical record often takes the form of a simple temporal "stack." Whenever a new test result is obtained and the test report is added to the medical record (at the top of the stack), the physician needs to interpret it in light of everything that came before (all the information beneath it in the stack). Program input might be summarized by only a few numbers—a previous probability of disease and the current test result to be analyzed, for instance. The output is a revised probability of disease, which becomes one component of the input for analysis of subsequent test results.

Critiquing systems. Often, a physician has formulated a test or treatment plan, but would like some advice concerning its suitability. Has something important been neglected (a potential drug interaction, for example)? Critiquing systems accept patient data along with the action contemplated by the physician as input, and then provide a criticism of that plan along with one or more proposed alternatives. Given a patient with atypical chest pain and left ventricular hypertrophy, it could remind the physician that the electrocardiographic (ECG) stress test he plans to perform can be misleading in the face of rest ST-T wave abnormalities, and could suggest an alternative or additional procedure (such as perfusion scintigraphy) to improve reliability.

Management systems. Sometimes the physician has a goal in mind, but not a plan. Management systems accept patient information and the physician's diagnostic or therapeutic goal as input and provide a plan tailored to that goal as output. For example, if the physician defined his goal as that of an accurate diagnosis regardless of cost, the optimal testing plan would be output. If monetary considerations were introduced, a more cost-effective testing plan would be output. The physician could change these goals or the input data at will, and thereby perform a series of "what if" analyses [43].

How Accurate Are Computer Decision Aids?

Standards of Performance

When an expert is faced with an unfamiliar problem, he readily recognizes his limitations. Computer decision aids are far less sophisticated; they don't know when they don't know. For this reason, their validation should be especially thorough. Few such studies have been conducted, however, and fewer still have attempted to define the standards by which such performances is to be assessed. The ultimate accolade for any computer decision aid is to have its advice taken as seriously as that of an expert medical consultant. One test of this rigorous standard is to determine if established experts are able to distinguish in any way between the advice offered by their human peers and that offered by the decision aid when both are presented in an identical format (as in written reports, for example). This simple but powerful "imitation game" is called a Turing test in honor of the British mathematician who first proposed it as an operational test of machine intelligence [44].

Whitbeck and Brooks [45] think that a computer decision aid should be judged not only in terms of its accuracy, but also with respect to the appropriateness of its conclusions and the scope of its considerations. One needs to know what alternative conclusions might have been drawn, the degree of confidence in each conclusion [46], and the consequences that might result from acting on the wrong conclusion. The best way to assess the performance or a computer decision aid, they say, is by assessing its ability to explain its "reasoning." This, however, is not an easy task. The quality of one's reasoning-clinician or computer—depends on both *rhetorical* (is the explanation relevant?) and *dialectical* (is the explanation logical?) aspects. A logical and relevant explanation is clearly more persuasive than one that is illogical and irrelevant, but we would have a difficult time choosing between the remaining alternatives.

Wasson et al. [47] recently proposed a number of standards that should be required of what they term "clinical prediction rules," and concluded that a majority of validation studies failed to meet these standards. Only 42% contained an adequately detailed description of the prediction rule, only 34% measured the rule's error rate, and only 6% determined the effect of the rule on patient care. In addition, investigators too often fail to distinguish between the promise of performance (*efficacy*) and performance itself (*effectiveness*) [48] and ignore the distorting effects of various biases [34,49–52]. As a result, what works under ideal academic conditions might not work in the community.

Computer-Aided Diagnosis of Coronary Artery Disease

CADENZA is a microcomputer program based on Bayes' theorem that was specifically developed to aid the physician in interpreting clinical data relative to the diagnosis and functional evaluation of coronary artery disease [27,53]. The program operates on an Apple II or IBM-PC computer. A FORTRAN version [54] is also available for mainframe use. The program's output consists of a two-page document containing a tabulation of the input data, a graphic statistical analysis, and a narrative summary regarding the patient's symptoms, the level of physical fitness relative to age and gender, the adequacy of exercise for diagnosis of coronary ischemia, the potential anatomic location and functional severity of coronary artery disease, and the risk of a coronary event over the next year. This document can serve as the official clinical report for a stress laboratory after overreading by the supervising physician.

CADENZA can analyze data from the patient's clinical history, from conventional coronary risk factors, and from a number of noninvasive diagnostic tests such as exercise ECG and radionuclide imaging. The program also allows the user to perform his own "what if" analyses. If he is thinking about ordering a stress test on a particular patient, for example, he can enter the data that are already available along with one or more anticipated test responses. The change in disease probability on the basis of these fictitious test results allows one to judge the relative contribution of as yet unavailable information.

Numeric Analysis

Sensitivity and specificity estimates used by the program are derived from the published medical experience encompassing over 60,000 patients [27]. When appropriate, these data are fitted to various frequency distributions to allow the analysis of each test observation as a continuous variable rather than as a dichotomous outcome [27,55,56]. These values are further adjusted relative to the amount of exercise performed. The data set for each test is then analyzed by serial application of Bayes' formula, resulting in an increase or decrease in the probability of disease. The final probability and standard deviation are used to construct a probability distribution, from which are calculated several indexes that quantify the degree of confidence in the assessment [27,46,55].

Test Interpretation

The set of observations that make up each test is interpreted as "normal," "abnormal," or "equivocal" according to a rule that compares the true positive rate (± 1 SD) with the false positive rate (± 1 SD). An interpretation of normal means that the observations are significantly more often encountered in the absence of disease, whereas abnormal means that the observations are significantly more often encountered in the *presence* of disease. The term equivocal means there is no significant difference between the true and false positive rates [56].

Clinical Validation

We validated CADENZA in a prospective study of 1,097 patients [27]; 170 of them underwent diagnostic coronary angiography and the remainder were followed up for one year from the date of testing to detect subsequent coronary events (death and nonfatal infarction). Three findings were noteworthy: 1) probability of disease predicted angiographic prevalence with an average error of only 3%; 2) the higher the probability of disease, the greater the severity of angiographic disease; and 3) the higher the probability of disease, the greater the incidence of coronary events. In a subsequent study [57], CADENZA probabilities also correlated with coronary events in 215 patients with previous myocardial infarction, and in an additional 491 patients with suspected coronary artery disease.

A number of other investigators have validated CADENZA. Wong et al. [58] showed that disease probability was highly predictive angiographic prevalence in 68 catheterized patients, and observed that the probability estimate for 253 patients correlated significantly with the beliefs of experienced clinical cardiologists. Greenberg et al. [59] compared the results of multivariate discriminant analysis with CADENZA in 113 patients undergoing ECG stress testing. They found that the two methods of analysis were equally accurate. Detrano et al. [39] reported similar results in 303 patients undergoing thallium scintigraphy and cardiac fluoroscopy in addition to ECG stress testing using logistic regression analysis and a Bayesian model very similar to that in CADENZA. Hlatky et al. [60] reported that CADENZA was slightly, but significantly, more accurate than the clinical judgment of 91 experienced cardiologists in the analysis of stress ECG and thallium scintigraphy. Melin et al. [61] reported that a probabilistic testing strategy based on CADENZA improved the cost-effectiveness of noninvasive testing in 135 women, whereas Detry et al. confirmed the utility of CADENZA in comparison with multivariate analysis in 387 men. Several other studies [63–68] have confirmed the accuracy of empiric Bayesian analysis with respect to the diagnosis of coronary artery disease, despite the potentially serious theoretical limitations inherent in the model.

Similar validations of several non-Bayesian algorithms have been conducted. For example, Lee et al. [69] recently compared the accuracy of a multivariate survival model with that of five expert cardiologists in predicting one and three-year survival in 350 patients with coronary artery disease. Clinicians were not consistent when confronted with a large number of variables. Consequently, the statistical algorithm was more accurate than were the clinicians in predicting survival.

Algorithms Versus Heuristics

Although the accuracy of algorithmic decision aids such as these can equal or exceed that of conventional clinical opinion. heuristic systems are often more practical whenever the requisite database is not available or when unacceptable violations of the assumptions inherent in the model occur. We recently developed the prototype of such an expert system [70] using a commercial development tool called RuleMaster (Radian Corporation). This tool contains an automatic rule generator, that translates declarative knowledge in the form of examples into procedural knowledge in the form of if-then-else rules. The resultant system interprets exercise ECG and exercise myocardial perfusion scintigraphy with respect to a diagnosis of coronary artery disease using only 13 such rules.

We compared these heuristic interpretations with probabilistic interpretations derived from CADENZA, and with the expert interpretations of 21 clinical cardiologists using 42 hypothetic test cases [71], each based on two exercise variables (peak heart rate and systolic blood pressure), two ECG variables (magnitude and slope of ST segment depression), and two scintigraphic variables (number and severity of myocardial perfusion defects). The clinicians and the heuristic program interpreted each case on a 7-point ordinal scale ranging from 1 (definitely normal) to 7 (definitely abnormal). Clinician interpretations correlated linearly with log

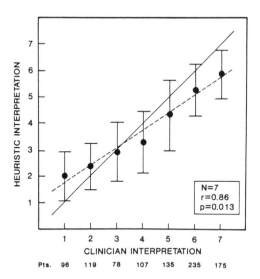

Figure 13.4. Heuristic interpretation versus clinician interpretation. Each **circle** represents a mean value (±SD). The number of patients (Pts.) included in each mean value is noted along the **bottom** of the illustration. The **solid line** is the line of identity and the **dotted line** is derived from linear regression. N = 7-point ordinal scale ranging from 1 (definitely normal) to 7 (definitely abnormal) [71].

odds of disease from CADENZA ($r = .91$, $p < .001$). Heuristic interpretations and clinician interpretations were highly correlated (Fig.
13.4); 36% of the clinician and heuristic interpretations were in precise
agreement and 35% differed by only a single grade. The overall accuracy
of the heuristic interpretations (referenced to the pooled clinician interpretations) was not significantly different from those derived from
CADENZA ($87 \pm 16\%$ versus $88 \pm 14\%$). These findings suggest that a
relatively simple heuristic system can perform almost as well as a complex
numeric algorithm [72].

Will Physicians Use Computer Decision Aids?

Published Surveys

New technology is always suspect. It was once feared that the invention
of papyrus would cause memory capacity to dry up if people could write
everything down, and that the invention of printing would prevent them
from thinking for themselves if they could read the thoughts of others. In
our own time. we are similarly warned that the use of electronic calculators in schools will cause the degradation of mathematical skills. Physicians, then, might well see the computer as some sort of "Big Brother"
that threatens to monitor their competence, to justify the denial of their
fees, and ultimately to replace them as decision-makers. Do they?

Singer et al. [73] recently surveyed the attitudes of 296 physicians regarding their use of computer data bases; 37% of these physicians were
not satisfied with their ability to keep up with new medical developments;
76% said that they wanted to implement or increase their use of computers in clinical practice; 69% thought that the computer would be useful as a source of published information; 42% thought that it would improve their access to the results of clinical trials; and 28% thought that it
could be very useful in providing probability estimates of successful treatment outcomes. In summary, these physicians indicated by a margin of 2
to 1 that computers could significantly improve their practice of medicine.
Similar encouraging attitudes have been reported by others [74–76].

A somewhat different perspective is provided from a survey of 933
physicians, residents, and medical students by Anderson et al. [77].
Although these subjects acknowledged the computer's potential for reducing the cost and improving the quality of care, they also expressed
concerns about governmental and hospital control of their practices.
threats to privacy, legal difficulties, and ethical dilemmas. For these
reasons, computer decision aids might end up being used only by those
who develop them [78]. Witness, for instance, an official response to the
suggestion that a respected professional decision analyst conduct a formal
multi-attribute analysis of the decision to locate a liquid natural gas stor-

age facility along the California coast [79]:"Absolutely not! And it's not because [he] isn't an excellent analyst, but because he doesn't work for me and therefore he would be out of my control."

Our experience is more gratifying. We recently surveyed 50 physicians who had been using CADENZA for 1,111 months (22 per physician) on 28,992 patients (580 per physician). Only 12% used computers frequently in their practice; 24% used them occasionally, 26% rarely, and 38% never; 78% said they use CADENZA to analyze the results of ECG stress testing, 52% to help decide who needs additional testing, and 30% to analyze the results of additional testing; 78% said they use the information in the computer report to supplement their own report, whereas 60% mail the report to referring physicians, and 24% use it as a replacement for their own report. Satisfaction with the program averaged 4.0 on a 5-point scale (where 1 is low and 5 is high); 25% rated the program a 5, 57% rated it a 4, 16% rated it a 3 and 2% rated it a 2; none gave it a rating of 1. These data indicate a relatively high level of acceptance of this computer decision aid by these practicing physicians.

Referral Patterns

Strategic planning is an important potential application for computer decision aids. Never before, for instance, has the physician caring for a patient admitted to the coronary care unit with a suspected acute ischemic syndrome had more options available beyond those provided by conventional ECG monitoring, serum enzyme analysis, and antiarrhythmia prophylaxis. The additional choices include Holter ECG, echocardiography, radionuclide angiography, thallium scintigraphy, pyrophosphate scanning, cardiac catheterization, coronary angiography, aspirin, heparin, nitrates, beta blockers, calcium channel antagonists, intravenous or intracoronary streptokinase, tissue plasminogen activator, counterpulsation, coronary angioplasty, and coronary bypass surgery. There are exactly 2^{17} or 131,072 combinations and 17! or 355,687,428,096,000 permutations among these alternatives (the actual number of choices probably lies somewhere between these extremes). Thus, just as the prudent driver uses a road map to plan the most direct or most scenic route, the prudent physician might want a road map of his management alternatives before setting out on an analogous journey.

To determine if physicians actually use such road maps, we analyzed the pattern of referral for scintigraphic stress testing in 2,213 patients with suspected coronary disease and compared this behavior with that predicted for 17 referring cardiologists by a questionnaire designed to elicit their strategic beliefs [80]. A total of 316 patients (14% were referred for a second test within 30 days of the first test (perfusion scintigraphy if radionuclide angiography had been performed first or vice versa). The

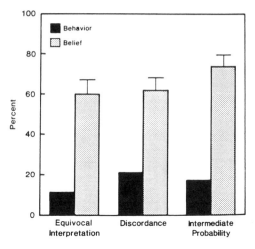

Figure 13.5. Behavior of 17 referring cardiologists compared with that predicted from their beliefs [80].

cardiologists identified three factors (each indicative of diagnostic uncertainty) they thought would most lead them to request a second test. They believed that they would refer 60% of patients with an *equivocal interpretation* of the scintigraphic test, 62% of patients with *discordance* between the ECG and scintigraphic responses (one interpreted as normal and the other as abnormal) and 74% of patients with an *intermediate probability* of disease after the first test.

The actual behavior of referring cardiologists was very different from that predicted from these beliefs (Fig. 13.5) Only 11% (61 of 517) of patients with an equivocal interpretation, 23% (118 of 566) with discordance and 17% (85 of 488) with an intermediate probability (between 0.1 and 0.9 using CADENZA) were referred for a second test ($p < .001$ for each). These values are not significantly different from the 16% referral rate in patients without evidence of diagnostic uncertainty. Thus, contrary to what these physicians believed, diagnostic uncertainty did not influence their testing behavior. Many patients who did not seem to need a second test received it, whereas an even greater number who did seem to need the test did not receive it. Computer decision aids, then, might improve these utilization patterns by calling such inconsistencies to the physician's attention.

In a similar study, Epstein and McNeil [81] compared the beliefs and behavior of 27 office physicians with respect to the ordering of common laboratory tests (ECGs, urinalyses, chest radiographs and blood counts) in 324 hypertensive patients. In contrast with our findings, beliefs and behavior were significantly correlated, and the most important reasons for ordering these tests were: 1) to help with treatment decisions. 2) to reassure the patient, 3) to assess prognosis, and 4) to establish a baseline. These data coupled with our own indicate that utilization patterns are likely to vary from disease to disease and from test to test.

Will Patients Accept the Use of Computers by Physicians?

In a recent British survey [82], 17% of patients opposed the use of computers by their doctors, the majority fearing a breach in confidentiality. A controlled field study [83] of patient reactions to computer use by their doctors during general practice encounters tends to contradict this view. The investigators observed no degradation in the patients' perceptions of the doctors' attentiveness and rapport, or their satisfaction with or their confidence in the treatment received. They concluded that the response of the patient to such encounters is influenced more by which doctor he sees than by whether that doctor uses a computer. An engaging anecdote serves to underscore this conclusion: on seeing her doctor using a computer decision aid, one patient is said to have exclaimed, "Isn't this wonderful? Now you doctors won't have to guess so much anymore!" (Weed, personal communication).

What Are the Legal and Economic Implications?

Federal Software Regulation

The Food and Drug Administration is currently developing a policy to regulate medical software systems as medical devices [84]. Candidate areas of importance include 1) the appropriateness of the underlying model (algorithms and heuristics); 2) evidence that the model was correctly implemented in software; 3) evidence that undesirable changes will not take place in copying, distribution and use; 4) a description of software safety; 5) proper labeling of the performance specifications and hardware requirements: and 6) documentation of software changes that affect safety and effectiveness. The contemplated policy is directed only at commercial systems, and FDA commissioner Frank E. Young has voiced his reassuring opinion that, "In principle, any time the physician's judgment can override the judgment of the computer. . . . then FDA has little or no [regulatory] responsibility" [85]. Nevertheless, in defining the minimal criteria of an acceptable medical decision *aid* (even if only in terms of marketability). the agency will simultaneously be defining the characteristics of an acceptable medical *decision*. This could have a material medicolegal impact on the entire profession.

Medicolegal Liability

Will the use of computer decision aids increase the physician's exposure to legal liability? Because the first case claiming personal injury resulting from the use of medical software has yet to be filed, one can only conjecture over the position the courts will take on this matter. According to Weistart [86], the legal test for liability is entirely dependent on the medical profession's standard of reasonable care, and not on an externally imposed norm. Computer decision aids can thereby reduce the physician's liability exposure by helping codify and disseminate such standards. Miller et al. [87] note that a physician who relies on the advice of a computer decision aid could be held as negligent as one who relies on the advice of a human consultant. but only if it is judged that he should have known the advice was substandard. As the availability of medical computers increases, they warn also of an equal potential for liability if the physician is judged to have failed to exercise reasonable care by *not* having consulted a computer decision aid.

Conflict of Interest

Conflict of interest is inevitable in any complex socioeconomic system [88,89]. Suppose, for example, that a physician and patient are considering whether or not to initiate a treatment that has some probability (p) of being effective, and $1 - p$ of not being effective. We denote G as the gain to the patient if he is given the treatment and it is effective, whereas L is the loss to the patient if he is given the treatment and it is not effective. If we assume that the losses associated with nontreatment are negligible, the patient's utility is represented by the net gain associated with effective treatment minus the net loss associated with ineffective treatment. $G \cdot p - L \cdot (1 - p)$. As long as this value is positive (gain outweighs loss), the patient should prefer to be treated, and this occurs whenever $p > L/(G + L)$. Similarly, g is the gain to the physician if he gives the treatment and it is effective, whereas l is the loss to the patient if he gives the treatment and it is not effective. The physician's utility then is $g \cdot p - l \cdot (1 - p)$, and he should prefer to initiate treatment as long as this value is positive. This occurs whenever $p > l/(g + l)$. If $l/(g + l) > p > L/(G + L)$; however, the preferences of the patient and the physician will be in conflict: the patient has more to gain by being treated, whereas the physician has more to gain by not offering the treatment. Thus, conflicts will occur any time the physician values his gains and losses differently than does the patient. It makes no difference what units each uses to quantify these gains and losses (the physician could be interested in survival, and the patient could be interested in quality of life), it is only the *ratio* of gain to loss that counts. In such cases, computer decision aids can expose the potential for conflict before it occurs. or can help adjudicate conflicts that do occur by requiring all parties to make their private utilities public.

Conclusions

A recent White Paper prepared by the U.S. Department of Commerce [90] predicts that

> the computer . . . . will redistribute worldly wealth in the form of knowledge. . . . [and] will alter human existence as profoundly as did the control of fire, the emergence of speech or the agricultural revolution.

Whether one accepts such hyperbole, computer decision aids—at the very least—promise the physician clinically applicable ways to deliver formal decision models to the bedside. If this promise alone is realized, the computer will 1) help us make hidden assumptions explicit, 2) allow us to determine whether a given clinical opinion is consistent with those assumptions and with the conventional rules of logic, and 3) provide us access to a relevant database, thereby supplementing our limited personal experience by placing it into a broader perspective. It will not compete with the practicing physician in the process of clinical decision making, but rather interact with him as a colleague in that process [46,91,92]. For this promise to be fulfilled. however, the physician must play an active role in developing the requisite software, in establishing the domain of its application and in defining the standards for its assessment [93,94]. The computer scientists and knowledge engineers, for their part, must assure that the software communicates effectively and conveniently with the physician (preferably using natural language), and that it is capable of convincingly explaining the reasoning behind its conclusions—something even the best of us sometimes has trouble doing. The following fanciful dialogue is faithful to this spirit:

> A: According to the clinical history, your patient has a 75% probability of angiographically significant coronary artery disease.
> Q: How sure are you?
> A: The standard deviation of my estimate is 11%. Therefore, the actual probability lies somewhere between 55 and 91% with 90% confidence.
> Q: What is the clinical significance of these numbers?
> A: An average man of this age has a $1.0 \pm 0.6\%$ chance of dying over the next year, and a median survival of 23.2 years (to age 78). This man's probability of coronary artery disease gives him a $3.2 \pm 1.2\%$ chance of dying over the next year, and a median survival of only 12.4 years (to age 67). This represents a 47% reduction in life expectancy.
> Q: Should I do an ECG stress test?
> A: For what purpose?

Q: Prognosis.

A: Exercise electrocardiography coupled with myocardial perfusion scintigraphy can revise the median survival of 12.4 years to as much as 23.1 years, or to as little as 7.8 years.

Q: What if the resultant median survival is only 10 years?

A: A formal decision analysis based on data at this institution supports a recommendation of myocardial revascularization to any man this age with a median survival < 10.6 years. A decision between angioplasty and bypass surgery depends on coronary anatomy.

Q: What assumptions are implicit in your judgment?

A: Well, to begin with, I believe in what I am doing. . . .

References

1. Freidson E. Profession of Medicine: A Study of the Sociology of Applied Knowledge. New York: Harper and Row, 1970, pp 168–9.

2. Hayakawa SI. Modern Guide to Synonyms and Related Words. New York: Funk & Wagnells, 1968; pp 508, 690–1.

3. Kong A, Barnett GO, Mosteller F, Youtz C. How medical professionals evaluate expressions of probability. N Engl J Med 1986; 315:740–4.

4. Robert WO. Quantifying the meaning of words. JAMA 1983; 249:2631–2.

5. Bryant GD, Norman GR. Expressions of probability: words and numbers (letter). N Engl J Med 1980; 302–411.

6. Kenney RM. Between never and always (letter). N Engl J Med 1981; 305: 1098–9.

7. Toogood JH. What do we mean by usually? (Letter). Lancet 1980; 1:1094.

8. Eisele JW, O'Halloran RL, Reay DT. Lindholm GR, Lewman LV, Brady WJ. Deaths during the May 18, 1980 eruption of Mount St. Helens. N Engl J Med 1981; 305:931–6.

9. Thomas L. Notes of a biology watcher. Information. N Engl J Med 1972; 287:1238–9.

10. Slovic P, Fischhoff B, Lichtenstein S. Facts versus fears: understanding perceived risk. In Kahneman D, Slovic P, Tversky A (eds): Judgment under Uncertainty: Heuristics and Biases. Cambridge: Cambridge University Press, 1982; 463–89.

11. McNeil BJ, Pauker SG, Sox HC, Tversky A. On the elicitation of preferences for alternative therapies. N Engl J Med 1982; 306:1259–62.

12. Tversky A, Kahneman D. The framing of decisions and the psychology of choice. Science 1981; 211:453–8.

13. DuPont RL. The nuclear power phobia. Business Week 1981 Sept 7:14–6.

14. Bakwin H. Pseudodoxia pediatrica. N Engl J Med 1945; 232:691–7.

15. Fischhoff B, Slovic P, Lichtenstein S. Knowing with certainty: the appropriateness of extreme confidence. J Exp Psychol 1977; 3:552–64.

16. Bordage G, Zacks R. The structure of medical knowledge in the memories of medical students and general practitioners: categories and prototypes, Med Educ 1984; 18:406–16.

17. Bordage G, Allen T. The etiology of diagnostic errors: process or content? An exploratory study. Proceedings of the 21st Annual Conference on Research in Medical Education, 1982; 171–6.

18. Blois MS. Clinical judgment and computers. N Engl J Med 1980; 303:192–7.
19. Thomas L. Notes of a biology watcher. The technology of medicine. N Engl J Med 1971; 285:1366–8.
20. Weisbrod BA. Economics and medical research. Washington, DC: American Enterprise Institute, 1983.
21. Gardner M. Mathematical Games. The Laffer curve and other laughs in current economics. Sci Am 1981; 245(6):18–31.
22. Shortliffe EH, Davis R, Axline SG, Buchanan BG, Green CC, Cohen SN. Computer-based consultations in clinical therapeutics: explanation and rule acquisition capabilities of the MYCIN system. Comput Biomed Res 1975; 8:303–20.
23. Bleich HL. Computer-based consultation: electrolyte and acid-base disorders. Am J Med 1972; 53:285–91.
24. Miller RA, Pople HE Jr, Myers JD. Internist-1, an experimental computer-based diagnostic consultant for general internal medicine. N Engl J Med 1982; 307:468–76.
25. Miller PL. Critiquing anesthesia management: the "ATTENDING" computer system. Anesthesiology 1983:58:362–9.
26. Swartout WR. Explaining and justifying expert consulting programs. In Clancey WJ, Shortiffe EH (eds): Readings in Medical Artificial Intelligence: The First Decade. Addison-Wesley, Reading, MA: 1984; 382–98.
27. Diamond GA, Staniloff HM, Forrester JS, Pollock BH, Swan HJC. Computer assisted diagnosis in the noninvasive evaluation of patients with suspected coronary artery disease. J Am Coll Cardiol 1983; 1:444–55.
28. Miller PL, Black HR. HT-ATTENDING. Critiquing the pharmacologic management of essential hypertension. J Med Systems 1984; 8:181–7.
29. Pozen MW, D'Agostino RB, Selker HP, Sytkowski PA, Hood WB Jr. A predictive instrument to improve coronary-care-unit admission practices in acute ischemic heart disease. N Engl J Med 1984; 310:1273–8.
30. Puccetti R. The case for mental duality: evidence from split-brain data and other considerations. Behav Brain Sci 1981; 4:93–123.
31. Diamond Ga, Forrester JS. Analysis of probability as an aid to the clinical diagnosis of coronary artery disease. N Engl J Med 1979; 300:1350–8.
32. Hlatky MA, Pryor DB, Harrell FE, Califf RM, Mark DB, Rosati RA. Factors affecting sensitivity and specificity of exercise electrocardiography. Multivariable analysis. Am J Med 1984; 77:64–71.
33. Diamond GA. Reverend Bayes' silent majority. An alternative factor affecting sensitivity and specificity of exercise electrocardiography. Am J Cardiol 1986; 57:1175–80.
34. Diamond GA, Rozanski A, Forrester JS, et al. A model for assessing the sensitivity and specificity of tests subject to selection bias: application to exercise radionuclide vertriculography for diagnosis of coronary artery disease. J Chronic Dis 1986; 39:343–55.
35. Fryback DG. Bayes' theorem and conditional nonindependence of data in medical diagnosis. Comput Biomed Res 1978; 11:423–34.
36. Russek E, Kronmal RA, Fisher LD. The effect of assuming independence in applying Bayes' theorem to risk estimation and classification in diagnosis. Comput Biomed Res 1983; 16:537–52.

37. Hilden J. Statistical diagnosis based on conditional independence does not require it. Comput Biol Med 1984; 14:429–35.
38. Afifi AA, Azen SP. Statistical Analysis. A Computer Oriented Approach. New York: Academic Press, 1979; 289–352.
39. Detrano R, Leatherman J, Salcedo EE, Yiannikas J, Williams G. Bayesian analysis versus discriminant function analysis: their relative utility in the diagnosis of coronary artery disease. Circulation 1986; 73:970–7.
40. Tversky A, Kahneman D. Judgment under uncertainty: heuristics and biases. Science 1974; 185:1124–31.
41. Duda RO, Shortliffe EH. Expert systems research. Science 1983; 220:261–8.
42. Zadeh LA. Fuzzy sets. Inform and Cont 1965; 8:338–83.
43. Patterson R, Eng C, Horowitz S, Gorlin R, Goldstein S. Bayesian comparison of cost-effectiveness of different clinical approaches to diagnose coronary artery disease. J Am Coll Cardiol 1984; 4:278–89.
44. Turing AM. Computing machinery and intelligence. Mind (1950). Reprinted in Hofstadter DR, Dennett DC. The Mind's I. Fantasies and Reflections on Self and Soul. New York: Basic Books, 1981, pp 53–68.
45. Whitbeck C Brooks R. Criteria for evaluating a computer aid to clinical resasoning. J Med Philos 1983; 8:51–65.
46. Diamond GA, Forrester JS. Metadiagnosis: an epistemologic model of clinical judgment. Am J Med 1983; 75:129–37.
47. Wasson J, Sox H, Neff R, Goldman L. Clinical prediction rules. Applications and methodological standards. N Engl J Med 1985; 13:793–9.
48. Diamond GA. Monkey business. Am J Cardiol 1986; 57:471–5.
49. Ransohoff DF, Feinstein AR. Problems of spectrum and bias in evaluating the efficacy of diagnostic test. N Engl J Med 1978; 299:926–30.
50. Diamond GA, Vas R, Forrester JS, et al. The influence of bias on the subjective interpretation of cardiac angiograms. Am Heart J 1984; 107:68–74.
51. Rozanski A, Diamond GA, Berman D, Forrester JS, Morris D, Swan HJC. The declining specificity of exercise radionuclide ventriculography. N Engl J Med 1983; 309:518–22.
52. Bobbio M, Rozanski A, Pollock BH, Diamond GA. Why do physicians estimate probabilities erroneously (abstr)? Clin Res 1986; 34:359A.
53. Sorting Out Software. CADENZA (software review). Comput Phys 1984; 2:11–2.
54. Diamond GA, Pollock BH. Computer-assisted diagnosis in noninvasive evaluation of coronary artery disease (letter). J Am Coll Cardiol 1984; 3:465–2.
55. Diamond GA, Forrester JS. Improved interpretation of a continuous variable in diagnostic testing: probabilistic analysis of scintgraphic rest and exercise left ventricular ejection fractions for coronary disease detection. Am heart J 1981; 102:189–95.
56. Rozanski A, Diamond GA, Jones R, et al. A formar for integrating the interpretion of exercise ejection fraction and wall motion and its application in identifying equivocal responses. J Am Coll Cardiol 1985; 5:238–48.
57. Staniloff HM, Diamond GA, Pollock BH. Probabilistic diagnosis and prognosis of coronary artery disease. J Cardiac Rehab 1984; 4:518–29.
58. Wong DF, Tibbits P, O'Donnell J, et al. Computer-assisted Bayesian analysis in the diagnosis of coronary artery disease (abstr). J Nucl Med 1982; 23:P83.

59. Greenberg PS, Ellestad MH, Clover RC. Comparison of the multi-variate analysisand CADENZA systems for determination of the probability of coronary artery disease. Am J Cardiol 1984; 53:493–6.

60. Hlatky M, Botvinick E, Brundage B. Diagnostic accuracy of cardiologists compared with probability calculations using Bayes' rule. Am J Cardiol 1982; 49:1927–31.

61. Melin JA, Wijins W, Vanbutsele RJ, et al. Alternative diagnostic strategies for coronary artery disease in women: demonstration of the usefulness and efficiency of probability analysis. Circulation 1985; 71:535–42.

62. Detry JMR, Robert A, Luwaert Rj, et al. Diagnostic value of computerized exercise testing in men without previous myocardial infarction. A multivariate, compartmental and probabilistic approach. Eur heart J 1985; 6:227–38.

63. Diamond GA, Forrester JS, Hirsch M, et al. Application of conditional probability analysis to the clinical diagnosis of coronary artery disease. J Clin Invest 1980; 65:1210–21.

64. Santinga JT, Flora J, Maple R, Brymer JF, Pitt B. The determination of the post-test likelihood for coronary artery disease using Bayes (sic) theorem. J Electrocardiol 1982; 15:61–8.

65. Dans PE, Weiner JP, Melin JA, Becker LC. Conditional probability in the diagnosis of coronary artery disease: a future tool for eliminating unnecessary testing? South Med J 1983; 76:1118–21.

66. Christopher TD, Konstantinow G, Jones RH. Bayesian analysis of data from radionuclide angiocardiograms for diagnosis of coronary artery disease. Circulation 1984; 69:65–72.

67. Detrano R, Yiannikas J, Salcedo EE, et al. Bayesian probability analysis: a prospective demonstration of its clinical utility in diagnosing coronary disease. Circulation 1984; 69:541–7.

68. Weintraub WS, Madeira SW, Bodenneimer MM, et al. Critical analysis of the application of Bayes' theorem to esquential testing in the noninvastive diagnosis of coronary artery disease. Am J Cardiol 1984; 54:43–9.

69. Lee K, Pryor D, Harrell F, et al. Predicting outcome in coronary disease. Statistical models versus expert clinicians. Am J Med 1986; 80:553–60.

70. Michie D, Muggleton S, Riese C, Zubrick S, RuleMaster. A second-generation knowledge engineering facility. Proceedings of the First Conference on Artifical Intelligence Applications, 1984; 591–7.

71. Pollock BH, Diamond GA. Heuristic and algorithmic interpretation of cardiac stress tests. Proc Am Assoc Med Syst Info 1986; 5:204–8.

72. Fox J, Barber D, Bardhan K. Alternative to Bayes? A quantitative comparison with rule-based diagnostic inference. Methods Inf Med 1980; 19:210–5.

73. Singer J, Sacks HS, Lucente F, Chalmers TC. Physician attitudes toward applications of computer data base systems. JAMA 1983; 249:1610–4.

74. Startsman TS, Robinson RW. The attitudes of medical and paramedical personnel twoard computers. Comput Biomed Res 1972; 5:218–27.

75. Melhorn JM, Legler WK, Clark GM. Current attitudes of medical personnel toward computers. Comput Biomed Res 1979; 12:327–34.

76. Teach RL, Shortliffe EH. An analysis of physician attitudes regarding computer-based clinical consultation systems. Comput Biomed Res 1981; 14;542–58.

77. Anderson JG, Jay SJ, Schweer HM, Anderson MM. Why doctors don't use computers: some empirical findings. J R Soc Med 1986; 79:144–6.
78. Friedman RB, Gustafson DH. Computers in clinical medicine: a critical review. Comput Biomed Res 1977; 10:199–204.
79. Linerooth J. The political processing of uncertainty. Acta Psychol 1984; 56:219–31.
80. Work JW, Pollock BH, Kotler TS, Berman DS, Diamond GA. Does diagnostic uncertainty influence referral for testing (abstr)? Clin Res 1986; 34:387A.
81. Epstein AM, McNeil BJ. Relationship of beliefs and behavior in test ordering. Am J Med 1986; 80:865–70.
82. Pringle M, robins S, Brown G. Computers in the surgery. The patient's view. Br Med J 1984; 288:289–91.
83. Brownbridge G, Herzmark GA, Wall TD. Patient recations to doctors' computer use in general practice consultations. Soc Sci Med 1985; 20:47–52.
84. Jorgens J. Schneider RH. Regulation of medical device software: role of FDA. Proc Am Assoc Med Syst Info 1986; 5:43–6.
85. Holden C. Regulating software for medical devices. Science 1986; 234:20.
86. Weistart JC. Legal consequences of standard setting for competitive athletes with cardiovascular abnormalities. J Am Coll Cardiol 1985; 6:1191–7.
87. Miller RA, Schaffner KF, Meisel A. Ethical and legal issues related to the use of computer programs in clinical medicine. Ann Intern Med 1985; 102:529–36.
88. Relman AS. Dealing with conflicts of interest. N Engl J Med 1985; 313:749–51.
89. Diamond GA, Rozanski A. Steure M. Playing doctor: application of game theory to medical decision-making. J Chronic Dis 1986; 39:669–77.
90. Wishard WVD. Dragments of 1985. Some events of 1985 that have been shaping the dimensions of a new time. U.S. Department of Commerce, 1986.
91. Goldman L, Waternaux C, Garfield F, et al. Impact of a cardiology data bank on physicians' prognostic estimates. Evidence that cardiology fellows change their estimates to become as accurate as the faculty. Arch Intern Med 1981; 141:1631–4.
92. Grundner TM, Garrett RE. Interactive medical telecomputing: an alternative approach to community health education. N Engl J Med 1986; 314:982–5.
93. McKinlay JB. From "promising report" to "standard procedure"; seven stages in the career of a medical innovation. Milbank Mem Fund Q 1981; 59:374–411.
94. Diamond GA. Meme machines. Ann Intern Med 1986; 105:788–9.

Chapter 14
Computerized Data Management and Decision Making in Critical Care
Reed M. Gardner

Care of the critically ill patient places unusual demands on the practicing physician. The critically ill are usually referred to intensive care units (ICUs) and are connected to sophisticated physiologic monitoring equipment. As a result of their illness or injury, these patients are subjected to a wide variety of laboratory tests. Their therapy is complex, its timing is critical, and careful documentation is essential. The large volume of resulting data must be stored, processed, and used for clinical decision-making. The tremendous growth of medical information, the demand for cost-effective care, and the need to document the justification for clinical decisions by patients, utilization review committees, third-party payers, and health care policy-makers have placed even more demands on physicians caring for the critically ill.

Concurrently, there has been a rapid development of computer technology. Critical care medicine and medical computing are both less than 25 years old. According to a recent article in *Scientific American*, if the aircraft industry had evolved as rapidly as the computer industry, a Boeing 767 would cost $500 today, would circle the globe in 20 min, and would do it on 5 gallons of fuel. The cost of computer logic is falling at the rate of 25% per year and the cost of computer memory at the rate of 40% per year. Computational speed has increased 200 times in 25 years, and energy consumption and computer size have decreased by 10,000 times [1]. It seems apparent, then, that as the complexity of critical care increases and the cost of computer hardware decreases, soon every critical care unit will have not one but many microcomputers.

The state of the art in critical care computing has advanced rapidly in the past decade. In the early phases of monitoring, computers were used

Adapted with permission from Surgical Clinics of North America—Vol. 65, No. 4, August 1985.

to acquire physiologic data such as blood pressure and cardiac output. After this, programs to communicate data from distant laboratories were implemented. Reports were generated from the more integrated data bases. Finally, closed-loop control and decision-making tools were added to assist the physician [2,3].

Whereas at first there was a reluctance on the part of physicians and nursing staff to use computers in the care of their patients, there is now a "cry for help" from these same health care providers. This change in attitude has come as a result of several developments in computing technology, particularly the advent of the personal computer.

Statement of the Problem

Barnett's recent review [4] of the application of computers to ambulatory practice quotes Florence Nightingale's 1873 book entitled *Notes on a Hospital*:

> In attempting to arrive at the truth, I have applied everywhere for information, but in scarcely an instance have I been able to obtain hospital records fit for any purpose of comparison. If they could be obtained, they would enable us to decide many other questions besides the one alluded to. They would show the subscribers how their money was being spent, what good was really being done with it, or whether the money was not doing mischief rather than good.

It is ironic that her comments are relevant more than a century later. They are true for records of ambulatory patient [4] as well as for those of the critically ill. The medical record remains the principal instrument for ensuring continuity of patient care. There is a real need to integrate and organize patient's records to optimize medical data review and decision making [2,4,5].

The traditional medical record has several limitations [4,5]:

1. It is physically inaccessible. Two examples will illustrate. For an emergency admission, the patient's previous record, although very valuable, can seldom be recovered and delivered in time to be of benefit. The complex and usually voluminous records of the critically ill are often "thinned." The process of recovering the "thinned" portion is often too slow to be of much use.
2. Information is available at only one location—where the chart is physically located.
3. The chart is usually poorly organized.
4. Illegible handwriting may make information unavailable or laborious and time consuming to retrieve.
5. There is no recording standardization, so even when charts are retrieved for review, it is difficult to compare them.

6. Retrieval of data for research is cumbersome (manual chart review) because the records must be read by trained personnel.
7. Data recorded from electronic instruments must be handwritten or manually attached to the patient's chart.

How the Computer Can Aid in Record-Keeping, Data Management, and Decision-Making for Critically Ill Patients

Table 14.1 shows a six-step sequence indicating how computers can be used to assist in solving record-keeping, data management, and decision-making problems encountered in ICUs.

Assistance in Data Collection

Digital computers are used almost exclusively in the newest bedside physiologic monitors. These microcomputer-based monitors help sort through the approximately 100,000 heartbeats that occur each day and identify those of interest (arrhythmias, asystole, and so on). The measurement of heart rate and arrhythmias and the ever-vigilant logging of these data have become hallmarks of intensive care monitoring. Indeed, the recent Concensus Conference on Critical Care Medicine acknowledged the importance of recognizing life-threatening arrhythmias [6].

In addition to the bedside monitoring tasks we take somewhat for granted, there are many other medical devices whose operation depends on microcomputers. For example, most of the instruments in the clinical laboratory are automated with microcomputers. Blood gas machines are highly dependent on computers to give prompt and accurate results.

Table 14.1. Uses of the Computer In intensive Care

1. Assist in data collection
2. Provide computational capability
3. Assist in data communication and integration or data
4. Record-keeping
5. Report generation
   Variable report format
   Available at multiple sites
   Data communications
   Eliminate redundancy
   More structured reports
   More accurate reports
   Current information
6. Assist in decision-making

Provision of Computational Capability

Just as pocket calculators have become pervasive in our everyday life, so will computers. Programmable computers relieve us from menial tasks. In contrast to humans, computers perform calculations just as well at 3 A.M. as at 9 A.M. Indeed the computer is the ultimate "slave" because it does exactly what it is told (programmed) to do, does it with great speed, makes virtually no mistakes, works 24 hr per day, and does not complain. Recently, there has been a widespread acceptance of small personal computers in critical care units to assist with the calculation and interpretation of hemodynamic monitoring, drug dosage, and blood gas data [7–9]. Examples of results of these programs are presented further on.

Assistance in Data Communications and Integration of Data

One of the most important tasks of physician and health care providers is to assimilate all data before making treatment decisions. Data on patients can be rapidly and accurately transmitted electronically from one computer system to another. Thus, data from the clinical laboratory can be received promptly by a critical care unit or surgical suite [10].

The importance of an integrated record was recently emphasized by the results of a study conducted in our department [11]. We examined the data used for the physician's decision-making during teaching rounds. We

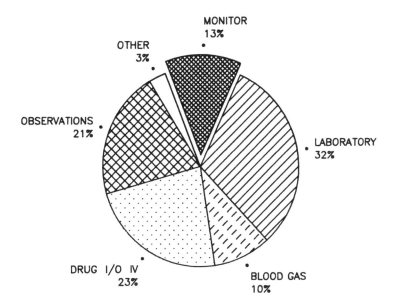

Figure 14.1. Pie chart shows data used for clinical decision-making by physicians during teaching rounds in our shock-trauma intensive care unit.

tabulated data used from our computerized shock-trauma unit into six categories: 1) bedside monitor; 2) laboratory; 3) drugs, input/output and intravenous; 4) blood gas laboratory; 5) observations; and 6) other. Figure 14.1 shows the findings of the study. We were surprised at the small percentage (13%) of the data contributed by the bedside monitor. Equally surprising was the large fraction (42%) that laboratory and blood gas data contributed to the decision-making process. It is clear from the information shown in Figure 14.1 that data from multiple sources must be combined to allow the physician to make effective treatment decisions. This study clearly showed the need for integrated record keeping. The computer is the ideal medium for such integration, since it can easily communicate with other computers and can archive data for quick review from multiple sites [12–15].

Record Keeping

The computer is an ideal record keeper because it can store and quickly recover vast amounts of information. A successful database management system should be "user-friendly," that is, easy to use after a few minutes of instruction. The recently introduced Apple MacIntosh with its "mouse" and the Hewlett-Packard model 150 with a "touch screen" are examples of computer hardware that is becoming more user-friendly.

In the real-time monitoring environment of a critical care unit, the computer system must also have high availability (no failures or down time). Fortunately, for medical computing, there are several other commercial applications of computers that have a similar need for high availability—telephone switching networks, air traffic control systems, nuclear and conventional power plant monitors, aerospace telemetry, and on-board control systems. As a result, there are a growing number of fault-tolerant computer systems [15]. We use a fault-tolerant system manufactured by Tandem Computer as our central system [2]. The system provides an availability of greater than 99.5% (down-time of less than 0.5%, or about 7 min per day), which has proved adequate for our clinical needs.

Report Generation

The ability of the computer to gain access to the data in its database and generate a variety of reports is a principal advantage of medical computing. The advantages Barnett [4] mentions for the record-keeping of ambulatory patients are even more impressive for that of critical care patients. These benefits are as follows.

Generation of report of variable formats. Flow charts, summary reports, unit reports, and similar reports must be readily available from patient data management systems. Figure 14.2 shows a specialized summary (rounds) report we are currently using. At any time of the day or night, a physician can get this report in less than 1 min. To generate this report, the computer searches the patient database and presents the most recent data by organ system. The data are to be reviewed and used for decision-making. Note that data from a wide variety of original sources are presented in a clear and legible manner. Cardiovascular data include hemodynamic monitoring information, laboratory data, and electrocardiogram (EKG) data, with computer-assisted interpretations. Respiratory data include blood gas data with computer-generated interpretations and corresponding ventilatory status. A wide variety of data from many different hospital locations are integrated to update the physician on the patient's laboratory, clinical, fluid balance, and medication status.

Data availability at multiple sites. Once the patient's record is in electronic (computer) form, it is simultaneously available at multiple sites. Physicians can review those data from any terminal connected to the system. Thus a critical care staff physician can review the same data on a terminal in his or her office as those simultaneously reviewed by the attending physician, who may be at the patient's bedside or at home using a personal computer. Fully one-third of the physicians on our staff have personal computers. As a result, the level of computer literacy and, consequently, of the physicians' interest in "phone-in" access to patients' records on our computer system is increasing.

Data communications. Data communication is essential because a patient's care is seldom limited to the primary care physician. Physician specialists, in addition to respiratory therapists, dieticians, nurses, and social workers, have become an integral part of the health care team, especially for trauma patients.

Elimination of redundant entry. As Florence Nightingale pointed out, seldom are data on patients used for just a single purpose. For example, administration of a medication must be documented to fulfill the medico-legal requirements of the hospital record, but more importantly it must be charted because it has an effect on the patient's medical recovery. Those concerned with management of costs and efficiency are also interested in what medications were given. To accomplish all of these tasks on paper requires either the redundant entry of data by a nurse or ward secretary or the creation of multiple copies of handwritten records, which are sent through the hospital's "communication system" and eventually archived (usually in a computer). By having the computer capture the record in electronic form and transmit the data to appropriate patient files, redundant and inefficient data entry can be eliminated. Thus, if a nurse charts a medication at the bedside terminal, the data are captured promptly and

```
NAME:                              NO.    65209    ROOM: E410                         DATE: SEP 01 06:05
   DR. REES.              SEX: M   AGE: 42   HEIGHT: 178   WEIGHT: 75.80   BSA: 1.94   BEE: 1709   MOF:  7
================================================================================================
CARDIOVASCULAR: 1                                    EXAM: _____
TIME         CO   CI   HR  SV  SI   VP  MSP  MP SVR LWI PW  PA  PVR  RWI    _____
SEP 01 05:36  8.20 4.22  82 100  51 7.0M  88  76  8  53  12  18  0.7  7.6
        SEP 01 05:35 DOPAMINE (INTROPIN)  3.00 MCG/KG/MIN
        LV PARAMETERS ARE WITHIN NORMAL LIMITS
                    SP   DP   MP   HR  :  LACT      CPK        CPK-MB      LDH-1       LDH-2
    LAST VALUES    101   62   76   78  :
    MAXIMUM        210  110   76  164  :  4.1 (12:30)    (    )      (    )      (    )      (    )
    MINIMUM         72   47   72   40  :
    HEART RATE = 100   QRS = 60   PR = 160   QRS AXIS =   20
        ++++ PHYSICIAN OVERREAD ++++
    NORMAL ECG
      SINUS TACHYCARDIA
    NO SIGNIFICANT ECG CHANGES SINCE 08/15/1984.20:00
================================================================================================
RESPIRATORY: 3
SEP 01 04    pH   PCO2  HCO3   BE   HB  CO/MT  PO2  SO2  O2CT  %O2 AVO2 VO2   C.O.  A-a  Qs/Qt PK/ PL/PP  MR/SR
01 05:18 V  7.45  37.1  25.6  2.5 10.0  1/ 1   33   71  10.0   40                                 /  / 5  16/
01 05:17 A  7.50  31.5  24.5  2.6  9.6  2/ 1   76   95  13.0   40  3.40               128   17    /  / 5  16/
        SAMPLE # 49, TEMP 36.1, BREATHING STATUS : ASSIST/CONTROL
        MILD ACID-BASE DISORDER
        SEVERELY REDUCED O2 CONTENT (13.0) DUE TO ANEMIA (LOW HB)
31 20:46 V  7.43  32.2  21.2 -1.6 12.1  1/ 1   43   80  13.6   40                              40/ 40/ 5  20/
31 20:45 A  7.45  34.2  23.6  0.9 11.9  1/ 1   89   98  16.4   40  3.06               111   12  40/ 40/ 5  20/
================================================================================================
NEURO AND PSYCH: 0
    GLASGOW 15 (00:15) VERBAL _____ EYELIDS _____ MOTOR _____ PUPILS _____ SENSORY _____
    DTR _____       BABIN. _____  ICP _____     PSYCH _____
================================================================================================
COAGULATION: 0
    PT:       (    ) PTT:      (    ) PLATELETS: 419 (05:10)  FIBRINOGEN:   (    ) EXAM: _____
    FSP-CON:  (    ) FSP-PT:   (    ) 3P:        (    )
================================================================================================
RENAL, FLUIDS, LYTES: 0
    IN   8720 CRYST  6360 COLLOID        BLOOD      NG/PO  2310 : NA  142 (05:10) K    3.3 (05:10) CL 112   (05:10)
    OUT  2945 URINE  1841 NGOUT          DRAINS  265 OTHER   839 : CO2  23 (05:10) BUN 21  (05:10) CRE  1.0 (05:10)
    NET  5775 WT   76.40  WT-CHG  0.00  S.G.  1.015              : AGAP 10.3       UOSM          UNA      CRCL
================================================================================================
METABOLIC --- NUTRITION: 0
    KCAL    2501  GLU  226   (05:10)  ALB   1.5 (05:10) :  CA   6.5 (05:10)  FE  (    )  TIBC     (    )
    KCAL/N2  158  UUN        (    )   N-BAL             :  PO4  2.7 (05:10)  MG  (    )  CHOL 106 (05:10)
================================================================================================
GI, LIVER, AND PANCREAS: 0                                                              EXAM:
    HCT    31.0 (05:10) TOTAL BILI   1.6 (05:10) SGOT  64 (05:10) ALKPO4 363 (05:10) GGT   209 (05:10) _____
    GUAIAC  (    )  DIRECT BILI  1.2 (05:10) SGPT  52 (05:10) LDH  344 (05:10) AMYLASE  (    ) _____
================================================================================================
INFECTION: 3
    WBC 22.6 (05:10) TEMP 39.3 (08:00) DIFF  34B, 57P,  4L,  5M,  E (05:10) GRAM STAIN: SPUTUM _____ OTHER _____
CULTURES:
    BLOOD _____ SPUTUM _____ URINE _____ CSF _____ CATH _____ WOUND _____ OTHER _____
================================================================================================
SKIN AND EXTREMITIES:
    PULSES _____ RASH _____ DECUBITI _____
================================================================================================
TUBES:
    VEN _____ ART _____ SG _____ NG _____ FOLEY _____ ET _____ TRACH _____ DRAIN _____
    CHEST _____ RECTAL _____ JEJUNAL _____ DIALYSIS _____ OTHER _____
================================================================================================
MEDICATIONS:

MORPHINE, INJ                    MGM  IV       8.0    DOPAMINE, INJ                      MGM  IV     525
ACETAMINOPHEN, ELIXIR            MGM  NG       650    METAPROTERENOL (ALUPENT), SOLUTION MGM  INHAL 75.0
METRONIDAZOLE,INJ                MGM  IV      2000    HEPARIN, INJ                       UNITS IV      0
NAFCILLIN, INJ                   MGM  IV     10000    OSMOLITE, LIQUID                   ML   NG D  2910
CEFOPERAZONE (CEFOBID), INJ      MGM  IV      4000
```

Figure 14.2. A rounds report generated by the computer is divided into sections by organ system or physiology. A multi-organ failure score (MOF: 7) indicates the severity of illness.

218

accurately for all clinical purposes as well as administrative and nonclinical management functions.

The implementation of computerized respiratory therapy charting at our hospital has increased therapist productivity by 18%. This increase came even in the face of having therapists take the time to enter their own procedures into computer terminals. When the therapists chart their clinical procedures by computer, the computer automatically acquires management information, bills the patient, and fulfills medico-legal documentation requirements. By reducing the manual paperwork, a higher percentage of the therapist's time was spent on patient care.

Increased structure in reports. As can be seen from Figure 14.2, computer-generated reports are highly structured. Because their format is standardized and predictable, structured reports are efficient for reviewing patients' data. Like a familiar newspaper, they are easy to scan. To illustrate the concept, I like to compare reviewing a patient's chart with scanning a newspaper. As long as I am reading a Salt Lake City paper. I know where to look to find the national, local, and sports news as well as the cartoons. However, when I am in San Francisco and pick up a newspaper, I have to struggle for a few days to find the items I am interested in, but eventually I adapt. The same follows with computerized patient charting. Another newspaper analogy also applies to computerized patients' records. This is particularly useful, since we tend to put far more information on a computer terminal or on a printed report than most people will review. We do this for much the same reason a newspaper does. The information is there if you want it and is acessible in "small print" promptly, at relatively low cost.

Greater accuracy of computer-generated reports. Computer data are generally entered by means of a conversational, or interactive, mode. The computer terminal prompts the user to enter data in a prescribed format. Thus, as data are entered, a predefined set of rules is applied to validate the data and prevent errors. If errors occur, such as transposed digits (for example, pH 4.7 instead of 7.4), immediate feedback is given to the user, and the data entry error can be quickly corrected. The increased legibility of computer records compared with handwritten records is not questioned.

Finally, there is an attribute of computer reporting that is especially applicable to the critical care situation.

The computer record as source of the most current information. The data flow into the critically ill patient's record takes place almost continuously. The task of updating a single conventional paper record is overwhelming, even with electronic communications and printers. Keeping track of and filing each new piece of paper in the patient's chart become an impossible burden. Thus, in our system, a physician or nurse wanting the latest information about a patient reviews the data from a computer terminal. Until recently, when we installed computer terminals at each patient's bedside, access to terminals was a problem. Now that terminals are located at the bedside, access is no longer a problem. In fact, having the terminals at the bedside allows us to make the data entry and review "patient-specific." For example, since the computer "knows" what drugs are prescribed for each patient, pressing a single key on the terminal will cause it to display only those drugs. Then a simple menu selection permits the drug, its dose, and route of administration to be "charted" promptly and easily while eliminating the need to search through a formulary of over 2,000 drugs. Bedside terminals with memory capability (similar to personal computers) can store current information about a patient in its local memory. Since patient-specific drug prescriptions and patient care plans are stored in this manner, nurses can quickly and efficiently chart electronically.

Assistance in Decision-Making

The hallmark of a good physician is the ability to make sound clinical judgments. As Bergman and Pantell [16] point out, this process has traditionally been considered artful and intuitive, rather than scientific. However, in recent years the use of computers to assist in medical decision-making has gained wider acceptance [17]. Indeed, the discussion of "artificial intelligence" is commonplace in medicine today.

McDonald [18,19] has shown that a computer reminder system applied in an ambulatory clinic reduced oversights by physicians. He attributed physicians' errors to "channel noise" or information overload rather than to practitioner ignorance.

The opportunity to use the computer to aid in the complex task of medical decision-making in critical care has just begun [10,20] Figure 14.3 is a block diagram of the HELP (Health Evaluation through Logical Processing) computer system operational at LDS Hospital in Salt Lake City, Utah. The system collects and integrates data from a wide variety of data sources. Data are automatically stored and processed by the HELP system to determine if the new information by itself or in combination with other data in the patient's record (such as another laboratory value or a previous computer-generated decision) can be used to make a medical decision. The medical decisions are based on criteria stored on magnetic disk. The decision criteria were established by knowledge gained from physicians, nurses, and literature and from analysis of our own computer database. Decisions made by the HELP system are of the following four types: 1) interpretations—for example, blood gas and hemodynamic interpretations (Fig. 14.2); 2) diagnose; (3) alerts, that is, notification of

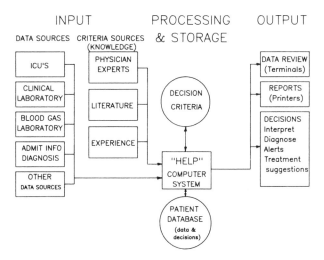

Figure 14.3. Patient data flows into the "HELP" decision-making computer system from a variety of sources. The decision-making criteria (knowledge base) are then automatically applied to the data, giving an output of computer-aided decisions. A variety of output is generated, including information for review on computer terminals, printed reports, and medical decisions.

life-threatening events such as critically low PO_2; and 4) treatment suggestions.

The application of protocols to treatment of patients was introduced several years ago in the ambulatory setting [18]. In recent years protocols have been applied to the care of hospitalized patients [21]. These protocols have been used to prevent adverse drug reactions [10] and to suggest fluid management [22] cardiac management of surgical patients [23], and therapy according to hemodynamic monitoring information [24].

Implementations Issues

A growing body of computer software tools and strategies is being developed for use with decision-making or "intelligent" systems [25]. Shortliffe [26] lists some excellent criteria for ascertaining which problems are appropriate for computerized medical decision-making. These include 1) demonstrated need for computer assistance; 2) recognized need for assistance by physicians; 3) core of formalized, readily available knowledge; 4) straightforward mechanism for introducing the computer-based tool into daily routine; 5) maintenance of the physician's role as ultimate decision-maker; 6) identification of highly motivated collaborators; and 7) avoidance of major theoretic barriers for the initial prototype system.

These criteria are idealized and cannot all be achieved. On the basis of Shortliffe's experience at Stanford University and our experience at LDS Hospital, however, these criteria are excellent guidelines.

Evaluation of the Computer System

As with computerized record systems for ambulatory patients, evaluation of cost and benefit of critical care computing is crucial. Unfortunately, there is no well-formulated technique for studying either manual or computerized medical records systems, especially those with medical decision-making capabilities. Shortliffe [26] mentions six guidelines for assessing the effectiveness of such systems. A system must 1) demonstrate that it is needed; 2) demonstrate that it performs at the level of the medical expert; 3) show that it is usable; 4) demonstrate its impact on management of patients; 5) show its impact on the well-being of patients, and 6) demonstrate its cost-effectiveness.

The computer will not solve all the problems of a modern ICU [27]. However, we need to harness its power to help us cope with the mass of detail required to manage the care of critically ill patients [28]. We must use the computer as a tool to assist us in integrating, evaluating, and simplifying data management, while at the same time using our human skills to make patient care more personal.

Summary

Computers are being increasingly employed in all levels of society. Computer applications in clinical medicine have lagged behind administrative and billing functions. However, computers are now finding an increasingly useful place in critical care medicine. The complexity of the patients' conditions and the large amount of data generated by critically ill patients provide an ideal area of application for computers. The computer can assist in collecting data, calculating derived parameters, speeding data communications, record-keeping, report generation, and decision-making. This article has discussed and illustrated how the computer can aid in the care of the critically ill.

References

1. Toong HD, Gupta A. Personal computers. Sci Am 1982; 247:87.
2. Gardner RM, West BJ, Pryor TA, et al. Computer-based ICU data acquisition as an aid to clinical decision-making. Crit Care Med 1982; 10:823.
3. Sheppard LC. computer control of the infusion of vasoactive drugs. Ann Biomed Eng 1980; 8:341.
4. Barnett GO. The application of computer-based medical-record systems in

ambulatory practice. N Engl J Med 1984; 310:1643.

5. Whiting-O'Keffe QE, Simborg DW, Epstein WV. A controlled experiment to evaluate the use of time-oriented summary medical record. Med Care 1980; 8:842.

6. Critical Care—Consensus Conference. JAMA 1983; 250:798.

7. Cottrell JJ, Pennock BE, Grenvik A. Critical care computing JAMA 1982; 248:2289.

8. Gardner RM. Information management—hemodynaminc monitoring. Semin Anesthiol 1983; 2:287.

9. Silage DA, Maxwell C. An acid-base map/arterial blood-gas interpretation program for hand-held computers. Resp Care 1984; 29:833.

10. Hulse, RK, Clark SJ, Jackson JC, et al. Computerized medication monitoring system. Am J Hosp Pharm 1976; 33:1061.

11. Bradshaw KE, Gardner RM, Clemmer TP, et al. Physical decision-making—evaluation of data used in a computerized ICU. Int J Clin Monit 1984; 1:81.

12. Asbury AJ, Lush K, Franks CI. Computers in high dependency units—ABC of computing. Br Med J 1983; 287:472.

13. Brimm JE, Peters RM. Applications of computers and other new techniques. In Berk LJ, Sampliner JE (eds): Handbook of Critical Care. 2nd ed. Boston: Little, Brown, 1982; pp 545–555.

14. Saunders RJ, Jewett WR. System integration—the need in future anesthesia delivery systems. Med Instrum 1983; 17:389.

15. Serlin O. Fault-tolerant systems in commerical applications IEEE comput 1984; 17:19.

16. Bergman DA, Pantell RH. The art and science of medical decision making. J Pediatr 1984; 104:649.

17. Warner HR. Computer-Assisted Medical Decision-Making. New York: Academic Press, 1979.

18. McDonald CJ. Protocol-based computer reminders, the quality of care and the non-perfectability of man. N Engl J Med 1976; 295–1351.

19. McDonald CJ, Hui SL, Smith DM, et al. Reminders to physicians from an in-rospective computer record—a two-year randomized trial. Ann Intern Med 1984; 100:130.

20. Gardner RM, Clemmer TP. Computerized protocols applied to acute care. Emerg Med Serv 1979; 7:90.

21. Shoemaker WC. Protocol medicine (editorial). Crit Care Med 1974; 2;279.

22. Shoemaker WC. Fluid management. Semin Anesthiol 1983; 2:251.

23. Rao TLK. Cardiac monitoring for the noncardiac surgical patient. Semin Anesthiol 1983; 2;241.

24. Marino PL, Krasner J. An interpretive computer program for analyzing hemodynamic problems in the ICU. Crit Care Med 1984; 12:601.

25. Lenat DB. Computer software for intelligent systems. Sci Am 1984; 251:204.

26. Shortliffe EH. Computer-based clinical decision aids: some practical considerations. First American Medical Informatics Association Conference Proceeding, San Francisco, May 2–5, 1982; pp 295–298.

27. Osborn JJ. Computers in critical care medicine. Promises and pitfalls. Crit Care Med 1982; 10:807.

28. Arnell, WJ, Schultz DG. Computers in anesthesiology—a look ahead. Med Instrum, 1983; 17:393.

Chapter 15
Performance of Computerized Protocols for the Management of Arterial Oxygenation in an Intensive Care Unit

Susan Henderson, Robert O. Crapo,
C. Jane Wallace, Thomas D. East,
Alan H. Morris, and Reed M. Gardner

Introduction

Adult respiratory distress syndrome (ARDS) is a form of respiratory failure characterized clinically by severe hypoxemia, diffuse infiltrates on chest radiograph. and decreased lung compliance. In its most severe form it has a survival of about 10%. In 1984, Gattinoni et al. reported a 77% survival in this subset of ARDS patients using a new form of therapy [1]. The new therapy included pressure controlled inverse ratio ventilation (PCIRV) and low frequency positive pressure ventilation with extracorporeal CO_2 removal (ECCO2R). Its goal was to reduce the peak and average pressures applied to the lungs by mechanical ventilators. The extraordinary survival reported with this new therapy and the fact that it was the result of an uncontrolled trial led to the design of a prospective randomized controlled clinical trial comparing PCIRV and ECCO2R with traditional positive pressure ventilatory support. The trial was executed at the LDS Hospital from 1987 to 1991. During the design phase of this trial it became obvious that the novelty of extracorporeal support could cause increased interest among the clinical staff, resulting in a difference in the intensity of care between patients receiving ECCO2R and patients receiving traditional ventilatory care. This created the possibility that differences in the intensity of therapy would bias the outcome of the study. To assure equivalency of care in both the control and new therapy limbs of the study, protocols were developed to control the management of arterial oxygenation in all study patients [2–4].

The protocols were first developed and tested as paper flow diagrams. The tested and refined protocols were then computerized, taking advan-

Adapted from an article published in the *Int J Clin Monit Comput* 8:271–280, 1992. Reprinted with permission of Kluwer Academic Publishers.

tage of a large, centralized computerized patient database at the LDS Hospital (the HELP system) [2,5–7]. Clinical data is routinely stored in this database; as a result, manual entry of data specifically needed to operate the protocols was minimized. The computerized protocols assessed elements of the patients' clinical status and laboratory data and automatically generated therapy instructions which were then displayed on bedside computer terminals. The protocols were used to care for patients 24 hr a day in a clinical intensive care unit (ICU) by the routine clinical staff and not by a research team. Once introduced into the clinical setting, the protocols have continually evolved in response to 1) the identification of errors in logic and programming, 2) unanticipated clinical circumstances, 3) disagreement between the clinical staff and the protocol instructions, and 4) an increase in the number of aspects of clinical care covered by the protocols. As expected. protocol evolution was most rapid in the start up phase (first eight patients) when the computerized protocols were untested and the clinical staff was adjusting to computerized protocol care. Thus, the logic used for the first patient was not identical to that used for the last patient. The changes in logic were, however, applied in parallel to both the control and new therapy groups ensuring the equivalency of care in the two groups.

Indices of computerized protocol performance for the first 16 patients were analyzed and reported in 1989 [3]. The clinical staff followed computerized protocol instructions 63.9% of the time for the first eight (start-up) patients, and 91.8% of the time for the remaining eight patients [3]. The major problem in creating the protocols was obtaining physician agreement on a standard protocol. This meant the physicians had to give up approaches to therapy that were a matter of style and agree on a detailed, standard approach to patient care. The purpose of this paper is to report on the performance of the computerized protocols on all patients in whom they were used. We will use information, with permission, from two earlier reports [3,4].

Methods

The HELP System

The HELP information system at LDS Hospital runs on a network of ten Tandem fault-tolerant computer processors using the Guardian Operating System with 3.4 gigabytes of disk storage distributed over 14 disk drives [5–7]. The eight drives handling clinical data are mirrored to reduce the possibility of data loss. Eighteen Charles River Data Systems (CRDS) minicomputers are interfaced to the Tandem, serving as multiplexers and pre-processors. All clinical and laboratory information on each patient is stored in the integrated database and is, therefore, available for review, report generation, and computer decision-making.

The data dictionary of the HELP system is a hierarchial representation of data elements known as PTXT. Patient demographic and clinical data is stored in coded form in a variety of active and archived files. Most of the programs which manipulate the database are written in PTXT Application Language (PAL) [6]. a structured programming language similar to Pascal. A few of the programs that require access to more fundamental operating systems functions (such as interprocess communication) are written in the Tandem Application Language (TAL), a structured programming language similar to C.

Protocol implementation

Paper-based protocols were developed by a team of 14 physicians and nurses from the pulmonary, critical care, and anesthesiology departments. The current protocols cover about 25 pages of flow diagrams and the computerized version has approximately 12,000 lines of PAL code.

Discrete values of arterial oxygen pressure (or, alternatively, bedside pulse oximetry data) trigger protocol execution, resulting in the generation of a specific instruction for therapy (Fig. 15.1). An example of a specific instruction is "Increase the inspired oxygen fraction (FIO2) by 10% from 50% to 60%." The instructions are based on patient data (e.g., vital signs, respiratory care parameters, and blood gas data) stored in the centralized database. Protocol instructions, which are also stored in the database, are reviewed at the patient's bedside terminal through the use of menus. These menus also allow the clinical care user to review data, manually activate the protocols and generate new instructions for therapy using the most recent patient data base, and to suspend protocol use when medical problems not addressed by the protocols demand atten-

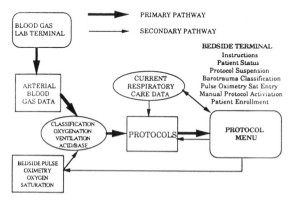

Figure 15.1. Basic organization of the computerized protocols. (Originally published in the proceedings of the Thirteenth Annual Symposium on Computer Applications in Medical Care, IEEE Computer Society Press, Los Alamitos, CA, 1989, pp 588–592 [3].)

tion. The protocol logic operates in the background and does not interfere with use of the bedside terminal for other tasks such as nurse and respiratory care charting.

Performance Evaluation

The protocols were used in an intensive care unit by the routine clinical staff, who would either follow or not follow an instruction. All instructions for 80 consecutive patients managed with the computerized protocols were reviewed and were categorized as 1) whether or not the instruction was correct and 2) whether or not the instruction was followed. Since the paper-based protocols created by the clinical team represented the desired medical logic, the therapy instructions derived from the paper diagrams were considered to be the "correct" instructions. When the computer instruction differed from the paper protocol instructions they were classified as "incorrect."

Instructions classified as "incorrect" and clinical actions which differed from computerized protocol instructions (correct instructions not followed) were examined by two individuals (S.E.H. and C.J.W.) and classified into one of the following categories:

Correct instructions (not followed by the clinical staff).

Clinical staff digressions from the protocol. Correct protocol instructions which were interpreted incorrectly or ignored or with which the clinicians disagreed. Clinicians at the bedside were allowed to override protocol instructions when the medical problem was not covered by the protocol, when the patient was unstable and required immediate intervention, and when it was thought to be medically justified to challenge the instruction. When physicians challenged the protocol logic, the issues were discussed by the entire team and the objection resolved.

Incorrect instructions (followed or not followed)

Software error. Error in the software code.

Nonrepresentative data. Data in the computer database that was incorrect or not "representative" of the patient's lung function, or missing at the time the protocol instruction was generated. For example, if changes had been made in the patients ventilator settings but had not been recorded and the protocols were activated, the instruction generated would be based on data that was not current and would be classified as "incorrect" because of non-representative data.

Undefined protocol logic (undefined logic). Decisions made in sections of the protocols that were in development or which had been instituted in the paper-based protocols but had not yet been computerized.

Cascade errors. Errors that occurred because a previous error had not been corrected before the next instruction was issued.

Other. Incorrect instructions caused by computer system problems or incorrect use of the computer protocols. Instructions where reasons for the error could not be identified were also included. Computer system issues included computer downtime, and problems with the data drive mechanism. The data drive is a system tool which initiates a particular process whenever a specific data item is stored in the database. This tool was originally used to activate the computer protocols whenever arterial blood gas data were stored for a protocol controlled patient. The tool proved to be unreliable and an alternate method of protocol initiation was developed and implemented after patient 3.

We will, with permission, also report some data from a subset of the study population (12 patients, Nos. 25 to 36) that was reported in 1990 [4] wherein we addressed the issues of whether compliance with the protocol instructions was affected by whether the instruction was correct, the direction of therapy (whether therapy intensity was increased or decreased or left unchanged) or the mode of ventilatory support. The term *compliance* is used only to indicate whether instructions were followed. The ventilatory support modes used in this clinical trial were CPPV (Continuous Positive Pressure Ventilation), CPAP (Continuous Positive Airway Pressure), PCIRV (Pressure Control Inverse Ratio Ventilation), and $ECCO_2R$ (Low-Frequency Positive Pressure Ventilation with Extracorporeal CO_2 Removal). Instructions in each of these modes were analyzed to determine if the mode of ventilation affected compliance with the computerized instructions. Individual patients may have been supported with more than one mode of ventilatory support.

Statistical Analysis

A chi-square test of independence was used to evaluate the frequency with which protocol instructions were followed or not followed as a function of instruction accuracy, direction of therapy, or the mode of ventilatory support. Significance was set at $p < .01$ because multiple comparisons were made. Mantel Haenszel chi-square analysis was used to evaluate compliance with protocol instructions as a function of time.

Results

Computerized protocols were used to manage arterial oxygenation in 80 ICU patients between September 1987 and May 1991. Fifty of these patients were not enrolled in the clinical trial comparing new and traditional ARDS therapy. Of 21,347 instructions issued on these 80 patients, 90.2%

Table 15.1. Protocol Performance Summary

Patients	Total instructions	No. followed	No. "correct"	Clinical staff digressions	Software errors	Causes of incorrect instructions Nonrepresentative data	Undefined logic	Cascade errors	Others
1–8	1,892	1,208	1,352	144	136	141	91	Unknown	172
(% total instructions)		(63.8)	(71.5)	(7.6)	(7.2)	(7.5)	(4.8)		(9.1)
9–80	19,455	17,949	18,056	99	154	813	20	314	98
(% total instructions)		(92.3)	(92.8)	(0.5)	(0.8)	(4.2)	(0.1)	(1.6)	(0.5)
All patients	21,347	19,157	19,408	243	290	954	111	Unknown	270
(% total instructions)		(89.7)	(90.2)	(1.1)	(1.4)	(4.5)	(0.5)		(1.3)

See the text for definitions.

were classified as "correct" and 89.7% were followed by the clinical staff (Table 15.1). Computerized protocols were used simultaneously with the paper based protocols for the first 16 patients (9/87 to 7/89) [3,4]. After July 1989, the computerized protocols were used exclusively with the paper-based protocols being used only when the computer was unavailable or as a reference. Protocol performance for the first eight patients in the study differed, as a group, from the following 72 patients. Of 1,892 instructions in the first eight patients, 1,352 instructions (71.5%) were classified as correct and only 1,208 instructions (63.8%) were followed (correct instructions and instructions followed were not always the same) (Table 15.1). In the subsequent 72 patients 92.3% of 19,455 instructions were followed and 92.8% were correct (Table 15.1) There were 243 digressions from the protocols by the clinical staff, over half of which occurred with the first eight patients.

There were 540 "incorrect" instructions with the first eight patients. Twenty-five percent of these incorrect instructions were caused by software errors and 26% by nonrepresentative data. For the subsequent 72 patients, there were 1,399 "incorrect" instructions; 11% were due to software errors and 58% to nonrepresentative data. The number of software errors expressed as a percentage of total instructions decreased from 7.2% in the first eight patients to 0.8% for subsequent patients. The percentage of incorrect instructions caused by nonrepresentative data decreased from 7.5% of total instructions for the first eight patients to 4.2% for the remaining 72 patients (Table 15.1).

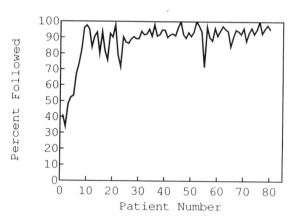

Figure 15.2. Percentage of computerized protocol instructions followed by the clinical staff calculated and displayed for each individual patient. Twenty-one patients were treated using paper based protocols before computerized protocols were instituted. Patient number one in this figure is the first patient in whom the computerized protocols were followed and the twenty-second patient treated with protocols.

Table 15.2. Effect of Instruction Accuracy, Type of Therapy Instruction and Mode of Therapy on Whether Instruction are Followed (12 Patients—all Instructions)[†]

	Total instructions n	Instructions followed, n (%)	Instructions not followed, n (%)
Effect of instruction accuracy*			
Instruction "correct"	2,337	2,278(97.5)	59(2.5)
Instruction "incorrect"	300	82(27.3)	218(72.7)
Effect of therapy**			
Intensity increased	829	741(89.4)	88(10.6)
Intensity decreased	1,284	1,111(86.5)	173(13.5)
No change—wait	524	508(96.9)	16(3.1)
Effect of mode of therapy***			
CPPV	1,914	1,705(89.1)	209(10.9)
CPAP	349	313(89.7)	36(10.3)
PCIRV	128	125(97.7)	3(2.3)
ECCO$_2$R	246	217(88.2)	29(11.8)

Modified with permission from material originally published in the Proceedings of the Fourteenth Annual Symposium on Computer Applications in Medical Care, IEEE Computer Society Press, Los Alamitos, CA, 1990, pp 284–8[4].

[†]The 12 patients were patients 25–36.

*$p < .001$ by chi-square test of independence

**$p < .001$ by chi-square test of independence. An instruction to make no change — wait is statistically different from the other two instructions ($p < .02$). The difference between increasing and decreasing therapy was not significant, $p = .06$

***$p = .02$

Figure 15.2 illustrates the percentage of instructions that were followed by the clinical staff for each individual patient in sequence. There was a highly significant increase in compliance with protocol instructions with time ($p < .00001$).

Results of the expanded analysis for the subset of 12 patients are summarized in Tables 15.2 and 15.3. The clinical staff was slightly more likely to follow an instruction to wait (make no change in therapy) than to increase or decrease the intensity of therapy (Table 15.2). There was a trend suggesting they would be more likely to follow an instruction to increase therapy over one to decrease it but it was not statistically significant. The mode of ventilatory support did not affect the likelihood that the clinician would follow an instruction (Table 15.2). As expected, instruction accuracy had the dominant effect. The clinical staff was clearly more likely to follow a "correct instruction" (97.5% followed) than an "incorrect" one (27.3% followed). Because of the strong effect of instruc-

Table 15.3. Effect of Type of Therapy and Mode of Therapy no Compliance With 'Accurate' Protocol Instructions (12 Patients—"Accurate" Instructions Only)[†]

	Total instructions n	Instructions followed n (%)	Instructions not followed n (%)
Effect of therapy*			
Intensity increased	742	723(97.4)	19(2.6)
Intensity decreased	1,102	1,062(96.4)	40(3.6)
No change—wait	493	493(100.0)	0(0.0)*
Effect of mode of therapy**			
CPPV	1,705	1,657(97.2)	48(2.8)
CPAP	303	298(98.3)	5(1.7)
PCIRV	123	121(98.4)	2(1.6)
ECCO$_2$R	206	202(98.1)	4(1.9)

Modified with permission from material originally published in the Proceedings of the Fourteenth Annual Symposium on Computer Applications in Medical Care, IEEE Computer Society Press, Los Alamitos, CA, 1990, pp 284–8[4].

[†]The 12 patients were patients 25–36.

*$p < .001$ by chi-square test of independence. The no change—wait instruction is significantly different from the other two instructions.

**$p = .52$ by chi-square test of independence.

tion accuracy on compliance with the protocols, we also examined the effect of the direction of therapy instructions and the mode of ventilatory support using only the "accurate" instructions (Table 15.3). The clinical staff was still statistically more likely to follow an instruction to "wait" than to increase or decrease therapy intensity. Though the difference for a wait instruction was statistically significant, the differences between the wait instructions and instructions to increase or decrease therapy were clinically insignificant. Compliance with the protocols did not change with the mode of ventilatory support when only accurate instructions were analyzed.

Discussion

Issues Relating to Whether or Not Instructions Were "Correct"

Protocol therapy instructions were classified as correct 90.2% of the time in all 80 patients (Table 15.1). and incorrect 9.8% of the time. The term incorrect is used only to indicate that a computerized instruction differed from what was intended based on the paper-based protocols; such instructions were not necessarily clinically inappropriate. The most common reason for an incorrect instruction was nonrepresentative data, and the primary reason for nonrepresentative data was delayed computer data entry by the clinical staff. Delayed data entry resulted in a database that was not likely to be representative of the patients true clinical state at the time the protocols were activated. Other causes of nonrepresentative data included data that was missing or incorrectly entered and data associated with transient instability of the patient. An interesting side effect of computer protocol use was an improvement in the accuracy of the patient's computerized medical record. Although the protocols were complex, the clinical staff learned to anticipate protocol instructions quite accurately, making it possible for them to recognize that a protocol instruction was based on erroneous data. It became common for the clinical staff to return to the patient's computerized medical record, edit the bad data, and generate a new protocol instruction using corrected data.

Occasionally a computer protocol instruction would be generated during a brief period of instability where the clinical data, though accurate, was not representative of the patient's steady-state conditions. For example, minor manipulations like suctioning or turning the patient can cause transient drops in arterial oxygen saturation. Protocol instructions based on the transient data were considered incorrect. The clinical staff was instructed to ignore them and to generate a new therapy instruction by bedside activation of the protocols once the patient had stabilized. The problem of nonrepresentative data was recognized early in the use of the protocols, and training programs were instituted to correct the problem. While improvement in the timely and accurate entry of data was achieved, the problem persists, and we expect the effect of training alone to be limited. In the complex and stressful setting of an ICU, patient care must retain the highest priority. Data entry of patient parameters may be delayed by urgent patient care needs. Automated data collection and recording is currently being tested in the ICU using a Medical Information Bus (MIB) system [8–10]. Implementation of the MIB may minimize this category of error. It will also alter the data collection environment, raising new possibilities and problems.

After the testing and debugging process that occurred primarily in the first eight patients, software errors proved to be insignificant. Software errors were associated with 7.2% of all instructions in the first eight patients and with only 0.8% of the instructions in subsequent patients. During the care of the first eight patients the software was being updated to correspond with the current versions of the paper based protocols and, at the same time, was being tested, corrected, and refined. For the first eight patients the clinical staff was actively using both the paper and computer versions of the protocol with the understanding that the paper protocol was to have precedence when conflicts were encountered. By the ninth patient the computerized protocols were sufficiently accurate to be used clinically and precedence was then given to the computerized protocol instructions. As new decision logic was added to the existing protocols, this process of testing and debugging the software was repeated.

Incorrect instructions which occurred because of undefined protocol logic were associated with 4.8% of all instructions in the first eight patients declining to 0.5% for the entire study group. Undefined logic refers to those areas of protocol logic that were not explicitly defined. For example, the current protocol logic contains the simple clinical question, "Is paralysis needed?" The patient parameters used and the clinical assumptions involved in answering this question have not been explicitly defined. Therefore, we have been unable to develop logic that would allow the computer to determine a patient's need for paralysis. One advantage of computerizing protocol logic is that it forces the careful examination of the factual and logical basis for every decision. In doing so, it forces the identification of underlying assumptions and deficiencies and becomes an effective method of clarifying the process of medical decision making.

Cascade errors were incorrect instructions which occurred because a previously counted error had not been corrected before another instruction was generated. For example: if the most recent value of PEEP was 25 cm H_2O, but the therapist erroneously charted 5 cm H_2O, an incorrect instruction would be generated. Additional incorrect instructions generated before the erroneous PEEP entry was corrected were counted as cascade errors. We did not isolate this category in the first eight patients. but in the subsequent patients it accounted for 22% of the incorrect instructions. We believe that the majority of the cascade errors occurred as a function of nonrepresentative data with fewer errors a result of software problems. We do not, however, know the exact breakdown of the cascade errors as a function of the original error.

The incorrect instructions categorized as "Other" included computer system problems, incorrect use of the computer protocols, and instructions which could not be categorized elsewhere. Incorrect use of the protocols included occurrences when the clinical staff incorrectly suspended or terminated suspension of the computer protocols. Protocol control is suspended for situations or processes which are outside the scope of protocol logic, such as patient transport, surgical procedures, dialysis, etc. We were able to find an explanation for all but 1.5% of the incorrect instructions.

The category "Clinical Staff Digressions" does not refer to incorrect instructions, but rather to correct instructions that were not followed. There were 144 (7.6%) such instances for the first eight patients, 99 (0.5%) in the subsequent patients, and 243 (1.1%) for the total population of 80 patients. Disagreements with protocol instructions and unexplained failure to follow instructions were considered to be a function of the clinicians' treatment preference or style; such instances decreased as confidence in the protocols grew. Increases in digressions would occur when new logic was computerized and when new staff members rotated into the ICU and were introduced to protocol controlled patient care.

The major problems currently confronting use of computerized protocols are logistical: 1) inaccurate and delayed data entry, 2) misunderstandings by the clinical staff of the elements of therapy covered by the protocols, and 3) failure to master the technical aspects of operating the protocols. Correction of these problems would eliminate practically all of the remaining incorrect instructions.

Clinical Staff Adherence to Protocols

Compliance with the protocols was evaluated by measuring how often the instructions were followed by the clinical staff. The percentage of protocol instructions followed improved with time (Fig. 15.2, Table 15.1). The transient drops in compliance seen in Fig. 15.2 are primarily a result of the introduction of new logic, rotation of new clinical staff into the ICU, and identification of previously unencountered clinical problems. They also occasionally occurred as a result of a small total number of instructions for a given patient. For example, patient 15 was under protocol care for only a short time receiving only five protocol instructions of which four instructions (80%) were followed.

In the subset of 12 patients (patients 25–36), 89% of all instructions were followed. Instruction accuracy was the most important factor associated with protocol compliance (Tables 15.2 and 15.3). Instructions directing an increase in therapy intensity were followed 89.4% of the time and instructions directing a decrease in therapy were followed 86.5% of the time (Table 15.2). This difference was close to statistical significance ($p = .06$). Further data might confirm a slight preference by clinicians to increase therapy intensity over reducing it. When the clinician was instructed to remain at the current level of therapy (a wait instruction) compliance increased to 96.9% (Table 15.2).

Since the effect of accuracy on compliance was so strong, we also analyzed the data using only the accurate instructions. When the instructions were accurate, when there were no software errors, and the data was current and correct, the percentage of instructions followed increased from 89.5% to 97.5% (Table 15.2). Analyzing only the accurate instructions, the pattern of compliance as a function of therapy intensity was unchanged (Table 15.3). The finding that wait instructions were followed more frequently than instructions to increase or decrease therapy is consistent with the feelings of the clinical staff that an instruction to wait is easier to follow than one to change therapy.

There was no difference in the degree of compliance with the protocols as a function of ventilatory support mode whether all instructions or only accurate instructions were analyzed [4] (Tables 15.2 and 15.3). There were slight differences among the modes in the distributions of the directions of therapy instructions, but the differences were small and should not affect the preliminary conclusion that compliance with the protocols was unaffected by ventilatory support mode [4]. The sample size is too small, however, to be certain of this conclusion.

Of the 300 instructions (11.4% of the total) classified as incorrect (Table 15.2), 82 (27.3%) were followed by the clinical staff. This could be interpreted to suggest that the clinical staff blindly followed protocol instructions. We think this is not the case for the following reasons: 1) Since our protocols represent only one way of approaching therapy, a computerized instruction that differed from the intended instruction may still have been clinically appropriate, 2) The therapeutic steps suggested by the protocol are small, for example, "increase PEEP by 2 cm H_2O," and, thus, are unlikely to cause objections by the clinical staff. 3) No clinical errors as a result of protocol use were reported. 4) The clinical staff is sophisticated and unlikely to follow an instruction that violates good clinical judgement. 5) The clinical outcomes were good (survival for the clinical trial patients was four times that of historical controls (39% vs. 9%) [11]).

In summary, the development of protocol logic and the subsequent computerization requires the medical care provider to examine carefully the assumptions, preferences, biases, deficiencies, and information involved in the decision-making process. The systematic and careful development of protocol logic and its acceptance by consensus are the most important factors in the success of our medical protocols. We believe that the most significant implication of this study is that protocol controlled care of critically ill patients is possible in spite of the complexity of the environment and the differing clinical styles of the clinicians.

Summary

Computerized protocols were created to direct the management of arterial oxygenation in critically ill intensive care unit (ICU) patients and have now been applied routinely, 24 hr a day, in the care of 80 such patients. The protocols used routine clinical information to generate specific instructions for therapy. We evaluated 21,347 instructions by measuring how many were correct and how often they were followed by the clinical staff. Instructions were followed 63.9% of the time in the first eight patients and 92.3% in the subsequent 72 patients. Instruction accuracy improved after the initial eight patients, increasing from 71.5% of total instructions to 92.8%. Instruction inaccuracy was primarily caused by software errors and inaccurate and untimely entry of clinical data into the computer. Software errors decreased from 7.2% in the first eight patients to 0.8% in subsequent patients, while data entry problems decreased from 7.5% to 4.2%. We also assessed compliance with the protocols in a subset of 12 patients (2,637 instructions) as a function of 1) the mode of ventilatory support, 2) whether the instruction was to increase or decrease the intensity of therapy or to wait for an interval of time, and 3) whether the instruction was "correct" or "incorrect." The mode of ventilatory support did not affect compliance with protocol instructions. Instructions to wait were more likely to be followed than instructions to change therapy. Ninety-seven percent of the correct instructions were followed and 27% of the incorrect instructions were followed. The major problem in creating the protocols was obtaining clinician agreement on protocol logic and their commitment to utilize it clinically. The major problem in implementing the protocols was obtaining accurate and timely data entry. We conclude that computerized protocols can direct the clinical care of critically ill patients in a manner that is acceptable to clinicians.

Acknowlegments

This work was supported by NIH grant HL36787, the LDS Hospital Deseret Foundation, and the Respiratory Distress Syndrome Foundation.

References

1. Gattinoni L, Pesenti A, Caspani ML, Pelizzola A, Mascheroni D, et al. The role of total static lung compliance in the management of severe ARDS unresponsive to conventional treatment. Intensive Care Med 1984; 10:121–6.
2. Sittig DF, Pace NL, Gardner RM, Beck E, Morris AH. Implemention of a computerized patient advice system using the HELP clinical int]formation system. Comp Biomed Res 1989; 22:474–87.
3. Henderson S, East TD, Morris AH, Gardner RM. Performance evaluation of computerized clinical protocols for management of artierial hypoxemia in ARDS patients. Proc Thirteenth Symp Comput Appl Med Care. New York: IEEE Comput Soc Press, 1989: 588–92.
4. Henderson S, Crapo RO, East TD, Morris AH, Gardner RM. Computerized clinical protocols in an intensive care unit: How well are they followed? Proc Fourteenth Annual Symp Comput Appl Med Care. New York: IEEE Comput Soc Press, 1900:284–8.
5. Gardner RM. Computerized management of intensive care patients. MD Comput 1986; 3(1):36–51.
6. Pryor TA. the HELP medical reasearch system. MD Comput 1988; 5(5):22–3.
7. Pryor TA, Gardner RM, Clayton PD, Warner HR. The HELP system. J Med Systems 1983; 7:87–102.
8. Hawley WL, Tariq H, Gardner RM. Clinical implementation of automated Medical Information Bus in an intensive care unit. SCAMC 1988; 12;621–4.
9. Gardner RM, Tariq H, Hawley WL, East TD. Medical Information Bus: The

key to future integrated monitoring [editorial]. Int J Clin Monit Comput 1989; 6:205–9.

10. Shabot MM. Standardized acquisition of bedside data; The IEEE P1073 medical information Bus. Int J Clinc Monit Comput 1989; 6:197–204.

11. Morris AH, Wallace CJ, Clemmer TP. Orme JF Jr, Weaver LK, et al. Extra-corporeal CO_2 removal therapy for adult respiratory distress syndrome patients. Resp Care 1990; 35:234–31.

Chapter 16
Acuity of Illness and Risk Prediction in Critically Ill Adults: The APACHE III Intensive Care Unit Management System

William A. Knaus and Carl Sirio

Overview

Providing patients with state-of-the-art, quality care has been a hallmark of 20-century medicine. Critical care units developed as an extension of postoperative recovery rooms and with the dissemination of effective electronic electrocardiographic cardiac monitoring, external cardiac massage, and respiratory support. Intensive care units (ICUs) proliferated worldwide in an attempt to improve patient outcome and overall quality of care by concentrating technology in the hospital environment.

Today, physicians admit patients to intensive care units with diverse disease processes and degrees of physiologic impairment. Admission is usually for intensive treatment of a severe illness, for expectant monitoring to detect and prevent complications, or for concentrated nursing care unavailable in other hospital settings. Despite the presumed utility of critical care therapy, the clinical literature highlights conflicting evidence regarding its benefit in various disease state [1,2]. As a result, a consensus on the appropriate use of intensive care resources does not exist [3–6].

Consequently, there is growing interest in accurately assessing severity of illness and other pertinent patient risk factors in order to estimate more exactly the probabilities for various outcomes. The most commonly studied outcome has been death. Other outcomes of clinical importance include the incidence of morbidity, and the overall length and quality of survival. These outcomes are listed in Table 16.1 with examples of specific endpoints subject to scrutiny.

Until recently little consideration was given by physicians, hospitals, third-party payers, government, and patients to the resources required in affording high-technology, high-intensity care. Following the introduction of the prospective payment system for hospitalized Medicare patients, the 1980s became rife with attempts to understand how and where hospital resources were expended and how physicians should best assess and

Table 16.1. Outcomes of Critical Care of Clinical Importance

Morality
Morbidity
 Nosocomial infection
 Re-intubation
 Self-extubation
 Re-admission to the intensive care unit within 24 hr
Length of survival following hospital discharge
Quality of survival
 Activities of daily living
 Satisfaction with quality of life achieved
 Return to work

monitor the quality of care provided. The professional mandate to perform appropriate and adequate peer review was thereby extended by other interested participants in the health care arena. The focus of these efforts has continued to concentrate on hospital based medicine, inclusive of patients admitted to the ICU, who are typically sickest.

Despite these demands for quality assessment, little published information exists on either reliable or efficient methods to assess quality, or the relationship between quality and the cost of health care. This is in large part due to the difficulty clinicians have had in determining the incremental value improvements and advances in diagnostic, therapeutic, and monitoring technology have had on outcome. This problem impacts equally on both actively treated and primarily monitored ICU patients. For both groups the fundamental questions remain: Who benefits from the higher level and intensity of care afforded in the critical care arena and how can that care be most efficiently provided?

The overriding focus of all quality evaluation is a continued search for excellence. Health outcomes must reflect a broad set of health status and health-related outcomes. In addition, this broad definition of quality recognizes the importance of professional responsibility to the individual patient within the context of the public's overall health.

Analysis of these complex questions is predicated on having effective measures of patient characteristics, the process of clinical care, and outcome. Measures of patient characteristics must include adequate and appropriate appraisals of the severity of illness, prior functional status, age, major diagnosis, and the location of treatment prior to admission to the ICU [7,8]. Evaluation of the process of care must include a consideration of both the clinical care provided to an individual and the institutional framework in which care is delivered. Assessing this framework includes scrutinizing the overall organization and management of the ICU [9].

Outcome assessment can begin with short-term events such as hospital mortality. Over time, however, this should expand to include long-term morbidity and mortality. Currently, the tools to measure long-term outcomes are limited.

To date, governmental and institutional efforts to evaluate quality of care using a retrospective analysis of hospital mortality and morbidity data derived from computerized administrative discharge information have met with skepticism. This skepticism is due mainly to the underlying limitations of the tools used for analysis [10–12]. Ineffective methods to control for differences in patient characteristics have been employed and the processes of care have been largely ignored. Similarly, traditional, labor-intensive methods of quality assessment including review of adverse occurrences, documentation of policies and procedures, infection control programs, and periodic focused chart audits have not satisfactorily placed adequate emphasis on overall quality of care and resource utilization.

This chapter will focus on the components of ICU care which must be incorporated into any discussion of quality and utilization review. This will include a description of severity of illness measurement and risk predictions of hospital mortality. The APACHE III (Acute Physiology, and Chronic Health Evaluation) prognostic scoring system and the Therapeutic Intervention Scoring System (TISS) will serve as the model. The discussion on the evaluation of care will concentrate on the major areas of decision-making faced by ICU clinicians and managers. These include decisions to admit a patient to the ICU, the components of care within the critical care unit subject to constructive scrutiny, and the assessment of outcome. Following each discussion of the major areas of ICU decision-making a portrait of the part of the APACHE III™ Management System designed to assist clinicians and managers in their daily activities will be provided.

In addition to providing useful clinical information to the practicing physician during the course of care, the information provided by this system will serve to improve ongoing quality of care and utilization review activities. The intent of this approach to patient data collection and retrieval is to improve both the quality and clinical relevance of the information in any ongoing analysis while minimizing the amount of work required to secure the information.

Why Should We Measure Severity of Illness and Predict Outcome?

There are four advantages to improved and accurate severity-of-illness and predictive models of outcome in critical care. Each of these benefits plays a distinct role in improving the delivery of health care.

First, these models allow physicians to focus aggressive intervention on those individuals most likely to benefit. As institutional resources become constrained physicians are confronted with determining which clinical problems are most likely to benefit from ICU care. The Task Force on Guidelines of the Society of Critical Care Medicine has suggested that objective measures of illness should play a part in ICU admission and discharge decisions [13].

Second, physicians caring for critically ill patients are often faced with the decision to limit or withdraw therapy. These decisions are replete with clinical uncertainties. Prognostic information, accurately predicting outcome, could serve as an adjunct for these difficult but unavoidable decisions. Work is ongoing that will facilitate their use in individual patient-care problems [14].

Third, prognostic scoring systems will facilitate the assessment of new technologies and allow for comparative analysis with established modes of therapy [15]. Clinical trials using accurate and reliable pretreatment risk-stratification controls will help us better to understand the value of critical care by reducing the amount of unexplained variation in patient risk.

The fourth benefit of precise prognostic assessments is to enhance efforts to compare the performance of ICUs. The quality of care provided and the resources expended to produce desired outcomes is an area of increasing research concentration.

The Apache III Management System—Scientific Underpinnings and Utility in Clinical Quality Assessment and Utilization Review

Severity-of-Illness and Outcome Measures in Critical Care

Current efforts to assess severity of illness in critical care began with the development of disease-specific prognostic indices. Examples of such indices include the Glasgow Coma Score, the Killip classification system, and Ranson criteria [16–18]. Although accurate in providing relative risk stratification, these systems have been limited by their disease specificity. This prevents useful comparisons across diseases or for patients with complex disorders [19]. Today, there is widespread recognition that general, not disease-specific, methods of assessing severity of illness are often more useful because of their generalizability across a broad spectrum of diseases.

Therapeutic Intervention Scoring System (TISS). An important step forward in the move toward generic evaluations of severity of illness came with the development of the Therapeutic Intervention Scoring System (TISS) [20]. TISS was designed to quantify the amount of skilled nursing care a patient received. Although resource utilization is influenced by many factors, such as medical and nursing organization, protocols, and

policies, by measuring 78 distinct nursing monitoring and procedural responsibilities, TISS serves as an *indirect* measure of the severity of illness
across differing diseases. In addition to providing information on nurse
staffing requirements for varying levels of patient severity, TISS allows
for an analysis of both the utilization of a critical care unit and the cost of
that care relative to the intensity of care provided. An important limitation of TISS is its inability to allow for a direct understanding of the relationship between a patient's specific illness and the impact of ICU care.

Acute Physiology, and Chronic Health Evaluation (APACHE). Progress
in the development of general severity of illness measures for the critical
care patients evolved further with the introduction of APACHE [21].
APACHE is predicated on the postulate that, prior to ICU therapy,
short-term hospital mortality in critically ill adults is influenced by five patient variables. These include the degree of physiologic deviation from
normal, age, chronic health conditions, disease, and the location of prior
therapy administration. In this manner one gets a more accurate understanding of the interrelationships between disease, physiology, and the
individual's ability to recoup from physiologic stress. The important
determinants of outcome are summarized in Table 16.2.

APACHE I and II. The original system consisted of two parts. The acute
physiology score (APS) was based on 34 physiologic measures designed to
capture the severity of an acute illness. In addition, APACHE consisted
of a preadmission health evaluation describing a patient's prior health status. The APS consisted of variables available near the time of admission
felt to be clinically important by an expert panel of intensive care physicians in predicting mortality. Relative weights were assigned to each variable signifying the degree of abnormality from normal for each variable
and the relative importance of that derangement when compared to the

Table 16.2. Determinants of Patient Outcome

Information available	Patient and treatment factors
Before treatment	Type of disease (diagnosis)
	Severity of disease
	Physiologic reserve
	Age
	Chronic disease
After treatment	Therapy available
	Application of therapy
	Timing
	Process
	Response to therapy

other variables. Studies evaluating the validity of APACHE in risk prediction demonstrated a direct relationship between the APS and the relative risk of death. The chronic health indicators were associated with an increased risk of death only for those patients with severe and failing health prior to admission.

APACHE II differed significantly from its predecessor. The number of physiologic variables incorporated in the initial assessment of severity was reduced to 12. In addition, several threshold values and weights for the physiologic measures were changed. For example, the importance of the Glasgow Coma Score and the importance attributed to acute renal failure were increased due to a better understanding of the impact of coma and renal failure on outcome. The impact of each of these changes was evaluated using multivariate comparisons to the original APACHE model.

The assessment of chronic health was changed as chronic health risk points were assigned for ongoing organ dysfunction. Chronologic age was incorporated into the APACHE II model, with increasing age being given an increasing number of risk points. In addition, the impact of emergency surgery was integrated into the analysis of outcome as investigation revealed this to be independently associated with an increased risk of mortality.

The resultant APACHE II score was a sum of the acute physiology, age and chronic health points. This point total, when combined with a patient's actual disease state in a multivariate logistic analysis, provided the basis for an assessment of severity of illness and risk of mortality. The APACHE II system was validated on 5,815 patients from 13 US medical centers and revealed a consistent relationship between APACHE II scores and observed hospital death rates. This relationship was found across the entire spectrum from a low to a high risk of death.

APACHE III. Until recently there has not existed a national benchmark for comparison of outcomes in critical care. The completion of the APACHE III study allows for the first time the establishment of a national, mortality-based performance assessment standard for all hospitals with more than 200 beds [22].

The objective of the recently completed APACHE III study was to refine APACHE methods in order more accurately to predict hospital mortality for severely ill hospitalized adults. Data was collected on 17,448 patients from medical, surgical and mixed medical/surgical ICUs from 40 US hospitals. The majority of these hospitals were randomly chosen to represent the breath of critical care services currently existing nationwide. Building upon the preexisting model of determinants of clinical outcome used in APACHE II, and using the reference database, APACHE III includes medical or surgical diagnosis, acute physiologic abnormalities, age, major co-morbidities, and treatment location prior to admission, to

Table 16.3. Components of Apache III Evaluation

Acute physiology	Chronic health
Vital signs	AIDS
Pulse	Solid tumor with metastasis
Mean blood pressure	Hematologic malignancy
Respiratory rate	Hepatic failure
Temperature	Cirrhosis
	Immunosuppression
Neurologic assessment	
Glasgow coma score (modified)	Age
Blood chemistry data	Disease
pO_2 or A-aDO_2	
pCO_2 and pH	Patient location prior to ICU admission
Creatinine	
Blood urea nitrogen	
Serum sodium	
Serum albumin	
Serum bilirubin	
Serum glucose	
Hemogram data	
Hematocrit	
White blood count	
Urine output data	
Urine output per 24 hours	

produce a risk estimate of a patient's hospital mortality [7]. The major components of this model are highlighted in Table 16.3.

The number of physiologic variables included in APACHE III have been increased to reflect the importance of additional physiologic measures in predicting outcome. These new variables include bilirubin, albumin, glucose, urine output, and blood urea nitrogen. The entire set of APACHE III physiologic variables is listed in Table 16.3.

In addition, the weights assigned to each variable employed were reexamined and set empirically. The importance of chronic health and age on outcome were reevaluated. The disease categories available for classification with APACHE II were expanded to include 79 major disease classifications.

The APACHE III prognostic system consists of two major components. The first includes an APACHE III score which can provide initial risk stratification for severely ill patients within defined homogeneous patient groups. The second element is the APACHE III predictive equation which uses the APACHE III score and the national reference database containing disease categories and treatment location prior to ICU admission to produce patient specific hospital mortality risk estimates.

Importantly, the study design allowed for simultaneous validation of the experimentally derived weights for physiology, age, and chronic health. The overall predictive accuracy of the first day APACHE III equation is such that for 95% of patients a risk estimate within 3% of the observed is produced within 24 hr of ICU admission. The first day APACHE III equation accounts for the majority of variation in observed death rates when applied to critical care units. The equation applied in this manner produces an R^2 of .90. Although severity of illness measures for critically ill patients attempt to capture all important variables related to outcome, some unmeasured variability still exists. As systems such as APACHE become more refined, and their underlying normative databases grow, the effect of these unmeasured variations will become even smaller.

APACHE III will improve the evaluation of the processes of clinical care as well as new therapeutic modalities. Physicians will be able to derive an accurate estimate of the number of excess deaths attributable to variations in quality of care and using the normative database identify areas in need of improvement and acknowledge areas of excellence [23]. Furthermore, physicians will have more reliable estimates of patient prognosis to incorporate into clinical decision-making.

The importance of this evolution in accurate patient description and risk stratification relates to a vital issue in quality assessment. The nature, characteristics, and risks of the patient population in question must be reliably and accurately documented, and well understood before useful statements regarding quality can be made.

ICU Decision-Making

Decisions in the intensive care sphere center around three distinct topical areas. The first set of decisions involve triage assessments. Triage decisions are followed by patient-specific diagnostic and therapeutic determinations made by the medical staff. The third and broadest topical area of decision-making involves the choice of an overall strategy for the organization, management, and structure of intensive care delivery. These decisions are often made in collaboration by the medical, nursing, administrative, and ancillary care leadership staffs.

Triage appraisals have an impact on the overall quality of care before, during, and after admission to the ICU. Diagnostic and therapeutic judgments, as well as the organization and structure of the ICU, affect the quality of care during the period of time spent in the critical care unit. Both triage and diagnostic or therapeutic decisions have clear immediacy regarding their impact on patient care.

Decisions regarding the structure, organization, and management of intensive care services which are delivered may also influence the overall delivery of quality care. These decisions impact on the care provided to all patients irrespective of the individual clinical situation. It is necessary to focus on all three areas of ICU decision-making and their potential for impacting on the quality of care. However, formal measures to evaluate the organization and management structure of intensive care units do not currently exist. Only recently have investigators begun to describe the important components of structure and management in the ICU [24]. Once the important organizational elements have been identified, our next challenge will be to develop the necessary tools to compare and contrast outcome as a consequence of these differences.

Within the context of providing high-caliber critical care, the value of assessing severity of illness for clinical decision-making, quality assessment and utilization review will become ever more apparent to the clinician at the bedside when information is provided in real time and can be used to assist ongoing patient care. The capability of prognostic systems to provide this information is becoming a reality as current efforts to automate APACHE III data collection are achieved. As databases continue to expand, improvement and refinement in the predictive ability of these systems will be possible.

System Overview

The APACHE III Management System (the System) is a currently available commercial system designed to provide real-time clinical information to physicians, nurses, and other clinical staff to support the effective treatment and management of critically ill medical and surgical patients. Using the APACHE III patient database, the System will enhance triage decision-making at the time patients are considered for admission to and discharge from the ICU. Furthermore, with the capability to produce daily updated predictions of risk of mortality for individual patients, the System will allow for more objective insights into the impact of ongoing diagnostic and therapeutic decisions. These capabilities will enhance the quality assurance and utilization review activities within an institution.

The System also provides doctors and other interested managers summary data regarding the utilization of and outcome from ICU services over time to further facilitate utilization review and quality assessment activities. This capability allows for improved short- and long-term planning and evaluation of critical care services. In addition, this will help institutions meet requirements for monitoring care posed by external review agencies such as the Joint Commission on Accreditation of Healthcare Organizations (JCAHO) [25].

To provide these capabilities as well as several others not specifically

Table 16.4. Apache III Management System User Modules

Data entry
Clinical decision support
Utilization management
Nursing resource management
System administration
Computer assisted instruction
Research and ad hoc reporting

discussed in this chapter the APACHE III Management System is designed around seven distinct user modules. The modules are listed in Table 16.4.

The *data entry* module allows the user to follow patients as they are admitted, discharged, and transferred from the ICU. All demographic, physiology, TISS, and occurrence information is entered into the system through this module.

The *clinical decision support* module provides risk predictions for individual patients and displays detailed information and trends on selected patients. The information provided by this module is essential for the discussions that follow on triage decision-making and ongoing diagnostic and treatment evaluations.

The *utilization management* module allows for direct comparison of the users' ICU and hospital performance compared to national normative data from the APACHE III database. The data provided by this module is integral to the System's ability to provide valuable information for both quality assurance and utilization review activities.

The *nursing resource management* module allows the user to project staffing requirements by relating a units' overall severity of illness to nursing intensity. This module is designed to play an important role in the organization and management of ICU nursing resources. In addition, this module helps streamline short- and long-term nurse scheduling.

The *system administration* module helps to maintain the System. It handles user identification, password, security, and data storage functions. This module also provides internal troubleshooting capabilities. The System has a *computer-assisted instruction* module that facilitates user training as well as a *research and ad hoc reporting* module that allows individual institutions to tailor the Systems' capabilities to their specific requirements.

The APACHE III Management System is based on a UNIX operating system and is currently ported to Sun Microsystems Sparcstation and IBM RISC 6000. The system can be linked with multiple workstations and utilizes a graphic laser printer. The System runs on Oracle Relational Data

Base Management software and uses the X Window System for a graphic user interface. The System is designed to be electronically interfaced with clinical laboratory information systems; patient monitoring systems and the hospital's admission, discharge, and transfer system. For multi-hospital institutions the decentralized application of the APACHE III Management System entails the installation of hardware and software at each hospital. Hospitals can be linked together electronically, or data can be transmitted by magnetic cartridge or floppy disk.

Clinical Decision Support and Triage Decision-Making

Triage is the medical screening of patients to determine their priority for treatment. In the critical care setting it involves decisions that affect both the admission and discharge of patients from the unit. A central issue in the triage of patients is the allocation of resources to maximize the potential for appropriate outcomes for individuals while utilizing total resources in the most effective overall manner.

The pressure to move patients into and out of the ICU can vary enormously between institutions, depending on a variety of factors. These include the size, location, and case-mix of a hospital as well as local practice styles regarding the utilization of intensive care resources. Bed availability and hospital protocols influence decisions to admit and discharge patients from the ICU [26–28]. In addition, physician-specific decisions based on personal heuristics can markedly influence the type of patients admitted into the critical care unit. In many hospitals coping with intense triage pressure, concern centers on how quality may be impacted when, potentially, patients are discharged prematurely [29].

In order to evaluate these issues fully an accurate assessment of patients' clinical characteristics is required at the time admission to the intensive care unit is considered. Recent work indicates that acute physiologic abnormalities are powerful predictors of the potential risk for a patient admitted for monitoring subsequently requiring and receiving active ICU therapies [30,31]. Using such a comprehensive evaluation of patient characteristics, physicians will be better able to determine which patients are in greatest need of critical care services. This will allow for a more objective determination of those most likely to benefit from admission to the ICU. These insights can help structure admission criteria for patients likely to receive active intensive care treatment as well as those likely to need solely monitoring.

For many of these patients for whom objective measures of physiologic status indicate they are "low-risk monitor" admissions there are legitimate questions as to whether they are best treated in an ICU, in a less intensive step-down unit, or on the general hospital floor. These are patients who typically have a less than 10% risk of death and a less than 20% risk of requiring active ICU interventions. In those instances where a patient is admitted, it would be helpful to know when discharge can be safely considered. The accurate and reliable identification of these low-risk monitor patients, and a measure of their eventual requirement for therapy, can serve as an excellent quality assessment activity.

There are also groups of patients for whom critical care is not successful in reversing the effects of an acute illness. Some patients are at a high risk of short term mortality despite aggressive intervention, while others fail to respond to treatment. Patients in these circumstances may be candidates for setting therapeutic limits or withdrawal of life-sustaining therapies. The decision to forgo critical care treatment is often complex and wrought with emotion. Nevertheless, such decisions are made with increasing frequency and are legitimate areas for quality assessment and assurance activities.

The decision to forestall intensive care for these patients will be enhanced by better assessments of the attendant risk of a decision either to provide or to waive intensive care. By providing objective estimates of the likelihood of hospital survival, the triage information provided by the APACHE III ICU Management System may lend support in formulating care plans for these desperately ill people. Precise estimates of the likely benefit derived from aggressive care will also allow clinicians to judge objectively comparative entitlements to care [32–34]. Explicit probabilities used as adjuncts and incorporated into decision-making, such probability statements could improve the overall quality of patient care [35–38].

The APACHE III Management System and Triage Decision-Making

The APACHE III Management System provides the capability to assist in the triage of patients into and out of the ICU. The system is designed to provide comparative patient information to the unit director, or appropriate designee, to supplement clinical impressions and experience when making admission and discharge decisions. This information is a part of the clinical decision support module.

The System displays the probability of ICU and hospital death as well as the remaining predicted length of stay for all current ICU patients. Patients are represented by a stylized bed symbol. Screen layouts are designed to assure System users easy-to-understand visual comparisons between patients.

Additional information—such as current APACHE III score, nursing work, patient classification as being at a low risk of death and at a low risk of requiring active treatment, and the probability of readmission to the ICU if discharged—presently is available. This information can also be displayed for patients being considered for admission to facilitate determinations of comparative entitlement to ICU care, especially during times of constrained resource availability when competition for beds is high.

The System highlights the patient's risk of both ICU and hospital death through the coordinated use of color-coded information. Patients at high risk of death will be indicated in red, those at intermediate risk in yellow and those at low risk in green. An example of the System's primary triage screens are depicted in Figure 16.1. The System has the capability to print hard copies of all visually displayed screen information in order to provide documentation for the medical record.

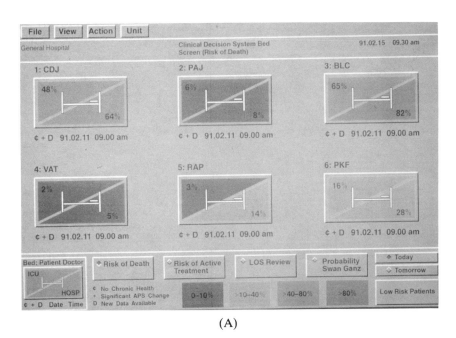

(A)

Figure 16.1. Clinical Decision Support—triage decision support.
(A) This displayprovides the APACHE III risk of ICU and hospital death for all patients in a 6 bed ICU. Information includes the patients' names and primary physicians. The risk of death is color coded by risk of death range. (B) This display provides the APACHE III predicted risk of active treatment and probability of discharge alive for the same 6 bed ICU. The indicated risks are color coded using a design paralleling that for Figure 16.1A. (C) This display provides further insight into the clinical details for two patients in the ICU. Information includes patient and primary physician, nurse, age, hospital and ICU length of stay to date, treatment catagory (low risk, active treatment), diagnosis, surgical status, and APACHE III component scores for admission and current acute physiology as well as chronic health. Predictions for current and future TISS and outcome are provided. Mortality risk trends are presented graphically.

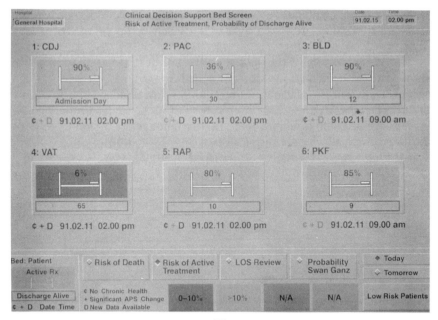

(B)

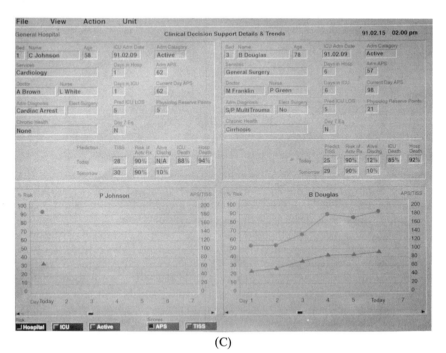

(C)

Figure 16.1. (Cont.)

Diagnostic and Therapeutic Decision-Making and the Process of Care—Issues for Quality Assessment and Utilization Review

A common tool currently used in quality assessment is the internal or external chart audit. The standards to which such charts are held vary depending on local standards of care as well as the abilities and knowledge base of the chart reviewer. The current process makes little provision for objective estimation of patient risk or severity of illness, much less the efficiency and efficacy of care. Selection of charts for review typically results from the identification of important sentinel events such as the need for mechanical ventilation or inotropic support. Charts may also be flagged for selective analysis of iatrogenic complications, nosocomial infections, medication errors, reintubation rates, readmission to the ICU after discharge to the floor, or other suspected markers of deficient process of care. Establishing protocols and standards by which charts are evaluated is helpful but more widely applicable benchmarks for review and evaluation are needed [39,40].

In order adequately to assess the significance on patient outcome of these and other sentinel events there must be quantifiable, reproducible, and validated means of estimating the a priori risk of these events occurring. There has been limited study coupling chart audit review with an objective judgment of patient risk [41]. When this is done the most frequently considered outcome is mortality. The aim of this type of analysis is to search for examples of "preventable deaths." Quantifying mortality during intensive care therapy and hospitalization for an acute illness will serve as a useful measure of quality if lower death rates clearly reflect differences in medical care.

When an analysis of patient hospital mortality has been used as a primary method to evaluate the quality of hospital care a persistent question has remained. Can hospital death rates be adequately adjusted for variations in the baseline risk of death of patients accurately to reflect the quality of care? Data to support the use of mortality as a marker for care is growing.

Recent studies suggest that there may be differences in the process and quality of care in hospitals identified as high- and low-death-rate outliers for patients with cerebrovascular accidents and pneumonia. The methods employed in the analysis included both objective and expert subjective analysis to reach conclusions regarding preventable deaths. The conclusion from these studies is that preventable deaths are more likely to be found in patients with an initially low risk of death when compared to those with intermediate or high risks [42,43].

In the intensive care arena data is coming to light that suggests risk-adjusted hospital mortality can be used to assess quality. A recent study was performed reviewing the outcome data for 13 US hospitals in which APACHE II scores and disease were used to control for variations in patient characteristics. Standard mortality ratios (SMR) of observed over predicted death rates were compared. An SMR of 1.0 signified observed performance equalling predicted performance. Two hospitals were identified as having actual death rates significantly different than predicted. One hospital had a standardized mortality ratio (observed death rate/ predicted death rate) of 0.59, whereas another hospital had a ratio of 1.59. Substantial differences were noted retrospectively in the clinical and organizational process of care between the two institutions. This study supports the hypothesis that the process of care can impact on outcome in both positive and deleterious ways [44].

These findings led to a prospective multi-institutional study evaluating the potential links between the process of care and patient outcome from critical care. The APACHE III study explicitly evaluated the impact that diversity in setting, organization, and operating protocols of ICUs have on patient outcome. The process of care was systematically explored to evaluate whether seven key components of organization and management interact to affect quality. These processes include perceived unit effectiveness, staff communication, coordination, conflict resolution, member satisfaction, organizational culture, and leadership.

This study reveals links between a hospital's organizational structure, management and process of delivering care, and risk-adjusted patient outcome. Specifically, the technologic capability of an ICU is associated with lower risk adjusted mortality rates. Furthermore, concentration of a unit's therapeutic efforts around a limited number of diagnostic conditions is also associated with lower than expected risk-adjusted death rates. Lastly, organizational and managerial excellence as measured by leadership, communication, coordination, and problem-solving skills is significantly associated with greater ICU efficiency as measured by lower than predicted total length of hospital stay. There now exists further convincing evidence that ICU quality is directly impacted by the manner in which health care is provided [9].

There are obstacles and limitations to making the use of risk adjusted mortality rates the sole technique in ICU quality assessment. First, solely as a consequence of statistical selection and random variation, a hospital could become a statistical outlier. Every patient's clinical course has some unpredictability associated with it, and this cannot be controlled for by using even the most comprehensive case-mix adjustment. This would be an aberration relative to the care being provided and would most likely be corrected in analyses over time.

Secondly, hospital discharge practices, patient and family preferences, the use of do-not-resuscitate orders, and the selection of alternative sites, such as nursing home or hospice facilities, for death can also impact on hospital mortality statistics. As a consequence, hospital mortality should be assessed within a context of post-discharge deaths because they may serve to uncover disparities in death rates because of the time selected for discharge.

Lastly, if mortality rates are tied to the quality of clinical care and clinical decision-making, what are the normative standards that are most appropriately applied to an institution? Should hospital outcome be compared only to outcomes for hospitals with similar characteristics such as size, geographic location, and teaching status, or should universal standards apply for all institutions? To date, no consensus to these questions has arisen.

The APACHE III Management System and Outcome Evaluation

The APACHE III Management System, through the utilization management module, uses APACHE III data from individual patients to facilitate a review of outcome. Using the information provided one can construct an effective quality assurance and utilization review program. The System produces graphic and tabular reports to facilitate tracking of outcomes over time. Significant flexibility is built into the formatting of results in order to provide the user the capability to individualize analyses and focus on institutional-specific concerns.

Outcome data includes summaries of actual ICU and hospital mortality compared to risk-adjusted APACHE III predictions of mortality. The outcome data is structured to allow for ready comparisons of observed mortality to predicted mortality for institutions having similar characteristics as well as all hospitals in the APACHE III database.

Aggregated, overall mortality data may not be completely indicative of the care provided within a hospital. There can be areas of both strength and relative weakness. The System is therefore designed to allow for more in-depth analysis of mortality performance. Outcome can be stratified by hospital service and diagnosis. Within a diagnostic catagory, mortality performance is provided for quintiles of risk. Additionally, outcome results can be stratified by periods of time, thereby allowing for measurement and evaluation of the impact of quality or utilization interventions over time. Examples of the mortality-outcome-reporting capabilities of the System are provided in Figure 16.2.

There is growing need to consider severity-adjusted outcomes other than mortality in an ongoing evaluation of quality in critical care. The occurrence of morbid events can have a profound impact on the length and quality of survival. To this end investigators are beginning to evaluate additional measures of outcome in order to study the process of care and the relationships to outcome and quality. These measures include an analysis of the association of length of stay and severity. The APACHE III Management System provides the ability to provide length-of-stay

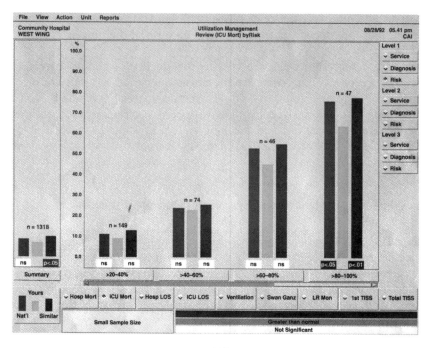

(A)

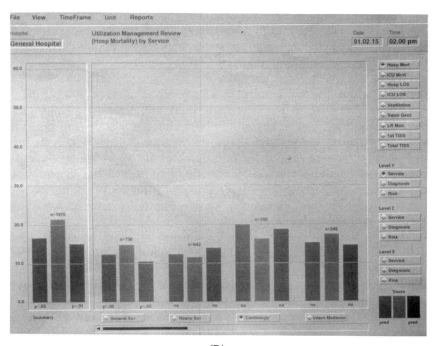

(B)

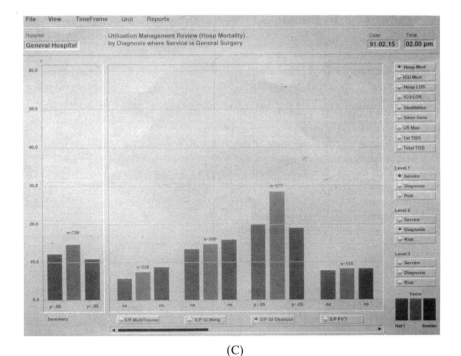

(C)

Figure 16.2. Outcome and utilization management.
(A) This display is an example of the APACHE III Management System hospital mortality review. The graphic display provides a hospital's actual mortality rate by risk ranges. The risk adjusted observed outcomes are compared to expected mortality rates for institutions with similar characteristics and all hospitals in the APACHE III comparative database. (B) This display subsets the information provided in the previous display by type of service. (C) This display provides outcome information for patients within specific diagnostic catagories (e.g. surgical).

data in a format analogous to the mortality information. Observed lengths of stay are compared to severity-adjusted predictions of hospital stay in aggregate and stratified by selected criteria.

The identification of patients at low risk of death, as well as their length of stay and outcome, is monitored for both quality assessment and utilization review activities. For all patients, nursing intensity, as captured by TISS, and first day and total resource consumption are tracked. The assessments can be subsetted by service, diagnosis, and risk range.

Additionally, the use of invasive technology such as pulmonary artery flow directed catheters (Swan-Ganz), rates of re-intubation after extubation or readmission to the ICU after recent discharge, and rates of nosocomial infection may have a bearing on quality of care. Using APACHE III controls for patient-specific illness, physiologic abnormali-

Table 16.5. Apache III Management System Adverse Occurrence Tracking List

Post-ICU admission bacteremia
Cardiac arrest
Reintubation with 24 hr of extubation
Self-extubation
Right mainstem intubation (prolonged)
Readmission to the ICU
Postoperative wound infection
Pneumonia, urinary tract infection or decubitus ulcer formation
Fall from bed
Medication error
Pneumothorax
Pulmonary embolus
Upper gastrointestinal hemorrhage
Transfusion error or reaction

ties, age, chronic health, and location of treatment prior to ICU admission, health care providers can monitor these events easily and make reliable comparisons between patient groups. Further, the total number of ventilator days expected for a patient can be predicted. Incidence rates for a variety of other adverse occurrences can be monitored. The spectrum of adverse occurrences that can be followed using the System are summarized in Table 16.5.

All reporting formats provided by the System can be used and structured as part of ongoing quality assessment and utilization review activities. The ad hoc reporting capability allows for specific analysis of potential problem areas or areas of institutional interest. The utilization management module also provides information to tie resource consumption to reimbursement reporting.

The APACHE III Management System also provides the capability to respond to external demands for quality and outcome information. For example, the JCAHO is currently evaluating the effectiveness of a hospital's quality assurance program through the suggested implementation of a ten-step program [26]. The System has the ability to monitor and produce reports that highlight compliance with these guidelines.

The Management and Utilization of ICU Nursing Resources

The preceding discussion has concentrated on measuring and evaluating patient characteristics, clinical care, and hospital outcome. As indicated earlier, critical care medicine is on the forefront of understanding the possible correlations between outcome and the organization, structure, and management of hospital care. This is because providing critical care requires the effective and coordinated activity of many individuals with a diversity of clinical skills. Consequently, the quality of care delivered could depend on the smooth interactions of the health care professionals providing direct bedside care as well as ancillary support.

Adequate, exemplary nursing plays a pivotal role in the care of critically ill patients. Moment-to-moment monitoring and assessment of a patient's condition can often alert physicians to significant changes in a patient's status. Nevertheless, nursing resources are at times limited or strained by the demands of patient flow and volume. Strategies to manage finite nursing resources effectively is a major component of the ICU management team's daily endeavors. The aim of these efforts is to streamline nursing staff planning to assure adequate coverage to meet anticipated patient care demands. The effectiveness with which these staffing issues are addressed is directly related to the overall organization and management of the ICU.

Investigators have recently used APACHE derived data accurately to forecast next-day nursing care requirements in patients receiving intensive care [45]. The relationship between patient risk factors on the first ICU day and therapy subsequently received on the second ICU day was analyzed. There was a strong correlation between a patient's Therapeutic Intervention Score (TISS) and subsequent therapeutic intensity across the spectrum of APACHE severity of illness ranges.

The APACHE III Management System and Nursing Resource Management

The APACHE III Management System links these areas together in the *nursing resource management module* to provide information aimed at streamlining nurse staffing in the critical care unit. The material provided in this section of the applications software is based on relationships between APACHE III predictions and TISS data. The 96 individual TISS elements are grouped into categories including *active treatment tasks*, *ICU monitoring tasks*, and *standard floor care tasks*.

The System uses either individual patient APACHE III scores and diagnosis or actual current TISS to predict future nursing requirements. This forecasting ability allows a manager user to calculate the number of nurses required to care for the unit's patients over the upcoming 24-hr period given the clinical status of current patients. This capability can help match an individual patient's nursing needs to staffing availability more exactly.

In addition, the data is utilized to document consumption of resources. These data allow for relative comparisons of resource utilization for each patient when controlling for severity of illness by comparing predicted and actual TISS. These data can be aggregated and displayed for the entire unit over time. This facilitates the determination of long-term staffing requirements up to one year.

Implement a Quality of Care and Utilization Assessment Program—Future Implications and Directions

Unfortunately, current efforts at quality assessment and assurance are often viewed as restrictive and punitive. They foster an attitude of contempt among physicians and sometimes serve to defeat the stated goal of improved performance in the best interest of patients. Despite frustration, physicians cannot abrogate their leadership role in the arena of striving for excellence in critical care. In addition, we cannot allow the fear of retribution or criticism to deter us from seeking ways to improve the smooth functioning of the ICU. Improvement can occur in an environment where people feel comfortable admitting mistakes, offering suggestions and seeking counsel when difficulties arise.

Although the provision of orderly and effective intensive care requires a physician team leader, the environment in which care is provided should foster a sense of individual accountability. Each participant in the delivery of an aspect of critical care should be guided by an institutional commitment to continued quality improvement. The leaders of the health care team have a responsibility to instill the belief in all participants that improvement in the quality of care delivered is a continuous and evolving process. This responsibility for self-scrutiny cannot be delegated to a committee or review panel but must be imbedded within the foundation of the ICU and hospital structure.

If quality of care and continuous assessment is a worthy goal in critical care, then methods for ongoing evaluation must be implemented. These methods cannot be overly labor intensive and must go beyond traditionally used formulas for evaluating care such as retrospective chart reviews [46,47].

Selective chart review may be of value in specific instances when suspected lapses in the process of care lead to deficient care. For example, patients determined to be at a low risk of death based on a physiologic assessment of severity who do in fact die during the course of care warrant explicit case review. Computerized identification of these patients will simplify the identification, tracking, and subsequent evaluation of care received by these patients.

If the quality of care is primarily affected by the process of care, then ongoing and overall monitoring of that care is needed. The most effective way to collect the needed information is with computerized data collection. This facilitates analysis and may help highlight subtle deficiencies that may not otherwise be apparent from the more conventional chart re-

Table 16.6. Model for Quality Assessment and Assurance in Critical Care Medicine*

Reliable and validated measurement of—		
Patient characteristics	Process of care	Outcomes
Disease[1]	TISS[1]	Short term measures[1]
Severity of illness[1]		Hospital mortality
Age[1]	Organizational structure	Low risk deaths
Chronic health status[1]	Management process,	Sentinel events
Location of patient prior to ICU admission (ER, OR/RR, floor, another hospital)[1]	policies and protocols	Morbid events, expected and unexpected complications of care
		Long-term measures:
		Mortality
		Functional status
		Patient satisfaction and preferences for quality of life

[1] Currently available for analysis using the APACHE III Management System.
* The assessment of quality in critical care requires an evaluation of the patient characteristics and the processes of care. This provides the information necessary to understand the implications of the measured clinical outcomes.

view process. Having this overall portrayal of the clinical process will then allow for a more focussed evaluation of individual case histories.

A model for continuous quality assurance and assessment in the critical care unit is presented in Table 16.6. This model is predicated on the concepts developed in this chapter. Included are measurements of selected patient characteristics, an evaluation of the process of care, and outcome assessments. The goal of this model is comprehensively to evaluate all aspects of clinical ICU care, including triage, diagnostic, and therapeutic decision-making, and the organization and management of the ICU.

Patient characteristics collected include acute disease, severity of illness, age, chronic health status, and patient location prior to ICU admission. This data is used to calculate a short-term probability of death using a representative, reliable, and validated comparative database such as the one collected for APACHE III. In this manner the observed and predicted risk-adjusted mortality rates can be compared.

In addition, this physiologically based patient data can be the basis for predicting other important aspects of care, including length of stay; requirements for resource consumption, including nursing care; and complications. When these predicted outcomes are compared to observed

Table 16.7. Examples of Equations for Standardized Mortality and Standardized Length of Stay*

Risk-adjusted outcome measures		
Patient risk-adjusted mortality ratio	=	$\dfrac{\textit{Predicted number of deaths}^{1}}{\text{Observed number of deaths}}$
Patient risk-adjusted length of stay	=	$\dfrac{\textit{Aggregate predicted length of stay}^{1}}{\textit{Aggregate observed length of stay}}$
Patient risk-adjusted nursing intensity	=	$\dfrac{\textit{Aggregate predicted TISS}^{1}}{\text{Aggregate observed TISS}}$

[1] All predicted values are derived from a normative, comparative data base. Using the normative data base a level of statistical significance for a particular ratio is determined. This allows for isolation of areas of potential strengths and weaknesses in an institution.
* Selected examples of using risk-adjusted severity of illness information to assess quality of care.

events, a portrait of care rendered will have been produced. Examples of the simple formulas for producing risk-adjusted outcome ratios for several outcome measurements are depicted in Table 16.7.

Over time it is anticipated that expanded databases will allow for predictions of long-term outcomes which will further enhance a comprehensive evaluation of the impact and quality of ICU care. The eventual inclusion of patient preferences and satisfaction into the outcome assessment model is an eventual goal requiring clinical instruments under development [48].

Evaluation of the clinical process of care is accomplished concurrently with the physiologically based assessment of outcome using a measure of bedside clinical intensity. TISS serves this function in the proposed model. In addition, an understanding of the organization and management of a critical care unit focuses on the overall process under which care is administered.

As part of the continued effort to improve health care delivery, the evaluation of quality will remain an area of focused attention within hospitals and among other interested third parties. A commitment to excellence remains a professional responsibility. External agencies will continue to mandate organized programs of quality assessment and assurance for ICUs. If these efforts are to have meaning to physicians and be of clinical utility in the process of evaluating critical care, an assessment of each patient's relative risk for the outcome in question prior to therapy is essential. By incorporating accurate patient risk stratification into the quality of care assessment we can help guarantee that information produced by these efforts is reliable and meaningful.

The process for achieving this form of comprehensive quality assessment and assurance in the intensive care setting is at an encouraging stage. Computerized programs such as the APACHE III ICU Management System already exist to aid in this evaluation. The evolution of well-constructed protocols for evaluating critical care will continue to develop as the methods to measure appropriate and meaningful outcomes become more sophisticated. The current state of the art requires experimentation and manipulation of quality assurance models in order to develop information that is useful to the medical community and the public. With the continued expansion of computerized data capturing, the task of collecting important information will be facilitated, quality assessment and utilization review activities will become less expensive, and the results will be more clinically meaningful.

References

1. Petty TL, Lakshminarayan S, Sahn SA, et al. Intensive respiratory care unit: review of ten years experience. JAMA 1975; 34:322–26.
2. Hook EW, Horton CA, Schaberg DR. Failure of intensive care unit support to influence mortality from pneumococcal bacteremia. JAMA 1983; 249:1055–1061.
3. Knaus WA, Wagner DP, Loirat P, et al. A comparison of intensive care in the U.S.A. and France. Lancet 1982; ii:642–46.
4. Zimmerman JE, Knaus WA, Judson JA, et al. Patient selection for intensive care: a comparison of New Zealand and U.S. hospitals. Crit Care Med 1988; 16:318–26.
5. Knaus WA, Wagner DP, Draper EA, et al. An evaluation of outcome from intensive care in major medical centers. Ann Intern Med 1986; 104:410–18.
6. Abizanda R. The facilities. In Miranda DR, Williams A, Loirat P (eds): Management of the ICU—Guidelines for Better Use of Resources. Dordrecht, The Netherlands: Kluwer Academic Publishers, 1990; pp 55–82.
7. Knaus WA, Wagner DP, Draper EA, et al. The APACHE III prognostic system: risk prediction of hospital mortality for critically ill hospitalized adults. (in press).
8. Escarce JJ, Kelley MA. Admission source to the medical intensive care unit predicts hospital death independent of APACHE II. JAMA 1990; 264:2389–2394.
9. Zimmerman JE, Shortell SM, Knaus WA, et al. An evaluation of outcome from 42 intensive care units: Risk adjusted mortality performance and factors associated with excellence. (in press).
10. Jencks SF, Williams DK, Kay TL. Assessing hospital-associated deaths from discharge data; the role of length of stay and comorbidities. JAMA 1988; 260:2240–46.
11. Park ER, Brook RH, Kosecoff J, et al. Explaining variations in hospital death rates—randomness, severity of illness, quality of care. JAMA 1990; 264:484–490.
12. Epstein AE. The outcomes movement—will it get us where we want to go? N Engl J Med 1990; 323:266–270.

13. Task Force on Guidelines-Society of Critical Care Medicine. Recommendations for intensive care unit admission and discharge criteria. Crit Care Med 1988; 16:807–808.
14. Zimmerman JE (ed). APACHE III Study Design: Analytic plan for evaluation of severity and outcome. Crit Care Med 1989; 17:S-169–219.
15. Kalb, PE, Miller DH. Utilization strategies for intensive care units. JAMA 1989; 26:2389–2395.
16. Jennett B. Resource allocation for the severely brain damaged. Arch Neurol 1976; 33:595–60.
17. Killip T III, Kimball JT. Treatment of myocardial infarction in a coronary care unit. A two year experience with 2150 patients. Am J Cardiol 1967; 20:457–464.
18. Ranson JHC, Rifkind KM, Roses DF, et al. Prognostic signs and the role of operative management in acute pancreatitis. Surg Gynecol Obstet 1974; 139:69–81.
19. Knaus WA, Nystrom PO. Severity scoring and prediction of patient outcome. In Tinker J, Zapol (eds): Care of the Critically Ill Patient, ed 2. London: Springer-Verlag, 1989.
20. Cullen DJ, Civetta JM, Briggs BA, et al. Therapeutic intervention scoring system: A method for quantitative comparison of patient care. Crit Care Med 1974; 2:57–63.
21. Knaus WA, Zimmerman JE, Wagner DP, et al. APACHE—Acute physiology and chronic health evaluation: A physiologically based classification system. Crit Care Med 1981; 9:591–96.
22. Zimmerman JE (ed). APACHE III study design: analytic plan for evaluation of severity and outcome. Crit Care Med 1989; 17:S169–S221.
23. Sirio CA, Knaus WA, Wagner DP, et al. Variation in risk adjusted hospital death rates: A national sample of intensive care units. Clin Res 1990; 38:281A.
24. Knaus WA, Draper EA, Wagner DP. An evaluation of outcome from intensive care in major medical centers. Ann Intern Med 1986; 104:410–18.
25. Examples of monitoring and evaluation in special care units. Joint Commission on Accreditation of Healthcare Organizations. Chicago, Illinois. 1988; 45–52.
26. Sax FL, Charlson ME. Utilization of critical care units: a prospective study of physician triage and patient outcome. Arch Intern Med 1987; 147:929–34.
27. Singer DE, Carr PL, Mulley AG, et al. Rationing intensive care: physician responses to a resource shortage. N Engl J Med 1983; 309:1155–60.
28. Strauss MJ, LoGerfo JP, Yeltatzie JA, et al. Rationing of intensive care unit: identifying patients at high risk of unexpected death or unit readmission. Am J Med 1988; 84:863–69.
29. Bloomfield H, Moskowitz MA. Discharge decision-making in a medical intensive care unit: identifying patients at high risk of unexpected death or unit readmission. Am J Med 1988; 84:863–69.
30. Wagner DP, Knaus WA, Draper EA, et al. Identification of low-risk monitor patients within a medical-surgical intensive care unit. Med Care 1983; 21:425–30.
31. Wagner DP, Knaus WA, Draper EA. Identification of low-risk monitor admissions to medical-surgical ICU's. Chest 1987; 92:423–28.

32. McClish DK, Powell S. How well can physicians estimate mortality in a medical intensive care unit? Med Decis Making 1989; 9:125–30.
33. Brannen AL, Godfrey LJ, Goetter WE. Prediction of outcome from critical illness; a comparison of clinical judgement with a prediction rule. Arch Intern Med 1989; 149:1083–86.
34. Chang RW, Lee B, Jacobs S, et al. Accuracy of decisions to withdraw therapy in critically ill patients: clinical judgment versus a computer model. Crit Care Med 1989; 17:1091–97.
35. Bion JF, Edlin SA, Ramsay G, et al. Validation of a prognostic score in critically ill patients undergoing transport. Brit Med J 1985; 291:432–39.
36. Chang RWS, Jacobs S, Lee B. Use of APACHE II severity of disease classification to identify intensive-care unit patients who would not benefit from total parenteral nutrition. Lancet 1986; ii:1483–90.
37. Ruark JE, Raffin TA. The Stanford University Medical Center Committee on Ethics: Initiating and withdrawing life support: Principles and practice in adult medicine. N Engl J Med 1988; 318:25–34.
38. Griner PF. The relationship between managerial and clinical decision making in the hospital. Med Decis Making 1988; 8:151–68.
39. Kellie S, Kelly JT. Medicare peer review organization preprocedure review criteria—an analysis of criteria for three procedures. JAMA 1991; 265:1265–1270.
40. Wennburg JE. Unwanted variations in the rules of practice. JAMA 1991; 65:1306–1307.
41. Dubois RW, Rogers WH, Moxley JH, et al. Hospital inpatient mortality: is it a predictor of quality? N Engl J Med 1987; 317:1674–80.
42. Dubois RW, Brook RH. Preventable deaths; who, how often, and why? Ann Intern Med 1988; 109:582–89.
43. Kahn KL, Brook RH, Draper D, et al. Interpreting hospital mortality data: how can we proceed? JAMA 1988; 260:3625–3628.
44. Knaus WA, Draper EA, Wagner DP, et al. An evaluation of outcome from intensive care in major medical centers. Ann Intern Med 1986; 104:410–18.
45. Draper EA, Russo M, Wagner DP, et al. Predicting tomorrow's therapy using today's APACHE II score. Clin Res 1990; 38:NEED.
46. Goldfield N, Nash D. Providing quality care: The challenge to clinicians; American College of Physicians, Philadelphia, PA, 1989; 159:452.
47. Sivak ED, Perez-Trepichio A. Quality assessment in the medical intensive care unit: evolution of a data model. Cleveland Clin J Med 1990; 57:273–79.
48. Murphy DJ, Cluff L (eds). SUPPORT: Study to understand prognosis and preferences for outcomes and risk of treatments: Study design. J Clin Epidemiol 1990:43(suppl);1S-123S.

Chapter 17
Automatic Extraction of Intensity-Intervention Scores From a Computerized Surgical Intensive Case Unit Flowsheet

M. Michael Shabot, Beverley J. Leyerle, and Mark LoBue

Intensive care currently accounts for approximately 20% of hospital expenditures in the United States [1]. While new modes of therapy and life support have become available, relatively modest progress has been made in quantifying the indications for and effectiveness of intensive care. In 1974 Cullen introduced the Therapeutic Intervention Scoring System (TISS), a method in which one to four points were assigned for each of 57 types of patient care interventions, depending on the intensity of the scored activity [2]. The TISS was intended to help determine appropriate use of intensive care facilities, provide information on effective nurse staffing ratios, validate a subjective classification of severity of illness, and analyze intensive care costs in relation to the amount of care offered.

Physiologic measurements were added by Knaus with the APACHE (Acute Physiology, and Chronic Health Evaluation) system in 1981, which scores 38 data items [3]. Using APACHE scores to normalize severity of illness, mortality rates have been compared for different hospitals in the United States [4] and between hospitals in the United States and France [5]. A Simplified Acute Physiology Score (SAPS) reported to be equivalent to APACHE was described by Le Gall in 1984 [6]. This system scores 14 ICU measurements, including age, heart rate, blood pressure, urine output, Glasgow Coma Score, and several basic laboratory tests. In 1985, Knaus introduced the APACHE II scoring system, which reduced the data gathering requirements to 12 acute physiologic parameters, five chronic health indicators, and an indicator for emergency or elective surgery. [7].

These measurement tools require that a manual scoring form be accurately completed by an individual familiar with the patient, the clinical re-

Adapted with permission from Shabot MM, Leyerle BJ, LoBue M: Automatic extraction of intensity intervention scores from a computerized surgical ICU flowsheet. Am J Surg 1987; 154:1,72.

cord, and ICU activities. Keene, in a 1983 update to the TISS which increased the number of scored interventions to 76, recommended that "data collectors should have a critical care background" [8]. This time-consuming activity required of highly trained and expensive personnel has likely limited the use of these scoring systems.

In order to automate the collection of patient acuity data, we have implemented a computerized intensity-intervention scoring system (CIIS). CIIS scores are automatically extracted from electronic flowsheets which are maintained by an ICU patient data management system [9,10]. The purpose of this study was prospectively to compare automatic CIIS scores with manual TISS scores and with outcome measures such as ICU mortality, hospital mortality, ICU length of stay, and hospital length of stay. In addition, CIIS scores were compared to a subjective classification of patients based on appropriate hospital location to receive care.

Methods

Patient Data Management System

Critical care flowsheets were maintained electronically by an on-line computer system (HP 78709A PDMS Patient Data Management System, Hewlett-Packard Company, Waltham, MA). In 1991, this system was replaced with the CareVue 9000 Clinical Information System (Hewlett-Packard Company, Andover, MA). These systems operate in two identical ten-bed Surgical Intensive Care Units (SICUs), located on different floors of the Medical Center. Physiologic data, including rates, pressures, urinary output, and core bladder temperature were captured by interfaces to bedside monitors and electronic urimeters. Clinical laboratory and blood gas results were automatically transmitted to the PDMS over data links from other hospital computers. All bedside data was validated by a nurse prior to posting on the electronic flowsheet. Vasoactive drug doses, derived hemodynamic variables, Glasgow Coma Scores, intake and output records, and results of bedside nursing activities were calculated or recorded by the system. Patient records were available at bedside video terminals, and permanent hard-copy flowcharts were printed by SICU laser printers every 12 hours [10].

Computerized Scoring System

A computer program extracted CIIS scores from the electronic flowsheets at 10 A.M. daily for the prior 24 hr period, ending at 7 A.M. The 3-hr scoring delay permitted inclusion of laboratory results for blood drawn before 7 A.M. Fourteen physiologic data items were scored according to the SAPS method of Le Gall [6], which assigns zero points for normal data and one to four points for progressively abnormal data (Table 17.1). In accordance with Le Gall's method, the scoring program searched for the

Table 17.1. Computerized Scoring System*

Physiologic variables scored by the method of Le Gall et al. [6]	
Age	Hematocrit
Heart rate	White blood count
Systolic blood pressure	Serum glucose
Body temperature	Serum potassium
Urinary output	Serum sodium
Blood urea nitrogen	Serum bicarbonate
Spontaneous respiratory rate or ventilation or CPAP	Glasgow Coma Score

Intervention variables in point scoring method	
Admission	4 points if present
Plan of care revision	4 points if present
Discharge	4 points if present
Arterial pressure catheter	3 points if present
Pulmonary artery catheter	4 points if present
Central venous pressure catheter	2 points if present
Intracranial pressure catheter	4 points if present
Oxygen source	
ventilator, ambu bag	4 points if present
T tube	3 points if present
mask, cool mist, heated aerosol	2 points if present
rebreathing or nonrebreathing mask	2 points if present
nasal prongs	1 point if present
room air	0 points if present
Different atrial arrhythmias (n)	points = n × 1
Different ventricular arrhythmias (n)	points = n × 2
Code blue's (n)	points = n × 4
Vasoactive IV drugs (n)	points = n × 4
Antiarrhythmic IV drugs (n)	points = n × 3
Miscellaneous IV drugs (n)	points = n × 2
Vital signs (n)	points = n ÷ 4
PA measurements (n)	points = n ÷ 2
Cardiac outputs (n)	points = n × 1
Neurologic checks (n)	points = n ÷ 6
Blood gases (n)	points = n × 1
Blood transfusions (n)	points = n × 1
IV bottles (n)	points = n ÷ 2
Hyperalimentation bottles (n)	points = n × 4
Enteral feeding bottles (n)	points = n × 2
Hemodialysis (n)	points = n × 4
Chest tubes (n)	points = n × 2
GI drainage tubes (n)	points = n × 1
Wound irrigations (n)	points = n × 2
Beside glucose checks (n)	points = n × 1
Transfers for tests (n)	points = n × 4
Seizure episodes (n)	points = n × 2
Weight measurements (n)	points = n × 2

*CPAP, continuous positive air-way pressure; GI, gastrointestinal; IV, intravenous; PA, pulmonary artery.

most abnormal validated data points available during the 24-hr measurement period.

Thirty-one indicators of nursing interventions were abstracted from the flowsheet and scored according to preconfigured formulas (Table 17.1). These formulas were designed to reflect the amount of nursing time required to accomplish the activity being scored. Thus, the original Cullen-Civetta TISS was enhanced with a quantitative component, known as the Quantitative Therapeutic Intervention Scoring System (QTISS). The SAPS and QTISS scores were summed to produce the CIIS score.

In 1991, coincident with the implementation of the CareVue 9000 system, it became possible routinely to collect the APACHE II chronic health and surgery indicators as part of the house staff s computer admission note. At that time, automatic APACHE II scoring was added to the severity extraction system. From that point on, independent SAPS, APACHE II, and QTISS scores have been collected from every patient, every day.

Manual TISS Scoring System

Manual TISS scores were collected quarterly on a hospital-wide basis for purposes of patient acuity measurement and nurse staffing adjustment. During measurement periods, a Cedars-Sinai modified TISS form with 113 check-off boxes was completed daily for each patient by SICU nurses. These TISS forms were scored remotely by an outside agency, and neither TISS scores nor CIIS scores were available to the SICU staff.

Patient Group I

A routine quarterly TISS study was scheduled for a seven day period, 1/2/86–1/8/86. During that interval consecutive SICU patients were scored with both the manual TISS and the PDMS CIIS. Data for 105 patient days were collected, and comparisons between daily TISS and CIIS scores were performed for both SICUs as a whole and for each ten-bed unit separately.

Patient Group II

CIIS scores, patient outcome, and patient classification data were collected prospectively on consecutive SICU patients for a 6-week period, 2/10/86–3/31/86. Outcome measures included SICU mortality, hospital mortality, SICU length of stay (LOS), and hospital LOS. For 533 of the 784 patient days, patients were classified by one of the authors (M.M.S.) according to the type of hospital care unit which would have been appropriate for the patient during the previous night. This classification was based on his physical examination, resident rounds, and review of flowsheet records. Appropriate care unit locations included the SICU, a surgical Stepdown Unit (unavailable at Cedars-Sinai) and the general Floor. The Stepdown Unit was assumed to have a nurse staffing ratio intermediate between the SICU and the Floor, and the capability for ECG monitoring without invasive monitoring or vasoactive drug infusions.

Statistical Analysis

TISS and CIIS scores for Group I patients were compared using linear regression analysis. For Group II patients, CIIS scores were compared to various outcome measures with the Kruskal-Wallis nonparametric analy-

8 SICU CSMC INTENSITY-INTERVENTION SCORE
From 18 Feb 93 07:00 to 19 Feb 93 07:00
12:37 PM Mon, 08 Mar, 1993

	1 8246	2 8250	3 8253	4 8258	5 8260	6 8262	7 8266	8 8268	9 8272	10 8276
Room										
Last Name										
First Name										
ID number										
Diagnosis or Procedure	OLTX	Craniotomy	S/P OLTX	Resection of AAA	Lumbar La minectomy	OLTX/Kidney Transplant	Tracheostomy, phar yngeal ab	Repair Rt. Femoral Artery A	Kidney Tr ansplant	ESLD
Days / Hours in ICU	7 24	1 15	65 24	2 24	1 10	60 24	5 24	2 24	1 16	2 24
Surgeon										
Service / Trauma	OLT	NS	OLT	GS	NS	OLT	ENT	VASC	VASC	GS
Age	48 1	72 3	57 2	72 3	73 3	44 0	68 3	79 4	36 0	55 1
Heart Rate	58 2	110 0	98 0	93 0	94 0	118 2	127 2	67 2	120 2	114 2
Systolic BP	162 2	165 2	130 0	179 2	138 0	108 0	188 2	123 0	167 2	130 0
Resp. Rate	26 1	VENT 3	VENT 3	36 3	8 2	VENT 3	44 3	38 3	30 1	24 0
Temperature	99.5 0	101.1 0	99.7 0	101.4 1	98.8 0	101.8 1	100.6 0	100.6 0	99.5 0	99.5 0
Glascow Coma Score	13 1	11 1	11 1	15 0	15 0	11 1	10 2	15 0	15 0	15 0
Urine Volume	2639 0	1622 0	1038 0	2621 0	4526 1	10 4	4692 1	986 0	12928 2	752 0
Hct	41.9 0	34.8 0	24.8 2	30.7 0	26.2 2	35.5 0	41.3 0	29.0 2	36.2 0	31.5 0
WBC	11.5 0	16.8 1	14.0 0	20.4 2	8.3 0	11.7 0	9.3 0	6.4 0	9.1 0	6.8 0
BUN	106.0 4	43.0 3	89.0 4	35.0 2	8.0 1	50.0 3	9.0 1	20.0 1	33.0 2	108.0 4
Glucose	195.0 0	296.0 1	163.0 0	116.0 0	251.0 0	126.0 0	290.0 1	88.0 0	343.0 1	126.0 0
Na+	140 0	143 0	141 0	140 0	137 0	129 2	137 0	138 0	139 0	137 0
K+	4.4 0	4.8 0	3.2 1	3.9 0	4.1 0	4.1 0	3.7 0	4.0 0	3.2 1	3.2 1
HCO3	24.0 0	20.0 1	29.0 0	20.0 1	25.0 0	15.0 1	26.0 0	20.0 1	25.0 0	15.0 1
Intensity score	11	15	13	14	9	17	15	13	11	9
Admission	no 0	yes 4	no 0	no 0	yes 4	no 0	no 0	no 0	yes 4	no 0
Plan of Care	no 0	yes 4	no 0	no 0	yes 4	no 0	no 0	no 0	yes 4	no 0
Discharge	no 0	no 0	no 0	no 0	no 0	no 0	no 0	no 0	no 0	no 0
Art. Line	yes 3	yes 3	yes 3	yes 3	yes 3	yes 3	no 0	yes 3	yes 3	yes 3
PA Line	yes 4	no 0	no 0	yes 4	no 0	yes 4	no 0	yes 4	no 0	yes 4
CVP Line	no 0	no 0	yes 2	no 0	no 0	no 0	no 0	no 0	yes 2	no 0
ICP Line	no 0	no 0	no 0	no 0	no 0	no 0	no 0	no 0	no 0	no 0
# of Diff. Atrial Arr.	1 3	...	...	...	2 6	...	...	1 3	1 3	...
# of Diff. Ventr. Arr.	...	...	...	...	...	...	...	...	...	...
# of CODE BLUE's	...	...	...	...	...	...	...	...	...	...
# of Vasoact. Drugs	1 4	...	1 4	2 8	...	2 8	...	1 4	1 4	...
# of Antiarr. Drugs	...	...	...	...	...	...	...	...	...	...
# of Misc. IV Drugs	...	...	...	...	...	...	...	...	...	...
# Vital Signs	24 6	24 6	22 5	24 6	10 2	33 8	23 5	25 6	21 5	17 4
# PA Measurements	24 12	...	...	24 12	...	33 16	...	25 12	...	14 7
# Cardiac Outputs	4 4	...	...	4 4	...	4 4	...	6 6	...	5 5
# Neuro Checks	9 1	13 2	6 1	7 1	6 1	10 1	13 2	9 1	8 1	9 1
# Art. Blood Gas	4 4	5 5	5 5	...	...	4 4	...	...	2 2	3 3
O2 Source	1 2	1 4	1 4	1 1	1 1	1 4	1 2	1 1	1 1	1 1
# Blood Transfusion	...	...	...	6 6	...	...	...	...	...	2 2
# of I/O Bottles	20 10	11 5	25 12	9 4	11 5	20 10	8 4	11 5	24 12	16 8
# Hyperal Bottles	...	...	...	5 20	...	...	4 16	3 12	...	4 16
Enteral Feeding	...	...	...	...	...	...	...	...	...	...
Hemodialysis	...	...	...	1 4	...	...	...	...	...	...
# of Glucochecks	5 5	3 3	6 6	...	2 2	6 6	5 5	1 1	3 3	4 4
# Chest Tubes	...	...	...	1 2	...	3 6	...	...	...	...
# GI Drain Tubes	5 5	4 4	5 5	1 1	1 1	3 3	...	...	1 1	2 2
Wound Irrigation	...	...	...	...	...	...	...	...	...	...
# Transfers for Test	...	...	...	3 12	...	...	...	...	2 8	4 16
Seizures	...	...	...	...	...	...	...	...	...	...
Daily Weight	...	...	1 2	...	...	1 2	...	...	...	1 2
Interventions score	63	40	93	50	23	95	30	46	53	78
TOTAL CIIS score	74	55	106	64	32	112	45	59	64	87
APS Points	10	15	12	13	4	20	12	9	12	12
Chronic Health Points	2	2	5	0	0	5	0	0	2	5
Age Points	2	5	3	5	5	0	5	6	0	3
APACHE II Score	14	22	20	18	9	25	17	15	14	20

8 SICU STATS	UNIT CENSUS	# TRAUMA PATIENTS	TOTAL CIIS	AVERAGE CIIS/PT	TOTAL APACHE	AVERAGE APACHE	AVERAGE AGE	# ADMITS	# VENTS	# ART LINES	# PA LINES	# ICP LINES	# IV DRUGS
	10	0	698	69.8	174	17.4	60.4	3	3	9	5	0	6

Figure 17.1. Computerized intensity-intervention score report.

sis of variance. Frequency distributions for patient care location classifications were analyzed with the Mann-Whitney U-test. The Bonferroni correction was used for all multiple comparisons.

Results

A CIIS report was generated daily for each SICU (Figure 17.1). Individual SAPS ("Intensity"), QTISS ("Interventions"), and APACHE II patient scores were calculated, and from them various ICU statistics were derived. The CIIS report requires many thousands of patient data file accesses, and currently uses about 2 min of background computer time. CIIS results were stored in a disk file for subsequent analysis.

Group I

A bivariate plot of manual TISS scores versus CIIS scores was constructed for the 7-day test period (Figure 17.2). Linear regression for data from all 20 SICU beds yielded the following formula: Manual $TISS = 0.51 \times CIIS + 16.1$, with a correlation coefficient of 0.77. However, regression analysis for each SICU separately yielded correlation coefficients of 0.89 and 0.60, indicating a significant difference between the SICUs in the way the manual TISS forms were completed ($p < .005$).

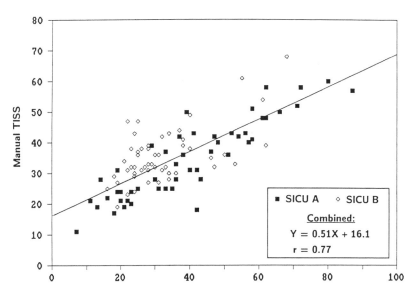

Figure 17.2. Manual TISS scores versus CIIS scores. SICU A, $r = 0.89$; SICU B, $r = 0.60$ ($p < .0005$).

Group II

CIIS scores were collected from 343 patients over 784 patient-days. A total of 323 patients had complete data sets, including the first SICU day. Outcome data for these 323 patients were compared to the CIIS score for each patient's first SICU day (day 1) and for the maximum CIIS score for a patient's entire SICU stay (Table 17.2). Statistically significant differ-

Table 17.2. Computerized Intensity-Intervention Score Versus Patient Outcome

	SICU death	Hospital death	Total deaths	Survival
Patients (n)	20	6	26	297
Day 1 CIIS[1] score	67.5*	35.8**	60.2*	33.3
Maximum CIIS score	74*	37.8**	65.6*	34.1
SICU LOS (d)	12***	3	9.9	1.8
Hospital LOS (d)	21.5***	45.3	27	13.6
Age (yr)	72.1****	54.5	68	63.6
Sex (male/female)	11/9	2/4	13/13	163/134

*$p \leq .016$ for SICU death versus all others and for total deaths versus survival.
** p not significant for hospital death versus survival.
Bivariate regressions (comparisons other than the following were not significant):
***$p \leq .001$ for surgical intensive care unit (SICU) length of stay (LOS) versus computerized intensity-intervention score (CIIS) and for hospital LOS versus CIIS.
****$p \leq .05$ for hospital LOS versus age.
[1] CIIS = computerized intensity-intervention scoring.

ences in the distributions of both day 1 CIIS and maximum CIIS scores were observed between those patients dying in the SICU and those who left the SICU alive ($p \leq .016$). No CIIS differences were detected for patients suffering late hospital death compared to patients discharged alive. Regressions of SICU LOS and hospital LOS against day 1 CIIS, max-

Table 17.3. System of Computerized Intensity-Intervention Scoring (CIIS) Versus Appropriate Patient Care Location

Appropriate patient care location	Patient days	CIIS	
		Mean	SD
SICU	371	50.7	17.5
Stepdown unit	148	24.3	6.4
Floor	14	15.1	4.1

*$p < .001$ for the difference between CIIS distributions.
SD, standard deviation; SICU, surgical intensive case unit.

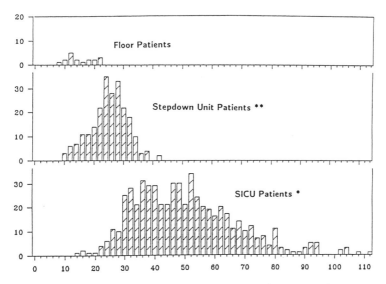

Figure 17.3. Frequency distributions of CIIS scores by appropriate care area. *p<.0001 for SICU versus Stepdown Unit. *p<.0001 for SICU versus Floor. **p<.0001 for Stepdown Unit versus Floor.

imum CIIS, age, and sex yielded strongly significant correlations only with CIIS scores (p ≤ .001). There was a modest association between age and hospital LOS (p ≤ .05).

Analysis of the 533 patients classified for appropriate patient care location revealed that 148 (27.7%) could have been cared for in a Stepdown Unit and that 14 (2.6%) could have received Floor care (Table 17.3). The CIIS scores for these patient care classifications were significantly different (p < .0001). Frequency distributions of CIIS scores per location revealed statistically significant differences for SICU patients versus Stepdown Unit patients, SICU versus Floor care patients, and Stepdown Unit versus Floor care patients (Figure 17.3).

Comments

There are several factors which favor the expanded use of intensity-intervention scoring systems for hospitalized patients. The cost of intensive care, coupled with limitations in health care funding, requires physicians, nurses, and administrative staff to evaluate potential ICU admissions critically. If safe and effective care can be provided in a less acute setting, there is little to be gained by admitting a patient to an

ICU. As patients are placed into graded levels of hospital care, it is becoming increasingly important to audit the results of this care. Is Stepdown Unit care as effective as ICU care for some patients? Which patients belong on the general Floor rather than the ICU or Stepdown Unit?

To answer such questions objectively, a quantitative scoring system is required. The results of care within a hospital and between hospitals can be accurately measured only when severity of illness is normalized or controlled. Knaus has stressed the importance of measuring the relationship between an ICUs case-mix and its death rate as an indicator of quality of care [11]. Control for severity of illness is also important in the evaluation of new critical care therapies. If patient study groups are not equally ill, the effect or lack of effect of a new therapy may be easily misinterpreted.

Financially it is now important for hospital management to understand the relationship between severity of illness and resource use within diagnosis related groups (DRGs). Horn found that the DRGs alone explained only 28% of the variability of resource use per case, while DRGs adjusted for severity of illness explained 61% of variations [12]. Acuity-based staffing has become important in order to deliver care which is both medically effective and cost effective.

While all these forces favor the establishment of standardized scoring systems, the skilled but manual labor involved has been a limiting factor. If these scores are used to determine staffing ratios, there is considerable risk of bias if bedside nurses complete the forms. Finally, the delay required to score manual forms and tabulate the results has precluded their use for real time staffing adjustments.

We have presented an automated system of extracting intensity-intervention scores in real time from a computerized SICU flowsheet. The method insures consistent scoring, freedom from observer bias, and it requires no manual labor. The system directly reflects the care that is recorded in the chart and in that sense it rewards good charting practices. These automated scores correlate well with manual TISS scores but do not suffer from ICU to ICU scoring variations. CIIS scores clearly reflect ICU mortality and length of stay. Of note is the fact that the CIIS score on the first SICU day is highly predictive in ICU and in-hospital deaths [13]. First day scores may thus be useful in normalizing prospective critical care research studies.

While our method was optimized for an electronic ICU flowchart, it could be extended to Floor care documents when these areas are converted to computerized charting. With a consistent electronic scoring system in place hospital-wide, it will be possible to allocate staff and other health care resources in real time based on severity of illness and intensity of interventions. Indeed, this enhanced management capability will likely be the driving force for the general introduction of computerized clinical charting systems.

Summary

Systems which objectively score severity of illness and intensity of patient care interventions have been used to guide the appropriate use of intensive care facilities, provide information on nurse staffing ratios, validate subjective classifications of patient illness, and normalize scientific and financial studies for severity of illness. Existing scoring systems require a well-trained observer to perform a thorough chart review to complete manual scoring forms. We have designed a new system in which computerized intensity-intervention scores are automatically extracted from electronic ICU flowsheets, eliminating both manual labor and potential observer variation. In prospective studies these computerized scores correlated well with manual TISS scores, ICU mortality, ICU length of stay, hospital length of stay, and a subjective classification of patients to graded levels of hospital care. Such automated scores may be used for real time allocation of health care resources and normalization of prospective studies for severity of illness.

Acknowledgments

The authors wish to recognize the expert statistical support of Moraye Bear and the Cedars-Sinai Scientific Data Center.

References

1. Russell LB. The role of technology assessment in cost control. In McNeil BJ, Cravalho EG (eds): Critical Issues in Medical Technology. Boston: Auburn House, 1982; pp 129–138.
2. Cullen DJ, Civetta JM, Briggs BA, Ferrara LC. Therapeutic intervention scoring system: a method for quantitative comparison of patient care. Crit Care Med 1974; 2:57–60.
3. Knaus WA, Zimmerman JE, Wagner DP, Draper EA, Lawrence DE. APACHE—acute physiology and chronic health evaluation: a physiologically based classification system. Crit Care Med 1981; 9:591–597.
4. Knaus WA, Draper EA, Wagner DP, et al. Evaluating outcome from intensive care: A preliminary multihospital comparison. Crit Care Med 1982 10:491–496.
5. Knaus WA, Le Gall JR, Wagner DP, et al. A comparison of intensive care in the U.S.A. and France. Lancet 1982 Sept 18; 2:642–646.
6. Le Gall JR, Loirat P, Alperovitch A, et al. A simplified acute physiology score for ICU patients. Crit Care Med 1984; 2:975–977.
7. Knaus WA, Draper EA, Wagner DP, Zimmerman JE. APACHE II: A severity of disease classification system. Crit Care Med 1985; 3:818–829.
8. Keene AR, Cullen DJ. Therapeutic Intervention Scoring System: Update 1983. Crit Care Med 1983; 11:1–3.

9. Shabot MM. Software for computers and calculators in critical care medicine. Software in Healthcare 1985; 3:26–29.

10. Shabot MM, Carlton PD, Sadoff S, Nolan-Avila L. Graphical reports and displays for complex ICU data: A new, flexible and configurable method. Comput Methods Programs Biomed 1986; 22:111–116.

11. Knaus WA, Draper EA, Wagner DP. Toward quality review in intensive care: The APACHE system. QRB 1983; 9:196–204.

12. Horn SD, Sharkey PD, Chambers AF, Horn RA. Severity of illness within DRGs: Impact on prospective payment. Am J Public Health 1985; 75:1195–1199.

13. Shabot MM, Leyerle B, LoBue M, Scarlata D, Bolus, R. First day intensity-intervention score predicts ICU and in-hospital deaths. Crit Care Med 1988;16:412.

Chapter 18
Quality Assurance and Utilization Assessment: The Major By-Products of an Intensive Care Unit Clinical Information System

M. Michael Shabot, H. Scott Bjerke,
Mark LoBue, and Beverley J. Leyerle

Introduction

The power of computerized Clinical Information Systems (CIS) has yet to be tapped by most hospital Quality Assurance (QA) and Utilization Review (UR) departments. The CIS provides an economical and reliable means by which key clinical data can be extracted from the electronic chart and utilized for quality and utilization analyses. In comparison with current manual methods of extracting data by chart audits, the electronic method is not only faster, it also allows for *every* chart to be audited against standards for efficiency and quality of care. The science of industrial quality management is well known and appreciated in most other industries—many agree that the time is at hand for using these techniques in health care institutions [1]. The Joint Commission for Accredation of Health Care Organizations (JCAHO), the Health Care Financing Authority (HCFA), and other regulatory agencies now require detailed information and trends about outcomes that can not be easily obtained by traditional, tedious methods of manual chart review. However, this volume of data can objectively be extracted from the electronic record provided by a comprehensive CIS. A reduction in the number of hours spent by QA and UR nurses culling data from charts could be channeled into more meaningful activities of data interpretation and reporting. In this paper we describe the use of CIS-derived data for secondary QA and UR activities. ICUs that have a CIS are ready to enjoy the benefits such a system can provide for daily monitoring of patient care and resource activities.

Adapted with permission from an article published by the American Medical Informatics Association, Inc., 1992.

The CIS as a Tool for Quality Assurance and Utilization Assessment

The Surgical Intensive Care Units (SICUs) at Cedars-Sinai Medical Center in Los Angeles, California, have utilized a CIS for routine patient care charting for the past seven years. The current system is the Hewlett Packard CareVue 9000 System (Hewlett-Packard Company, Waltham, MA). In 1986, we wrote patient data management system (PDMS) software which filtered through all flowsheet data daily in order to extract patient-specific indices of severity of illness and resource utilization [2]. These indices have been combined with information extracted from other hospital databases, including hospital outcome and nosocomial infection data [3]. At the present time, this database contains the records of over 10,000 consecutive SICU patients requiring 27,000 days of care. Analyses of many indicators of quality of care and utilization have been performed on this data.

Severity Scoring

Intensive care unit quality control requires a continuous quality improvement program with ongoing assessment of outcomes. In order to measure outcomes and appropriateness objectively for ICU care, it is necessary to determine the severity of illness of patients on admission to the ICU and during their stay. Several measurement tools have been introduced for this purpose. Although the APACHE II scoring system is popular, in 1985 we selected for our SICU the Simplified Acute Physiology Score (SAPS) as described by Le Gall [4]. SAPS scores 14 common ICU measurements, including age, heart rate, blood pressure, urine output, Glasgow Coma Score, and results of several basic laboratory tests. All 14 SAPS parameters were already being charted by our nurses as part of the routine electronic flowsheet. Therefore, we could perform SAPS calculations automatically with no extra data entry and no dedicated personnel. At the same time, we began to calculate a quantitative version of the Therapeutic Intervention Scoring System (QTISS)[2]. The QTISS provides a measure of intensity of services delivered to a patient. When summed, the severity and intensity scores produced the Computerized Intensity-Intervention Score (CIIS). In 1988, we reported that the CIIS on the first ICU day was a reliable predictor of ICU and in-hospital deaths [5].

In 1989, The French Multicenter Group of ICU Research reported the pooled SAPS-adjusted mortality rates for 3,687 patients from 38 French ICUs [6]. For the first time, the scores of surgical patients were separated from medical patients so that distinct subgroups could be examined. This provided an opportunity to compare our ongoing outcome analyses

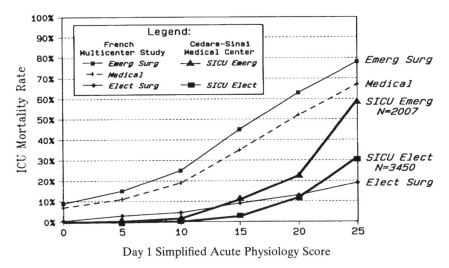

Figure 18.1. Severity-adjusted survival curves for Cedars-Sinai SICU and French multicenter study patients.

with the French experience. Figure 18.1 compares the severity-adjusted outcomes of approximately 5,500 Cedars-Sinai SICU patients with the French outcomes. There are likely to be differences in case selection, management, and ICU admission and discharge policies which account for some of the differences between our outcomes and the French experience. However, the data provide an ongoing standard that the SICU can use in future years to monitor the severity of patients admitted to the unit and the efficacy of the care delivered. Patient's are concerned about the overall outcome of the process of care, e.g. *death and survival*, and these scoring methods provide a way of monitoring that process as a whole. If a decline in severity-adjusted survival is observed for a certain period of time, detailed review for contributing factors may be undertaken. The contribution of automated, CIS derived scoring is that these analyses of

Table 18.1. Severity and Utilization Trends 1986–90

Fiscal Year	1986–87	1987–88	1988–89	1989–90
Admissions	2,521	2,393	2,062	2,227
Days of care	5,710	6,066	6,216	6,144
Trauma days	1,313	1,409	1,752	1,920
Mean ICU stay (days)	2.27	2.53	3.02	2.77
Mean SAPS	10.0	10.8	11.0	11.3
Mean QTISS	27.7	28.8	29.8	30.9
Mean CIIS	37.7	39.6	40.8	42.2

total quality assurance can proceed in the background and, in a continuous manner, provide both periodic reports and more urgent warnings if unfavorable trends are detected.

These standardized scores have also provided a way for us to monitor global trends in severity of illness and utilization of resources for our patients. Over the past several years, we have noted a progressive rise in severity of illness, a trend which has been appreciated by many but documented only occasionally (Table 18.1).

These data indicate that severity of illness is rising year by year and that trauma care days are increasing, but that length of stay has begun to decrease. To some degree the recent improvement in efficiency is a result of feedback from our prior CIS generated experience with outcome and utilization information.

Glucose Control Study

In 1990 the SICU was asked by the Nutritional Support Committee to determine whether problems with glucose control were occurring in patients receiving IV alimentation in the perioperative period. It was well known that perioperative disturbances in endogenous catacholamine and glucocorticoid metabolism impair the body's ability to handle a glucose load. The committee wondered whether it might be better to forgo nutritional support in the perioperative period than to risk "wide fluctuations in serum glucose," The question was a good one, but one which would formerly have been impossible to answer without manually reviewing hundreds or perhaps thousands of charts. However, we were able to provide a definitive answer with simple queries of our CIS and laboratory in-

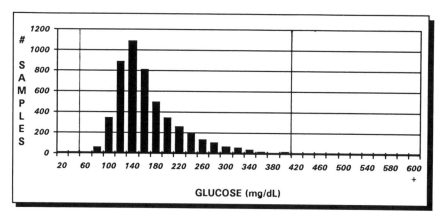

Figure 18.2. Histogram of blood glucose values for 1,189 consecutive SICU patients.

Table 18.2. Incidence of Critically Abnormal Glucose Values

	No. Patients	No. Glucoses	>400 mg/dl	<40 mg/dl
IV nutrition	89	996	17 (1.7%)	0 (0.0%)
No IV nutrition	1,040	3,989	28 (0.7%)	3 (0.1%)
p value			.003	NS

formation system (Flexilab, Sunquest Information Systems, Tucson, AZ). These queries collated laboratory blood glucose results with CIS information on each patient's IV alimentation status and severity of illness.

We examined glucose values of all patients cared for in the SICU over a six-month period from October 1, 1989, to March 31, 1990. We found a total of 4,985 glucose determinations taken on 1,189 consecutive patients. Only 48 (0.96 %) of the glucose values were found to be in the critically abnormal range, over 400 mg/dl or below 40 mg/dl (Figure 18.2). Nearly all critical values represented hyperglycemia, as shown in Table 18.2. While the incidence of hyperglycemia was greater in patients receiving perioperative IV nutrition, no detrimental effects occurred which would support discontinuing nutrition prior to surgery. Of the 23 patients who had one or more critical glucose values, only 9 patients were on IV alimentation. These 9 patients had a mean SAPS of 15.2, while the 14 hyperglycemic patients not receiving IV alimentation had a mean SAPS of 10.8 (p < .001). We then stratified all measured glucose values by the SAPS severity of illness on the day of sampling. This revealed that higher glucose levels correlated directly with increasing severity of illness (Figure 18.3). This suggests that the relative glucose intolerance noted in total

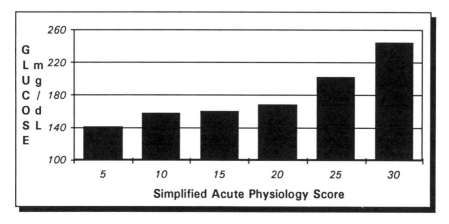

Figure 18.3. Relationship between glucose level and severity of illness.

parenteral nutrition (TPN) patients may be due to their underlying severity of illness rather than TPN per se. These results confirm the benefits of the CIS, which in a short time answered a specific clinical question, and enhanced our understanding of patients at risk for serious glucose problems.

Outcome Control Chart

Control charts are commonly used in industrial quality control, but seldom seen in hospitals. The charts, which depict outcome measurements over time, are valuable indicators of trends, favorable or otherwise. Signifiicant adverse deviations from the long-term average demand closer investigating. The following graph (Fig. 18.4) is a control chart for SICU mortality over the same period as the severity-adjusted outcomes above. The upward peak in mortality noted in the summer of 1988 was probably related to an outbreak of nosocomial infections, in part identified by this and corresponding infectious disease data.

Realized and Potential Benefits of an ICU CIS

An ongoing program of ICU quality improvement must begin with objective measurements of the processes and outcomes of care. This is in contrast with traditional methods of medical quality assurance, in which individuals, rather the processes, are analyzed [7]. Mortality control charts, analyses of severity adjusted mortality and correlation of adverse clinical events with severity of illness are starting points for effective quality assurance. Many other aspects of ICU care can and must be evaluated,

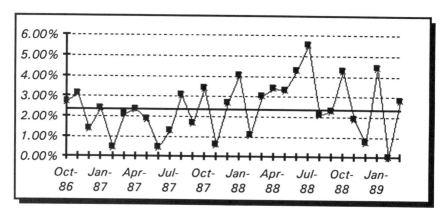

Figure 18.4. SICU mortality rate control chart, 1986–1989.

but first they must be measured. It is for this reason that a comprehensive ICU CIS is so valuable: as it automatically gathers crucially needed census, intensity and intervention data in a hectic environment that is otherwise poorly suited for administrative data collection.

Although many feel that the primary benefit of an ICU CIS is the maintenance of a well-organized, legible patient care flowsheet, we believe that this represents only the most superficial level of CIS functionality. We have programmed our CIS automatically to provide a second level of function in the daily measurement of severity of illness and intensity of interventions. We find these assessments to be invaluable in the daily management of a busy ICU, including triage of patients into and out of the unit and allocation of nursing/physician resources. Finally we have utilized CIS-derived analyses to provide a third level of ICU data management, the evaluation of long-term outcomes (Figure 18.5).

The ongoing mass of severity and intensity data, when combined with mortality, nosocomial infection and other available hospital data, is a powerful tool in the assessment of quality of care. We have utilized this data to effect changes in practice which provide more efficient and effective care.

There are potential benefits which have not yet been realized by our CIS and most others. Although our CIS is networked to data producing systems such as the clinical laboratory, the blood gas lab, and many bedside measuring devices, it does not have automatic access to the outcome data in other hospital computers. Thus, we periodically cull outcome data from other systems manually to perform outcome analyses on personal computers and hospital mainframe systems. We look forward to the time when all our systems are fully networked so that automatic analyses of severity-adjusted outcome can be carried on in the background. All the severity data available in a given month could be automatically compared

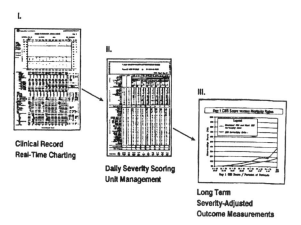

Figure 18.5. The three levels of operation.

to all available outcome criteria, so that both routine reports and nonroutine alerts could be issued. Such a system would provide earlier warning for adverse events and trends than are provided by current QA methods. Full use of the capabilities of a comprehensive CIS will provide more medically-effective and cost-effective ICU care.

Summary

In 1985 we developed a method of automatically extracting indices of severity of illness and intensity of interventions from CIS charts daily. These indices, when combined with outcome measures such as length of stay and mortality, provide a powerful new tool for quality management in the ICU. In this paper we describe our ICU's severity-adjusted survival rates as compared to internationally published norms. In addition we provide a detailed analysis of glucose levels in our ICU, which suggests that glucose control in surgical ICU patients is more closely related to measured severity of illness than administration of intravenous alimentation per se. CIS extracted indices provide a new basis for continuous quality measurement and improvement in the ICU.

References

1. Laffel G, Blumenthal B. The case for using industrial quality management science in health care organizations. JAMA 1989; 62:2869.
2. Shabot MM. Automatic extraction of intensity intervention scores from a computerized Surgical ICU flowsheet. Am J Surg 1987; 154:72.
3. Leyerle BJ, LoBue M, Shabot MM. Integrated databases for data management beyond the bedside. Int J Clin Monit Comput 1990; 7:83.
4. LeGall et al. The simplified acute physiology score. Crit Care Med 1984; 12:975.
5. Shabot MM, Leyerle BJ, LoBue M, et al. First day intensity-intervention score predicts ICU and in-hospital deaths. Crit Care Med 1988; 16:412.
6. The French Multicenter Group of ICU Research: Factors related to outcome in intensive care: French multicenter study. Crit Care Med 1989; 17:490.
7. Albright JM, et al. Outcome reporting to target areas for quality improvement. SCAMC 1990; 14:276.

Chapter 19
Nursing Decision Support: The Challenges Facing Nursing in Regard to Computerization

Judy Blaufuss and Beverley J. Leyerle

It is the purpose of the authors to acquaint other health care professionals with the evolving role of computers in nursing. With the introduction of computers at the bedside, technology has bolstered the nurse's ability to collect, correlate, interpret, and monitor thousands of pieces of information per patient. The computer provides immediate access to information that will complement the nurse's decision-making process.

The current shortage of nursing resources coupled with an increased demand for health care delivery are major issues facing nursing in the 1990s and beyond. This crisis has led to the development of new care-delivery models and reevaluation of how nurses spend their professional time. Three approaches have been identified in the literature as having potential benefit for better utilization of nursing time. The first is *nurse extenders*, or human extenders, such as orderlies for transporting patients or nursing service technicians for nonprofessional tasks which consume much of a nurse's time. The second approach is the employment of *technological extenders*, specifically the use of computers to handle the information-intense environment better. A third approach is the use of computer systems for *nursing decision support*. Computer systems support the nursing process through the interaction and integration with other hospital information systems to bring all information together at a single point for nursing decision support at the bedside.

This chapter will not address the role of nurse extenders or service technicians. The use of technological extenders to handle information and the use of computers to improve the decision-making process will be discussed from the viewpoint of the authors, relating the experiences of two major institutions.

Technology Extenders

The first area in hospitals to utilize technological extenders was the critical care environment. The critical care setting is the most information-intense environment within a hospital. The care of critically ill patients require nurses to have special skills and to make prompt, accurate treatment decisions. ICU nurses and physicians collect large amounts of information through frequent clinical observation, diagnostic testing, and the continuous monitoring of acquired physiological parameters. The computer is becoming a necessity in the ICU environment due to the large volumes of data generated and the limited amount of time nurses and physicians have to respond to life threatening situations [1].

"Most nurses might not recognize that the first step toward automation is not to address hardware or software requirements but to define the information requirements" [2]. If nursing is to benefit from computer technology, nurses in the clinical areas need to define what information requirements should be automated. Grobe emphasized that a "true nursing system should provide more than relief from repetitive time-consuming clerical and transcription responsibilities. Genuine nursing systems furnish automated support for nursing planning and patient care. A nursing system should maintain a database to serve as the focus for monitoring, delivering, managing, and evaluating quality nursing care" [3]. In essence, the key to having a successful nursing information system (NIS) is to have all aspects of documentation of the nursing process included.

The nursing process is the application of the scientific method of problem solving to nursing practice. It represents a comprehensive and systematic approach to nursing [4]. Essential components of the nursing process include data collection, or client assessment, diagnosis of problems amenable to nursing intervention, establishing desired outcomes, planning interventions to attain desired outcome, and evaluating these outcomes by collecting more data [5]. The nursing process is an ongoing process that continues throughout the course of care, with the major goal being coordination of available health care delivery services to ensure quality patient care.

In 1973, the American Nurses' Association established standards for nursing practice based on the nursing process framework. These standards are applicable across various care settings and clinical specialties. It should be noted that each standard involves the management and interpretation of nursing information; thus these are implications for developing criteria for automated nursing information systems.

Standard I: The collection of data about the health status of the client/ patient is systematic and continuous. The data are accessible, communicated, and recorded.
Standard II: Nursing diagnoses are derived from health status data.
Standard III. The plan of nursing care includes goals derived from the nursing diagnosis.
Standard IV: The plan of nursing care includes the priorities and the pre-

scribed nursing approaches or measures to achieve the goals derived from the nursing diagnosis.

Standard V: Nursing actions provide for client/patient participation and health promotion, maintenance, and restoration.

Standard Vl: Nursing actions assist the client/patient to maximize his/her health capacities.

Standard VI: The client's/patient's progress or lack of progress toward goal achievement is determined by the client/patient and the nurse.

Standard VIII. The client's/patient's progress or lack of progress toward goal achievement directs reassessment, reordering of priorities, new goal setting, and revision of the plan of nursing care [6].

In 1988 the Commission on Nursing recommended the development and use of automated information systems as the means of supporting nurses and other health professionals. The commission's decision is supported by the fact that "computers have been used in other health service industries to perform well-defined repetitive tasks and to free valuable human labor for high-level tasks that require the ability to interpret, integrate, and interpolate" [7]. With the nursing shortage, any reduction in time spent in recording, tracking, retrieving, and communicating information can reduce the demands on nurses' time and enhance an organization's nursing resources.

The need for effective information management is also growing under the pressure of evolving hospital policies, government regulations, Joint Commission on Accreditation of Hospital Organizations (JCAHO) and American Nurses Association standards, third-party payer requirements, and consumers' demands for improved quality and greater accountability in all aspects of health care. Ultimately, the computer is seen as a tool that can help to organize and communicate this voluminous amount of information.

Nursing's challenge is to use computer technology to innovate and to transform the manner in which nursing care is delivered [8]. The decisions made today about computer applications in critical care have a direct impact on the future of nursing practice. Nurses need to steer technology in the right direction and in the process revolutionize how nursing care is delivered.

The Implementation of Two Systems

The authors would like to share their experiences with the implementation and development of a computerized clinical information system oriented to nursing. Each has approached the use of computer systems in her institution from a different perspective.

Cedars-Sinai Medical Center, Los Angeles, California

Since 1984, the Surgical Intensive Care Units at Cedars-Sinai Medical Center (CSMC) have used a computerized clinical information system. The initial system was a Hewlett-Packard Patient Data Management System (HP78709A PDMS), in 1991 this systems was replaced with a Care-Vue 9000 Clinical Information System (HP9000 700 Series Hewlett-Packard Company, Andover, MA). The success of the clinical information system (CIS) can be attributed to the joint efforts of the CIS team and the nursing staff in the system design and implementation.

CIS is currently interfaced with 20 bedside physiological monitors (Merlin M1116A, Hewlett-Packard Company, Andover, MA), 20 urimeters, (Bard Urotrack Plus, C.R. Bard Company, Murray Hill, NJ), the clinical laboratory (which runs on VAX hardware with FlexiLab software by Sunquest Information Systems, Tucson, AZ) and blood gas laboratory, (VAX Hardware with Cedars-Sinai Medical Center software written in Forth),and Puritan-Bennett 7200a ventilators (Puritan-Bennett Corp., Carlsbad, CA). These interfaces provide for the collection and systematic organization of information at the bedside. Access to patient information from bedside terminals allows nurses and physicians to assess, evaluate, and make decisions on interventions in real-time.

Access to real-time patient information impacts directly on patient outcomes. Nurses and physicians no longer wait for results to be phoned to the unit, as has been the traditional form of communication. At the time of initial patient encounter an assessment for additional therapies can be determined at the bedside and initiated without delays caused by missing or pending data. Time spent caring for the patient, directly impacts length of ICU and hospital stay as well as the allocation and use of resources.

The initial effort of the CIS team was to optimize data retrieval, data display, calculations, and documentation, replacing the manual flowsheet with an electronically generated medical record. The initial computer-generated record utilized data for the sole purpose of producing the ICU chart. As a greater familiarity developed with the computerized system, it became apparent that data captured by CIS could be used for a variety of other purposes. Information contained in the electronic flowchart could also be used to evaluate such variables as severity of illness, alerts, length of stay and outcome, SICU resource utilization, and continuous quality improvement indicators [9].

The CIS became a powerful tool in establishing a multipurpose database. Since 1986, the CIS has stored information on 35,000 consecutive days of care delivered to over 13,000 patients for the two 10-bed SICUs. On a daily basis, the CIS scans an average of 30,000 data items and provides a severity-of-illness score for each patient in the SICU. The CIS team has coined the term "computerized intensity-intervention score" (CIIS). This scoring systems has been discussed in detail in Chapter 17.

LDS Hospital, Salt Lake City, Utah

Nursing at LDS Hospital has been actively involved in the computerized clinical information system since 1980. Initial use of the computer in the critical care units was for physiological monitoring, recording intake/ output volumes, and medication documentation. Nursing's first interface was in generating nursing care plans. This was implemented in late 1980.

In 1985 nursing implemented bedside nursing documentation in a 16-bed medical-surgical intensive care unit. By May of 1986, all four adult intensive care units (60 beds) had been brought on-line with bedside terminals. This allowed immediate access to patient information for assessment, evaluation, and/or decisions on interventions in real-time.

Since 1987, efforts have been directed toward the development of the remaining elements of nursing documentation, specifically, software applications for admission history, assessment, revision of current nursing care planning based on Gordon's Functional Health Patterns and Nursing Diagnosis, medication scheduling and charting, and finally a planner that would link all applications so that the nurse can coordinate all patient related activities.

Decision Support

Once nursing process documentation has been computerized, the next challenge presents itself. That is having the computer facilitate nursing decision support. Decision support can be demonstrated in various ways:

- Formatting tools, e.g., spreadsheet programs
- Analyzing systems e.g., decision trees
- Advisory systems e.g., expert systems

Basically, the goal is to support the nurse clinician and facilitate the smooth transfer of information necessary to make appropriate decisions. "A decision support system for nursing practice is intended to support nurses by providing them with information. . . . decision support systems help nurses to maintain and maximize their decision-making responsibilities and to focus on the highest priority aspects of patient care" [10].

Ozbolt [11] defined two factors contributing to the delay in development of decision support systems for the nursing process. The *first* is that of knowledge representation in nursing. What are the key concepts and issues with which nursing is concerned, how are the concepts and issues related, and how should nursing express them? Nurses as professionals need to agree on standardized language to describe what nurses do. Work is occurring in three areas of standardization: Nursing Minimum Data Set [12], Nursing Diagnosis [13], and Functional Health Patterns [14]. Standardization is necessary for automation and comparability within and among health care organizations.

The *second* factor contributing to the delay in the development of nursing decision support systems is the lack of knowledge about how nurses make decisions [11]. Wessling has observed that, more often than not, nurses are guided by intuition and subjective thinking that brings inconsistency to their data-gathering process. Wessling feels that "working with a computer forces the nurse to define and analyze nursing and to delineate functions logically" [15]. Blaufuss [4] confirmed similar findings during implementation of a computerized bedside charting system. Computerization caused nursing to develop a logical data file that facilitated charting of the nursing process. Once implemented, the system improved documentation of the nursing process significantly when compared with pre-implementation studies.

A key factor in the development of information systems with decision support capabilities is that the system must be interactive and integrated with the hospital information system (HIS). If the NIS is separate from the HIS, nurses will be forced into the same roll they perform in a manual system—pulling all the information together and trying to establish the

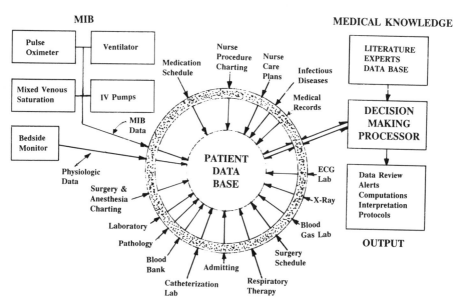

Figure 19.1. HELP computer system. Diagram of computerized intensive care unit data collection and decision-making system. Note wide variety of data sources and how data from there services are integrated into one patient database also illustrated schematically in the diagram is a medical decision support system. As data are collected, they are analyzed by the decision-making processor, illustrated by ring surrounding database. (Reprinted from Gardner RM, Bradshaw KE, Hollingsworth KW. Computerizing the intensive care unit: Current staus and future directions. *Cardovasc Nurs* 1989; 4(1):70, with permission of Aspen Publishers, Inc., (c) 1989).

inter-relationships. If the standalone NIS approach is adopted, the nurses' workload for information handling may actually increase.

Shown in Figure 19.1 is a diagram of the HELP (Health Evaluation through Logical Processing) computerized intensive care unit data collection and decision-making system in place at LDS Hospital in Salt Lake City, Utah. There a wide variety of data sources, and data from these sources are integrated into one central patient data file. As the data are collected, they are analyzed by the decision-making processor [16]. The HELP Patient Care System is designed to provide a global approach to health care information, using knowledge from every relevant source to assist in the evaluation and care of each patient. Paperwork is reduced to a minimum, data is are captured only once, and crucial patient information is always available to nursing, health care professionals, and ancillary departments [17]. The nursing application provides expert support for each step of the nursing process: assessment, diagnosis, planning, intervention, and evaluation. Figure 19.2 shows how specific functions of Nursing and other HELP System applications can provide clinical assistance at each phase of the nursing process. Individual software functions are shown in italics.

Like other applications throughout the HELP System, the Nursing application provides far more than the simple data collection and reporting found in typical health care software. The system can apply hospital-

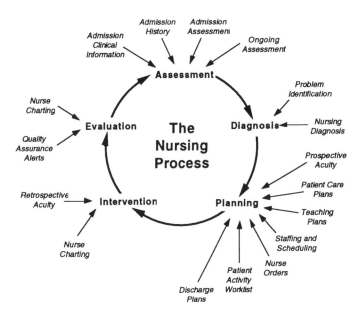

Figure 19.2. The HELP (Health Evaluation Through Logical Processing) computerized ICU diagram, (Reprinted with permission of 3M Health Information System, 1993).

specific decision logic to patient data, acting as an interactive consultant at the patient's bedside. This is a form of an expert system. Bloom et al. define an expert system as "a set of computer programs that serve as an aid in decision-making and problem-solving activities of an end user" [18]. The intent is that the system will assist the user in attaining higher levels of performance in the specific problem area addressed by the system. Of primary importance in the design of expert systems is the provision for accumulation and codification of a knowledge base. This allows for future retrieval, enhancing nursing's ability to conduct research and thus improve existing decision logic.

Clinical applications of Nursing Decision Support Systems

Computer systems allow nurses to apply decision logic to automatically acquired patient data. The amount of data retrieved and the application of the nursing process provides for the framework by which decision logic and multipurpose databases can be established. As noted by Brennan, computers should augment the decision process. The computer augments the nurse by collecting, organizing, displaying, and interpreting data in a fraction of the time it would take a nurse to attempt the establishment of inter-relationships.

At CSMC, CIIS scores and demographic data are compiled and stored by the computer system, but analysis of data is done off-line. As shown in Figure 19.3, data is stored on the clinical information system in ASCII "flat" file format. Data is periodically exported from CIS to an IBM-compatible PC and imported into a commercially available relational database (dBASE IV, Borland Co., Scotts Valley, CA). From the dBASE file data is exported into spreadsheet and graphical packages for analysis and presentation. CSMC has experienced a positive growth in computer technology and provides a model environment on the cutting edge for other areas to pattern after.

More complex and sophisticated statistical analyses are performed on the hospital's mainframe systems. Data subsets are selectively transferred over Ethernet to the hospital's VAX cluster. Demographics, admit-transfer-discharge data, procedural coding, diagnostic coding, and final discharge status from the hospital's mainframe HIS is integrated into the database for analysis. A biweekly fiscal accounting of the units of service (UOS) provided, nursing hours per patient day (NHPPD), and budgeted versus actual "averaged" acuity is integrated into the database. Periodically, parts of the VAX database are transferred back to the PC for detailed analyses [19].

The CIS stores data into two major databases. The first database contains information on every patient admitted to the SICUs. This database contains selected demographic data, Simplified Acute Physiology Scores

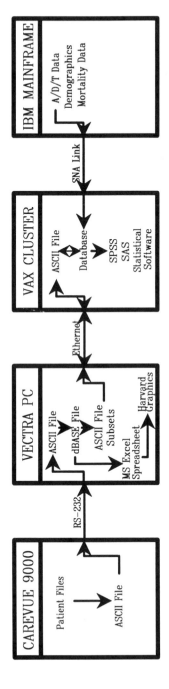

Figure 19.3. Transfer of data from Hewlett-Packard CareVue 9000 system to a distributed data network with two way distribution between a PC-based system and the Hospital Information System.

Table 19.1. Quantitative Therapeutic Intervention Scoring System Variables

Age	Heart Rate	Systolic BP	Temperature
Urinary Output	Blood Urea Nitrogen	Resp or ventilator rate	Hematocrit
White blood count	Serum glucose	Serum potassium	Serum sodium
Serun bicarbonate	Glasgow coma scale	Admission	Discharge
Revision to care plan	Arterial line	PA catheter	CVP
ICP Line	O² source	# Arterial arrhythmias	# Vent Arrhythmias
# Code blues	# Vasoactive drugs	# Antiarrhythmic drugs	# Misc IV drugs
# Vital signs	# PA measurements	# Cardia outputs	# Neuro checks
# Blood gases	# Blood transfusions	# IV bottles	# Hyperal bottles
# Eternal feedings	# Hemodialysis runs	# Chest tubes	# GI drainage tubes
# Wound irrigations	# Glucochecks	# Transfers for test	# Seizures
# Weights			

refers to the *number* of each of these events.

(SAPS), Quantitative Therapeutic Intensity Scoring System (QTISS), and Acute Physiology, Age and Chronic Health Evaluation II(APACHE II) scores, medical admitting service, and other unique indexes. A second database contains consecutive daily information for every patient admission. Between these two databases a variety of queries can be made. Single data sets may not provide enough information for all situations, and a more detailed query may be needed for example the explanation of a budget variance. Table 19.1 represents the type of information that can be extracted from a CIS database. All variables are available daily at the time of data extraction by CIIS. The use of simple database query's provides real-time information for unit based statistics and analysis of utilization.

Nursing Alerts

Nursing forms the hub of the patient care process, the central point that connects the information needs of the patient, the physician, and auxiliary departments (Figure 19.4). Nursing, as coordinator of patient care, plays a crucial role in identifying potential areas of risk!

Currently the Nursing Joint Venture Group at LDS Hospital, IHC,

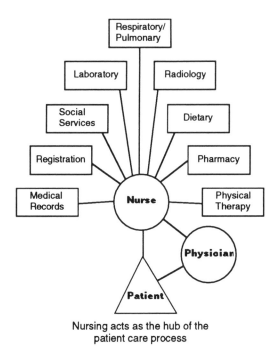

Nursing acts as the hub of the
patient care process

Figure 19.4. Nursing specific functions and other applications of the HELP System. (Reprinted with permission of 3M Health Information System, 1993.)

and 3M have identified six areas where the HELP Patient Care System has the potential to support nursing in delivering quality nursing care. These include subsystems that alert, interpret, assist, critique, diagnosis, and manage. Work has begun to structure decision logic based on current and ongoing nursing research, so that the NIS will be able to meet its identified goal. To support nurses with integrated patient data so as to improve efficiency and productivity of the nurse caring for the patient.

On the HELP system, decision logic is applied to patient data automatically as the data are entered by admitting clerks, nurses, physicians, and other health care professionals. Working with a complete profile for each patient, including data collected during past admissions, the Nursing application is able to act as a silent expert partner capable of reinforcing decisions at each step of the nursing process.

For example, when a patient is admitted, the system already has access to demographics and vital information from other previous admissions. This may include information that directly impacts the nursing care plan, such as a previous history of falls. Based on previous patient data and new information entered, the HELP system might predict a higher risk factor for a patient to fall. The system helps guide the user to appropriate interventions. The system's decision logic can actually spot potential trouble before it occurs, providing an alert that describes the problem and suggests alternative courses of action [20]. These alerts are created by expert clinicians who can describe the clinical indicators and the logic to assess indicators for specific patient problems. This system also monitors cost issues, pointing out equivalent treatments that maybe less expensive for both the patient and the hospital.

Another example of how the computer is being used to support nursing decisions is with our Skin Care Task Force. In May of 1992 the agency for Health Care Policy and Research (AHCPR), U.S. Department of Health and Human Services published "Clinical Practice Guidelines, Pressure Ulcers in Adults: Prediction and Prevention" [21]. The purpose of these guidelines is to help identify adults at risk of pressure ulcers and to define early interventions for prevention. The task force has incorporated these guidelines into standard protocols which were easily computerized. The team is currently conducting research first to validate these recommended standards and secondly to assess the computer support capabilities in alerting the nursing staff to patients at risk. Part of the evaluation piece is to evaluate costs saving of such an alerting mechanism and the impact on patient outcomes.

Cost of Quality Care

Cost and quality of care are the issues that most concern health care professionals today. Any computer system that helps facilitate the care delivery process by alerting nurses to potential problems before harm has occurred will favorably impact patient outcomes by avoiding complications and lead to decreased length of stays. By insuring quality, the institution also receives the benefit of cost savings.

Besides defining which information requirements need to be automated, nursing also needs to articulate the cost-benefit ratio of computerization. Until recently, only pharmacies or laboratories have been able to demonstrate a cost savings [22]. As Walker and Schwartz [2] noted, it is not easy to identify the cost-benefits of nursing interventions. They gave the example of the difficulty of quantifying "turning" a patient to prevent decubitus ulcers. Good nurses intuitively know which nursing actions prevent complications, but our challenge is to articulate those actions so that analysis can be achieved and a cost-benefit ratio determined. Hopefully, our research with the Skin Care Task Force will be able to do this.

When selling nursing informatics software, vendors often say that computerization will decrease full-time employees (FTEs) or the number of nurses required to care for the patients. Recipients of such a sales pitch are cautioned to evaluate such "cost" savings in a realistic way. Is the goal to decrease needed nurse staff or better utilize limited resources? Time saved by automation should allow the nurse to prioritize care requirements better and enhance such responsibilities as patient education and case management. These responsibilities currently are occurring infrequently or in a limited way because the nurse is expected to do so many other tasks that time is the limiting factor. The nurse's ability to quantify "cost" savings is imperative, but nursing, not financial analysts who quantify FTEs, needs to determine the "value" component. Impact on length of stay and decrease in complications better evaluates the impact of spending up-front time and resources with the patient, than does measuring staffing ratios at a given moment in time to determine if computerization has saved dollars. Patient outcomes should be a major variable in evaluating the costs of computerization.

Given today's health care environment of increasing and changing regulatory restrictions, cost containment and quality-of-care issues, as well as the nursing shortage and the increased severity of illness of patients, an automated acuity system has immense value to both the nursing service and hospital administration. The ability to identify nursing costs, resource utilization, and nursing contributions to hospital revenue has become essential to preparing and monitoring hospital budgets effectively [23–27].

This represents a very different approach to monitoring quality compared to traditional retrospective chart reviews to determine problem areas. In traditional monitoring, the harm has already occurred and the cost realized. Change occurs after the fact. An "expert system" has the capability of issuing warnings (alerts) concurrently as potential problems occur. An example is a nephrotoxic medication such as Gentamycin ordered by a physician for a renal failure patient. The decision logic looks at laboratory findings such as the creatinine clearance and alerts the care giver to the fact that the ordered dosage is too high or too frequent for adequate clearance. If given as ordered, the renal failure period maybe be prolonged. The physician can override the alert or change the dosage or frequency the drug is to be administered. Either way the potential for harm has been recognized at the time of prescribing the medication rather than after treatment has been initiated.

Staffing Patterns

Many systems classify patients into one of several levels of care and use the number of patients on each level to determine staffing needs [19,24,25]. However, staffing at LDS Hospital is determined by each patient's actual nursing-care hours. The total nursing-care hours for each unit per shift is divided by the number of hours worked by one nurse to determine the number of nurses required to deliver that care. In the Critical Care units, the computer uses this information to project the number of nurses needed for the upcoming shift. This projection is adjusted for admissions, transfers, and discharges. Since nursing hours or acuity hours are calculated each shift, rather than once a day, staffing decisions can be further refined by the charge nurse and staffing office on a shift-to-shift basis as needed, in order to respond to changes in patient acuity or census [28].

This has proven to be a reliable method for determining the appropriate number of staff for each nursing division. This staffing system has been very well accepted by the nursing staff, nursing administration, and hospital administration.

Cedars-Sinai uses a decentralized staffing strategy identifying the number of nurses needed per shift by patient acuity. Patients' acuity is determine by a housewide classification system. Patients are assigned to one of four categories of care. These category classifications are defined as minimal, medium (unit norm), extensive, and acute care. The differentiation between classes are based on the frequency of clinical observations, vital signs, laboratory data, surgical dressing changes, and administration of vasoactive drugs and blood products. The majority of these parameters are automatically captured by CIS and are incorporated into the daily CIIS. The SICU managers use CIIS as an adjunct in projecting needed staffing.

In addition to the daily use of CIIS, the computer system can be programmed to generate a biweekly summary report of unit based statistics (Fig. 19.5). The Nurse Mangers are provided the CIIS Summary report every two weeks in accordance with the nursing pay period. The report summarizes unique events, i.e., admissions, length of stay, number of patient days, number of trauma days, etc., in addition to total daily acuity.

At times it is not feasible to staff according to acuity, and additional staff are required to deliver safe/quality care over the "budgeted" acuity

```
                          CSMC - 8 SICU
           Computer Intensity - Intervention Score Summary
             for 14 days from 10/26/92 through 11/08/92
```

	Total	Avg/Day
# Patient Days	132	9.4
Admissions	27	1.9
Discharges	30	2.1
Length of Stay		3.7
# Trauma Admissions	8	0.6
# Trauma Days	29	2.1
SAPS Points	1606	114.7
TISS Points	5224	373.1
CIIS Points	6830	487.9
# Transfers for Test	46	
A-Lines - # Patient Days	92	
PA-Lines - # Patient Days	29	
CVP-Lines - # Patient Days	39	
ICP-Lines - # Patient Days	3	
Ventilator - # Patient Days	74	
# Vasoactive Drugs	36	
# Antiarrythmic Drugs	16	
# Miscellaneous Drugs	7	
# Liver Transplant Days	33	
# Blood Transfusions	79	
# Hyperalimentations	131	
# Glucocheks	251	
# Spun Hematocrits	239	
# Chest Tube Days	12	
# Dialysis Days	1	
# Code Blues	0	
# Central Line insertions	6	
# Peripheral Line insertions	28	

8 SICU Date	# pts	Total CIIS	AvgCIIS /Pt	#Patients Admit D/C		# A-Line	# PA-Line	# Vents	# HyperAl	# IV Drugs
10/26/92	9	534	59.3	2	2	8	3	5	11	2
10/27/92	10	568	56.8	3	2	9	2	6	9	5
10/28/92	10	593	59.3	1	1	9	2	5	15	7
10/29/92	10	513	51.3	3	3	8	2	5	18	3
10/30/92	10	517	51.7	4	4	7	1	6	18	3
10/31/92	10	570	57.0	2	2	7	2	7	14	3
11/01/92	10	501	50.1	2	2	7	2	6	9	3
11/02/92	8	411	51.4	0	2	5	2	6	8	1
11/03/92	6	377	62.8	0	2	4	1	4	8	5
11/04/92	6	564	94.0	0	0	6	3	5	7	6
11/05/92	5	501	100.2	1	2	6	3	5	4	9
11/06/92	7	414	59.1	4	2	6	3	4	3	3
11/07/92	5	361	72.2	3	5	5	2	4	3	5
11/08/92	6	406	67.7	2	1	5	1	6	4	4

```
8 SICU    Summary Sheet by: M. Michael Shabot, M.D., Dept of Surgery
Source: SICU CareVue 9000 CIS, 11/08/92 11:25
```

Figure 19.5. Biweekly summary of unit based patient acuity, produced by the CIS at Cedars-Sinai Medical Center, totaling the number of interventions, acuity indexes with by day of week breakdown. Copyright (c) CSMC 1991–1992

level. In order for this type of staffing need to occur, the patient mix is higher in acuity or some unusual circumstance has presented its self. During the summer of 1988, the SICUs experienced an outbreak of an unusual nosocomial infection. Patients identified to be at greatest risk were patients requiring greater than 72 hr of pulmonary intubation. In general, these were all ventilated patients. All patients intubated and on a ventilator were isolated from each other. At times the patient mix did not provide for appropriate pairing of patients and all patients were staffed 1:1.

For the three consecutive pay periods involved, acuity information was logged into a database file provided by CIS. With the aid of both actual and predicted nursing hours worked, for the same pay periods, the degree of deviation from the norm could be determined. These variance reports are prepared and distributed on a monthly basis. The variance is seen in Figure 19.6; between July 10, 1988, and August 20, 1988, the SICUs required 1,185 additional nursing-hours of nursing care. The comparison of CIIS points showed a deviation from an otherwise strong correlations of NHPPDs to CIIS scores.

The ability to perform these types of comparisons and correlations

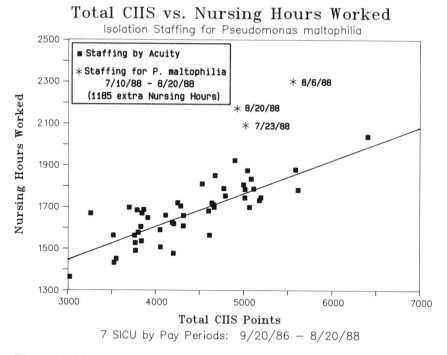

Figure 19.6. Nursing hours per patient day (NHPPD) plotted against patient acuity for three consecutive pay periods. Showing the increased acuity and staffing required to meet a specific incidence of patient related/required care.

would not be possible on a unit basis, if not for the database that CIS allows for.

Staff Billing and Productivity Management

Historically, nursing charges and costs have been included in the hospital room rate with other hospital overhead. This makes it difficult to identify where nursing resources are being utilized, their actual cost, and the nursing contribution to overall hospital revenue [24]. At LDS Hospital, a care-based patient classification system (PCS) is used for staffing, billing, and productivity measurement [29]. This PCS is a modification of a tool developed by Hudson et al.[30]. It is a care-based system that identifies the actual nursing care delivered to each patient rather than categorizing patients into levels of care. This process was developed at the hospital as part of the nursing component of the HELP Patient Care System [29].

Prior to implementation of variable billing for nursing services in April 1986, nursing care was included in the room rate, and all patients were charged a standard fee regardless of their need for nursing care. Generally, less acute patients subsidized the care of those who were more seriously ill. The implementation of care-based variable billing meant that each patient received a much lower room rate, covering room, board, and hospital overhead, and a nursing rate based on the actual minutes of nursing care provided.

The computer calculates the time spent on nursing care for each patient and stores it in a billing file. Nursing care time is then transferred to the hospital's financial system once a day, where it is multiplied by the nursing rate to determine the nursing care charge for that day. This charge then appears on the patient's bill along with the room rate and other daily hospital charges [29].

Third-party payers and the general health care consumer are demanding more accountability of health care providers. They are interested in itemization that allows them to scrutinize all hospital charges carefully. This benefits nursing but also poses challenges. The profession is now more directly accountable to patients and insurers for the services they provide.

Demands are placed on nursing for precise documentation of the care given to each patient and justification for standards of practice and the costs associated with those standards. In fact, one of the incidental benefits that occurred at LDS Hospital as part of variable billing was a dramatic improvement in the quality of nurses' documentation.

Billing information is downloaded to a microcomputer along with nursing costs each pay period as a part of routine monitoring of the nursing department budget. Nursing costs are divided into three categories for each nursing unit:

1. unit constants, which included the head nurse, clinical specialist, assistant head nurse, unit clerks, and equipment aides;
2. variable or direct nursing hours, which include the unit nursing staff (Nurses and LPNs) and any float pool or outside agency personnel used to staff the unit; and
3. overhead, which includes nonproductive hours (sick time, vacation, etc.), FICA, education hours, and nursing administration salaries.

Non-salary overheads are not included in the nursing department cost, but are included in the room rate as hospital overhead.

Nursing costs are broken down into average cost per acuity minute (or minute of nursing care) in each category (i.e., constants, variable and overhead) and total cost per acuity minute. Cost per minute are then compared to charges to determine each unit's productivity. Enough detail is included in each unit's salary budget report each pay period to identify specific areas that may have a major impact on overall unit productivity. Data include actual and budgeted dollars, the cost of agency personnel, cost of regular unit personnel, average salary rates, overtime hours, sick time, etc. Costs, revenue, and productivity are tracked throughout the year by unit, by specialty, and for the nursing department as a whole [29]

Productivity measurement has provided valuable information which is utilized for budget preparation, monitoring, and for determining areas where modification of work organization or management practices may improve department efficiency and/or minimize costs—e.g., reduction in sick time or overtime. Productivity information by staff members can also identify efficient nurses as well as tracking orientation process for new staff members.

The automated acuity system has dramatically changed the character of the nursing department. Staffing decisions are straightforward, easy to justify, and acceptable to staff nurses. Variable billing has made the nursing department a revenue center rather than a cost center. This has had major impact on budget preparation, as staff nurses are now revenue producers whose positions are not considered for budget reductions. Finally, the ability to link costs to revenue for department productivity measurements has allowed the nursing department to look objectively and precisely at its organization in order to become more efficient and cost-effective without compromising quality of care.

Limitations of the current system are its focus on tasks that the nurse completes rather than an analysis of tasks that could be provided by a nurse extender in place of a Nurse. The ideal acuity tool should measure all aspects of patient care needs and nursing process components, with the capability of determining or predicting the required ratio of RNs, LPNs, aides, or nurse extenders necessary to meet those needs. The ideal acuity system should automatically extract information from the patient care plan as well as assessment and charting. This would better measure the role of the nurse as coordinator of care and help the nurse manager evaluate the impact of case mix change. Such an enhanced system has the potential of developing outcome predictors which could be linked to case management in real time.

Computerized Records

Nurses notes at LDS Hospitals are computerized. As the nurse performs routine documentation of the care given to patients, the computer automatically flags key patient care activities and sends them to an acuity file. Time is also automatically given for indirect care such as report, charting, care planning, discharge planning, etc. All nursing care times were initially assigned using standard management engineering techniques. A hospital-based management engineer was actively involved in the development of the PCS [29].

At the end of a nursing shift the time allotted for all the nursing activities, both direct and indirect, are totaled in the patient's acuity file. This then determines the nursing care minutes needed for each patient that shift. Nursing care minutes for individual patients are then grouped by nursing unit to determine nursing hours per unit. The portion of a nurse's shift each patient requires is also computer determined (patient's hours of care are divided by hours worked by nurse). Nursing care hours are then reported for each unit by shift for a 24-hr period. This information is then used to determine staffing needs based on patient acuity rather than simply the census.

CSMC Severity of Illness Scoring

In an effort to measure severity of illness, much time and energy has been directed in the development of patient classification systems and systems like APACHE, SAPS, TISS [31–33] that measure acuity. These manual systems require that individuals knowledgeable in critical care (usually a nurse) review the medical record and score each patient. The manpower to perform this task is not available in a majority of institutions. Neither are the scores available on a daily basis for use by the nursing staff in the allocation of resources or decision-making. Due to the manpower and time involved in scoring patients, most institutions opt to score severity or intensity on a periodic or quarterly basis and project acuity and census based upon these periodic findings.

The SICU CIS has been programmed to extract from the patient's chart a computerized intensity-intervention score (CIIS) daily [34]. At 7 A.M. the system automatically generates a CIIS report. The assistant nurse managers or primary resource nurses can utilize CIIS scores in conjunction with shift report to identify those patients requiring 1:1 care and to make assignments matching nurses' skill levels to patient acuity. The

Table 19.2. SICU Utilization and Severity of Illness Trends

	86–87	87–88	88–89	89–90	90–91	91–92
Admissions	2,521	2,392	2,059	2,273	2,217	2,175
Days of Care	5,710	6,066	6,216	6,164	6,043	5,941
Trauma Days	1,313	1,409	1,752	1,920	1,262	1,258
Mean LOS (days)	2.27	2.53	3.02	2.71	2.73	2.73
Mean QTISS	27.9	28.9	29.9	30.9	33.1	38.2
Mean SAPS	10.1	10.8	11.0	11.3	12.5	12.7

LOS, length of stay; QTISS, quantitative therapeutic intervention scoring system; SAPS, simplified acute physiology score

use of a severity-of-illness score has provided Nursing with an objective parameter by which to support their clinical judgment. Severity-of-illness scores have proven to be a tangible means of patient classification and has been incorporated into the SICU operating standards as an additional criteria used to establish the need for 1:1 nursing care.

Nursing has been provided with a unique insight into nursing care delivery through the use of relational databases, acuity- and severity-of-illness scoring, and the ability to cost-out care. The importance of early recognition of trends in care and an increase or decrease in the number of admissions or severity in a unit, can directly impact the number of FTEs that a nurse manager requires. Clinical information systems now provide a much more timely and cost-effective means by which to monitor trends in real-time.

As shown in Table 19.2, unit census may fluctuate from year to year. But the continued rise in severity of illness over time reflects the unit activity. Between 1988–89-and 1989–90, the number of trauma patients rose due to changing geographical boundary shifts. Inspited of the increase in trauma days, the days of care and length of stay went down. This would normally indicate a need for fewer nurses. But the trend in severity of illness of patients reflects a truer picture of the unit acuity. Managers have the information necessary to support the maintainence of current staffing patterns with the addition of support for additional staff should the numbers indicated. This type of information can assist managers and administrators in assessing the impact a new programs play on existing ICU resources.

Future

Computerization will have its greatest impact on the decision-making process of the staff nurse and the function of the nurse manager. No longer will nursing practice focus on the assessment and care planning phase.

Rather, it will emphasize the implementation phase. McCormick and McQueen noted in 1988 that "diagnosis and prognosis based on systematically collected and collated data are more accurate than those based on clinical judgment and intuition alone. Decision-making can become more scientifically based as the probabilities of outcomes associated with alternative means of treatment can be compared" [35].

The science of nursing can be confirmed. The ability to have large data banks of nursing information that computer analysis is applied to assess nursing actions, independent decision-making, and patient outcomes may help to identify which combinations of variables are powerful predictors of patient outcomes. Specific predictors of individual or group data on patients can assist the staff nurse in evaluation and decision-making [35,36]. This gives the staff nurse a sense of control and helps to transform the complex health care environment into a more logical structure.

The nurse manager's role will also be impacted by computerization. Because of the increased flow of information from the patient level to administration, the manager will need a solid understanding of statistics and cost data and must have the ability to articulate the cost/benefit ratio of programs instituted. The key will be to deliver safe and quality care within monetary constraints [37,38].

Staffing and scheduling patterns that in the past created problems can better be analyzed and controlled. Costing-out nursing services will allow the nurse manager the opportunity to demonstrate what and how much nursing does and that nursing is a revenue generating department of the hospital. This will give the nurse manager control at budget time and evaluation of programs [37,38].

Use of an integrated system in which all applications programs share a common patient data file is more efficient than repetitive data entry into a variety of subsystems which are only partially linked by a communication function. The focus will shift from a Nursing Care Approach to a Patient Care Approach. Ball [39] points out that there is a paradox since we are in an age of increasing specialization, while the integrated computer systems focus on centralization of patient care functions. "Few health care organizations will be able to support five or six separate and distinct administrative departments to provide one service—patient care. For example, nursing, physical therapy, occupational therapy, dietary, respiratory therapy, and social service may need to be consolidated into nursing in order to provide more efficient, coordinated patient-centered care" [39]. Health care organizations will have decentralized management and centralized care delivery. This can only happen with the assistance of an integrated HIS. It also demonstrates the needed changes that must occur to nursing's current delivery of care structure.

Gardner asks whether computers can successfully match the needs of the ICU? He feels the answer revolves around two issues: "First, is there a critical mass of patient information in the computer data file and second, has the ICU developed an adequate computer user base with the maturity to live through the change in style of patient care required by computer implementation?" [40]. Both issues must be resolved for ICU computer systems to be implemented fully. These issues point out the work yet to be done and challenge nursing to take the leading role in steering computer technology in the right direction and, in the process, to revolutionize the way quality patient care is delivered.

References

1. Blaufuss J. Computer Technology. In Spicer JG, Robinson M (eds): Managing the Environment in Critical Care Nursing. Baltimoce: Williams & Wilkins, Publishers, 1990, p 93–104.
2. Walker MB, Schwartz C. What Every Nurse Should Know About Computers. New York: JB Lippincott, 1984.
3. Grobe SJ. Computer Primer and Resource Guide for Nurses. Philadelphia: JB Lippincott, 1984.
4. Blaufuss JA. Promoting the Nursing Process Through Computerization. In Salamon R, Blum B, Jorgenson M (eds): MEDINFO 86. Amsterdam: North-Holland Elsevier Science, 1986, p 585.
5. Yura H, Walsh MB. The Nursing Process (5th Ed.) East Norwalk, CT: Appleton and Lange, 1987.
6. Zielstorff RD, McHugh ML, Clinton J. Computer Design Critieria For Systems that Support the Nursing Process. Kansas City, MO: American Nurses' Association, 1988.
7. Secretary's Commission on Nursing Final Report. Washington, D.C. Department of Health and Human Services, 1988; 1:24.
8. Romano CA. Development, implementation, and utilization of a computerized information system for nursing. Nurs Administration Q 1986; 10:1–9.
9. Leyerle BJ, LoBue M, Shabot MM. The PDMS as a focal point for distribute patient data. Int J Clin Monitor Comput 1988; 5:155.
10. Brennan PF. Decision support for nursing practice: the challenge and th promise, In Hannah KJ, Guillemin EJ, Conklin DN, et al. (eds): Nursing Uses of Computers and Information Science. Amsterdam: North Holland, 1985; pp 315–319.
11. Ozbolt JG. Developing decision support systems for nursing. Comput Nurs 1987, 5:105.
12. Werley HH, Lang NM, Westlake ?. Brief summary of the Nursing Minimum Data Set Conference. Nurs Management 1986; 17:42.
13. McLane An (ed). Classification of Nursing Diagnosis: Proceedings of the Seventh Conference. North American Nursing Diagnosis Association. St. Louis: CV Mosby, 1987.
14. Gordon M. During Diagnosis: Process and Application, 2nd ed. New York: McGraw-Hill, 1987.
15. Wessling E. Automating the nursing history and care plan. J Nurs Administration 1972; 2:34.
16. Gardner RM, Bradshaw KE, Hollingsworth KW. Computerizing the inten-

sive care unit: current status and future opportunities. J Cardiovasc Nurs 1989; 4:68.

17. 3M article on HELP Patient Care System Nursing Applications. 1993.

18. Bloom KC, Leitner JE, Solano JL. develpment of an expert system prototype to generate nursing care plans on nursing diagnoses. Computers in Nursing 1987; 5(5):140–145.

19. Leyerle BJ, LoBue M, Shabot MM. Integrated computerized databases for medical data management beyond the bedside. Int J Clin Monit Comput 1990; 7:83.

20. Blaufuss J, Tinker A. Computerized Falls Alert—A new solution to an old problem. SCAMC November, 1989; 12:69.

21. U.S. Department of Health and Human Services: Pressure ulcers in adults: Prediction and prevention, AHCPR Publication No. 92-0050, May 1992.

22. Reider K, House M. Identifying requirements for a nursing systems. SCAMC November, 1983; 6:475.

23. Shaffer FA. Costing Out Nursing: Pricing Our Product. New York: National League of Nursing, 1985.

24. Didkers M, Paradise T. PCS: One system for both staffing and costing. Nurs Management 1986; 17(i):25.

25. Ethridge P. The case for billing by patient acuity. Nurs Management 1985; 16(8):38.

26. Strasen L. Standard Costing/Productivity Model for Nursing. Nurs Economics 1987; 5(4):158.

27. Adams R, Johnson B. Acuity and staffing under prospective payment. J Nurs Administration 1986; 16(10):21.

28. Shabot MM, Leyerle BJ, LoBue M. Automatic extraction of intensity-intervention scores from a computerized surgical intensive care unit flowsheet. Am J Surg 1987; 154:72.

29. Budd M, Propotnik T. A computerized system for staffing, billing and productivity measurement. J Nursing Administration 1989; 19(7):17.

30. J. Hudson et al. Intensive care nursing requirements: Resource allocation according to patient status. Crit Care Med, 1979; 7:2;69.

31. Knaus WA, Zimmerman JE, Wagner DP, Draper EA, Lawrence DE. APACHE-acute physiology and chronic health evaluation: a physioloigcally based classification system. Crit Care Med, 1981; 9:591.

32. LeGall JR, Loirat P, Alperovitch A, et al. A simplified acute physiological score of ICU patients. Crit Care Med, 1984; 12:975.

33. Cullen DJ, Civetta JM, Briggs BA, Ferrara LC. Therapeutic intervention scoring system: Method for quantitiative comparison of patient care. Crit Care Med 1974; 2:57.

34. Shabot MM, LoBue M, Leyerle BJ. Use of automatic computerized intensity-intervention scores to measure the appropriateness of ICU utilization. SCAMC 1987; 11:671.

35. McCormick K, McQueen L. New Computer Technology. In Series on Nursing Administrtion Vol. 1. Menlo Park, CA: Addison-Wesley Publishing Company, 1988; p 58.

36. Saba VK, McCormick KA. Essentials of computers for nurses. Philadelphia, PA: J.B. Lippincott Co., 1986.

37. Budd M, Blaufuss J, Propotnik T, Maynard J, Klingle C, Pryor A. An automated patient classification system for staffing, billing, and productivity
measurement. SCAMC 1988; 12:785.
38. Budd MC, Blaufuss J, Harada S. Nursing: A revenue center, not a cost center. Comput Health Care November 1988; p 24.
39. Ball MS, Hannah KJ, Jelger UG, Peterson H. Nursing information where
caring and technology meet. New York: Springer-Veriag, 1988.
40. Gardner RM, Sittig DF, Budd MC. Computers in the intensive care unit:
Match or mismatch? Textbook of Critical Care Medicine, 2nd Ed. Philadelphia: W.B. Saunders, 1989; ch 26.

Chapter 20
Anesthesia Support Systems
Omar Prakash and S. Meiyappan

Introduction

Rapid growth in computer technology in producing high-performance systems with superior ergonomic design has opened new avenues in various application areas in different segments of engineering which demand visual presentation and communication capabilities in addition to excellent number-crunching power. Incidentally, most of these applications are related to a category of monitoring, real-time model simulation, intelligent alarm annunciation, and maintaining a record of events. This new trend has very recently diversified into medical monitoring and computing. Cost is a major criterion from the point of widespread acceptance, and these systems were not economical until recently. Today, many high-end personal computer systems can provide an excellent platform for many concepts in medical monitoring to become a reality. The promises of such progress is phenomenal. With good cooperation among industries and between industries and users and with well-defined set of standards, computerized monitoring can certainly become, in a couple of years, the nucleus of support systems for anesthesia.

Computerized Monitoring

With the proliferation of noninvasive measurement techniques, which undoubtedly have clear merits, monitoring the various equipment has become a key issue. The pieces of information delivered by this equipment certainly help to improve the standard of delivering anesthesia. But when

Adapted from an article published in the *Int J Clin Monit Comput* 9:131–139, 1992. Reprinted with permission of Kluwer Academic Publishers.

monitoring this information itself becomes a hindrance, it strongly suggests the need for equipment to simplify the task of monitoring and improve the efficiency of the use of the information. In that context, computerized monitoring should not be viewed as yet another device pushed into intensive and critical care areas. Computerized monitoring is a new generation of technology; it is a platform, in a field where ease-of-use and quality of care are all that count. With the possibility of connecting various different standard pieces of equipment from different manufacturers and presenting the physiological state of the patient in a simple and coherent manner, computerized monitoring represents a milestone in support systems for anesthesia.

Use of computerized monitoring may not appear to directly fulfill any real demands in the intensive care or critical care environments, but it can improve the quality and efficiency of patient care. An analogy here is worth mentioning: When word-processing entered offices to improve productivity, there was reluctance and opposition to accept it. But today the view has totally changed and its contribution to productivity is unquestioned. The trend will be roughly the same in monitoring. The potential benefits of computerized monitoring may not be readily apparent, but as its use becomes more and more common, its full potential will be realized.

Recent Developments

The current trends in computerized monitoring are strongly characterized by the recent developments in computer technology. Graphic presentation and communication capability would be the key factors in deciding which monitoring system to choose. Graphic presentation refers to displaying data in a form easily comprehensible at a glance, for instance, as bar graphs or curves. Communication capability refers to the possibility of connecting one computerized system with another with support for remote and central monitoring. With these as major supporting features, the chief functions of a monitoring workstation will be—

1. To interface with various medical instruments and coalesce the data to form a device-independent description to have a single, common physiological state description that can be exchanged between different functional modules for analysis and alarm detection.
2. To achieve real-time graphic display schemes to facilitate quick identification of abnormalities at a very early stage.
3. To have powerful network communication capabilities between the workstations to facilitate remote monitoring and online analysis of patient data for research investigations and to generate high-quality graphic print-out of selected portions of the real-time and trend data on a central printer for record keeping.

The minimum set of monitoring functions for both hemodynamics and respiration would include the following:

1. Front-end monitoring of real time curves and the trends:
   a. Hemodynamic monitoring: blood pressure, SaO_2, analysis of ECG changes.
   b. Respiratory monitoring: end-tidal CO_2, shunt and dead space calculation, pressure-volume and Flow-volume loops.
2. User-callable decision support analysis functions:
   a. O_2-CO_2, Iso-shunt diagrams
   b. Hemodynamic derivatives like cardiac indices, peripheral resistance, etc.
   c. Acid-base disorders evaluation

Apart from monitoring tasks, the system can easily provide record-keeping functions e.g., maintaining a record of drugs given at different times, blood and fluid losses, laboratory reports on blood gas analysis, and other of remarks and comments.

Figure 20.1 shows, functionally, how one such system would appear. The bottom of the picture shows various medical instruments from which the data are collected and distributed. The top of the picture shows com-

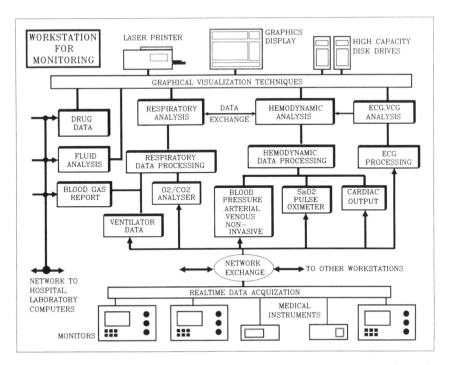

Figure 20.1. The functional layout of various modules in a workstation for real-time monitoring in anesthesia.

puter output devices. Various blocks, in the middle, represent the software modules which perform the specified task. The term *workstation* is used in the context of a computer used for a specific application, as in this case for monitoring.

The Transformation

Today there are not many systems for computerized monitoring. There are a few in-house or prototype systems, but as mentioned, the cost of such systems is the major factor, and with current rapid growth in computer technology, new such systems, economically priced, should be arriving soon in the marketplace. There are presently few entry-level products in the market, and most of them are for managing the trend values and to do record keeping (We shall discuss later in this chapter the usefulness of such record-keeping systems for anesthesia.) The concern is that these systems do not exploit sufficiently the potential capabilities of the computers that are used. But, assuming that versatile computerized monitoring systems become available in the not-too-distant future, various pieces of invasive and non-invasive equipment should be purchased with care to ensure that they support standard computer interfaces or, at least, that they will support them in the future. Every device, apart from the reliability and accuracy of the data it presents, should have connectivity to outside world. There should be a trade-off between an excellent, self-contained system with no external connectivity and normal, standard equipment with a good external interface to computers. In the future, every computerized monitoring system will provide an interface with all the different types of equipment in the high dependency area. Such interfaces will be a matter of major concern for the manufacturer of computerized monitoring systems. Eventually, the systems which survive in the market will be those which support connectivity to equipment of various different manufacturers. But from a maintenance point of view it would be preferable to have a common supplier for all medical monitoring equipment and computerized monitoring systems.

Automated Anesthesia Records

Automated anesthesia Records are entry-level systems for computerizing monitoring in anesthesia. Though automated records represent only a subset of an integrated computerized monitoring system, they addresses a real demand that exists today in anesthesia and other high-dependency areas. Also, interestingly, dissemination of experience has been quite extensive in this area, but with conflicting views. It is worthwhile to discuss the history and importance of automated records. [1–20]

History

Anesthesia records, though they were prescribed as a normal method for keeping track of an anesthesiologist's interaction with the patient, were given a low profile in what has always been one of the more action-oriented medical specialities. For a long time, they were used as an *aide memoire* for the anesthesiologist, as a "personal use record." But today, the growing complexity of pharmacological interventions with the patient demand more sophisticated physiological monitoring, which has created a strong demand and the necessity for a legible, well-documented, self-complete, more informative anesthesia record. In recent times, there have been considerable advances in overall health care delivery, especially in postoperative care. This has made the anesthesiologist's personal record even more important, as the record now becomes more common property, as a template of the physiological-state profile of the patient. Consequently, this lays profound emphasis on the quality, clarity, accuracy, and visual presentation of the data in the anesthesiologist's record.

Today, if anesthesia monitoring were to be compared to cockpit monitoring in an airplane, the anesthesia record would prove to be the "black-box" of the cockpit—a vital source of information.

In the following paragraphs, we will present a concise account of the purpose and clinical use of automated anesthesia records, their contribution to quality patient care, and experts' views and anesthesiologists' reaction to their most often debated pros and cons.

Automated Anesthesia Records

The major problems confronted when building an automated anesthetic record are multiple. In fact, even before the actual design of the system, considerable analysis of fundamental and practical issues surrounding the anesthesia record will be necessary. Such an analysis should address the following issues:

Purpose of the record
- What should it contain?
- Who needs to have access—to what information?
- When does the information need to be available?

Format of the record
- In what form should the data be recorded?
- In what form should data be presented?
- In what levels of detail?
- What text information should be included?
- What form of graphical presentation should be included?
- How should all the information be displayed?

Input of the data
- What are the sources of data and information?
- Which can be input automatically?
- How can integrity and accuracy of input be assured?
- What are the time-dependent constraints for input?
- What are the practical human-interface considerations for nonautomated input?

Clinical Use of Automated Records

During a routine anesthetic procedure, the anesthesiologist's major clinical functions are to anesthetize the patient safely (the primary task) to monitor and manage the patient's medical condition, and to maintain a current record of the procedure. Perhaps, most of the time, the record may just serve as a *memoire*, but irrespective of its usefulness at later time, it is an important requirement for quality patient care. Just as it is important to determine the exact nature of the patient's status at any moment, so too is it helpful to be able to plot the trend of this information over time to gain a broader perspective on the patient's progress through the anesthetic procedure. It can even prove critical should an alarm state requiring a detailed review of what has occurred up to that moment. Furthermore, during induction and other times when the patient demands the undivided attention of the clinician, it is difficult or impossible manually to maintain a record of even the simplest and most basic information [1]. The paradox of an incomplete to nonexistent record during the very time it is most important to be aware of the significant and rapid changes known to occur during such periods, and during which more physical and pharmacological manipulation of the patient is occurring has been commented on previously by Lerou et al. [15] While the handwritten record has historically served as an *aide memoire* reasonably well, the frequent and more detailed monitoring required for modern anesthetic procedure makes even the clerical portion of this function increasingly difficult. The proliferation of various monitors used during anesthetia makes it challenging enough for the anesthesiologist to maintain a handwritten record in an integrated, meaningful format even at the coarse time resolution of normal, manual record-keeping, let alone at the finer resolution that might later be desired in the analysis of critical event. It is quite strange to notice that despite the significant increase in monitored parameters since the mid-1970s, there has been little change in the number of average entries per manual anesthetic record to date [14].

Anesthesia records will find even greater importance when preparing for repeat anesthesia (either during the same admission or at a future time). It is from this point on that the clarity, completeness, accuracy, and detail of the record play a major role, if only because the attending clinician may not be available to supplement the record with unrecorded information.

The Anesthesia "Cockpit"

In the publication *Information Management in Anesthesia* [1] a striking comparison between the growing complexity of the anesthesia environment and the cockpit in aviation technology was presented. From its inception, the practice of anesthesiology has been characterized by a particularly intimate relationship between man and machine, such that anesthesiologists have long been among the more technology-literate physicians.

The parallels between the anesthesia environment and its aviation counterpart are indeed remarkable, from the long hours of sheer boredom penetrated by moments of abject terror, to the emphasis on quality assurance and the excellence of the overall safety record. In aviation technology, as more and more data was delivered to the cockpit, the point was reached at which, paradoxically, the pilot became less efficient and actually less vigilant, a situation ultimately relieved by greater computerization of the cockpit.

The Critiques

Since the introduction of automated anesthesia records, the merits of their use have been debated frequently. Manual record-keeping has been supported as a process that helps the anesthesiologist to be fully aware of anesthetic procedure. "The act of recording information on the chart forces the anesthesiologist to be aware of the time course and detail of anesthetic events" [16]. Similarly there is little written on the appropriateness of reliance on this clerical task as a means to apprise the clinician of what is happening to his or her patient. When one considers the problems of boredom and distraction during manual record-keeping, it is questionable whether removing the need for this clerical function would indeed have an adverse effect on vigilance. In a review of 6,000 anesthetias performed with automated record-keeping the sole method of charting, Edsall and colleagues found vigilance enhanced rather than impaired! [11]

Another concern that surfaces very often during discussions on automated anesthetic records are artifacts. Artifacts are probably inevitable in clinical monitoring, whether they are due to true transient physiological changes or whether they are due to interference with monitor input or output. Disregarding the values corresponding to artifacts is another common contributor to "smoothing" of the record. The justifications given for smoothing are many, ranging from the scientifically valid concern that inclusion of an aberrant value has some potential for distorting trend analysis, to the fear that such an aberrant value will be regarded by others as physiologically true and thereby be the cause of embarrassment at the least or impeachment at the worst.

It should be strongly emphasized that artifacts are in fact problems of monitoring rather than record-keeping. Good record-keeping is designed to report rather than obscure what was observed. If it fails to perform this function, then the record itself becomes an artifact.

Third-party oversight of a well-made automated anesthesia record is a frequent topic of discussion in the literature. This is where the clarity and completeness of the automated anesthesia record, which eliminates the clinician's ability selectively to record readings, faces unspoken resistance, presumably on the premise that Big Brother might detect something untoward in the record that might harm the interests of the record creator. The Big Brother issue is one of philosophy rather than technology [1]. In fact, it has been found that clinicians respond positively to the Big Brother issue; they see the clarity and completeness of automated anesthesia records as an opportunity to document the quality of their anesthesia care.

Practice of Automated Charting in the Thorax Centre, Erasmus University

Realizing the benefits of automated recording, researchers developed a microprocessor-based automated charting system at the Thorax Centre, Erasmus University, Rotterdam, in early 1970s. This charting was upgraded when newer technology became available. Over 10,000 records have been produced to date. Use of the automated charting system is a *de facto* routine procedure in the Thorax Centre. In fact, during breakdown and maintenance periods of the charting systems, severe complaints have been raised by practicing anesthesiologists that the lack of a charting system has caused considerable inconvenience in his or her attention to the quality of patient care. With the advent powerful personal computers, laser printers, cheap and efficient network communication capabilities, fast and large-capacity storage mediums, the whole complexion of automated anesthesia recording systems can change drastically. Presently, at the Thorax Centre, Erasmus University, we are developing a powerful computerized anesthesia recording systems based on an IBM Personal Systems/2 platform on a Token Ring network with the experience we gained in our earlier implementation of the automated charting systems.

Future Issues

High technology has become a hallmark of most areas of medical practice in the last third of the 20th century. In the operating room, as in other data-intensive areas of medical practice, its introduction has been particularly rapid. To derive maximum benefits from new advances in modern anesthesiology and to focus on quality of patient care, the automation of certain peripheral tasks should be cultivated.

The primary concern in the 1990s should focused not just on whether automation of anesthesia recording is necessary, but on setting standards for the functional specifications, quality, reliability, and uniformity of presentation. Lack of such standardization may lead to an outburst of too many different types of automated recording systems.

At the Thorax Centre, Erasmus University, we are presently working on possible standardization schemes. We will present here a short description of our standardization philosophy. We expect that the rapid growth in processing capabilities of personal computers will eventually bring "supervisory" monitoring (all-in-one screen monitoring compared to monitoring the different instruments directly), intelligent alarm techniques, real-time data record management, network communication for remote monitoring, and the automated recording systems all on one platform. With this general structure as our design framework, we are studying the following development approach to "fuse" various monitoring-related medical computing techniques so that as and when different

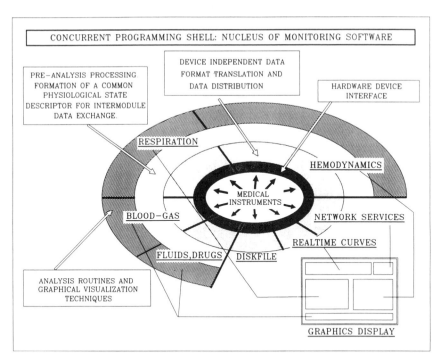

Figure 20.2. Standardizing the processing of data from various equipment. The shell diagrammatically illustrates the flow of information from the instruments to the user through different layers.

pieces are developed they can be quickly integrated within the general framework to produce a versatile monitoring workstation.

In Figure 20.2, the shell describes various monitoring-related software functions at different levels or layers with interconnection to various medical instruments as its central part. The picture represents the dynamic state of the software that will be running on the workstation. Concurrent programming will be the key element of the software. The different activities in various sectors will appear to progress concurrently from the centre along the radial direction, through different layers. The layers are formed for standardization convenience so that future changes could be limited to a small part of the software rather than the entire program.

Conclusions

The merits of a workstation-based approach to monitoring are many. Quick adaptability to new requirements, ease of upgrade, remote monitoring, and network capabilities are just a few. Such a workstation built on a standard hardware platform will assure evolutionary growth of the system's intelligence as new techniques that can substantially improve the monitoring standards become available.

With these ambitious objectives for computerized monitoring, one might wonder whether an economically viable solution exists using computers that are simple to operate. The answer is quite positive—it is very possible today to develop such a workstation using the powerful personal computers with high resolution and fast graphics display available in the market. Such a workstation can significantly improve the standard of patient care with early-warning "smart" alarm techniques and can also provide a convenient platform for various research activities. Software to utilize fully the capabilities of these systems for such purposes will be a major area of development in medical monitoring in the coming years.

Discouraging experiences in the past with in-house or commercial automated anesthesia recording systems cannot be a basis for judging future systems. Computer technology is far more advanced today than it was few years back, and now it can provide excellent performance to meet diverse real-time application areas for a smaller price. For rapid assimilation of these advances in medical monitoring, clinicians who use automated systems should freely express their opinions and constructive criticisms about such systems in the literature. This will be of great help not only to other clinicians but will also aid the industries in developing mature and intelligent systems.

References

1. Communicore Inc.: Information Management in Anesthesia—Issues and opportunities in the development and adoption of automated record keeping

as a standard practice. (Published by Communicore. Inc. under an educational grant from Diatek Patient Management System Inc. California, USA.)

2. Lunn JN, Vickers MD. A new anaesthetic record. Anaesthesia 1982; 27:651–7.

3. Middleton HG. A cumulative anaesthesia record system. Anaesthesia 1982; 37:1121–5.

4. Borden SG van der, Prakash O, Meij SH. A microcomputer based charting system for documentation of haemodynamic respiratory parameters and drug administration during cardiac anaesthesia. In Prakash O (ed): Computing in Anaesthesia and Intensive Care. The Hague: Martinus Nijhoff 1983; pp416–22.

5. Paull JD. Humanising the computer. Anaesth Intensive Care 1982; 10:191–6.

6. Baetz WR, Schneider AJL, Apple H, et al. The anesthesia keyboard system. In Gravenstein JS (ed): Monitoring surgical patients in the operating room. Springfield, IL: Charles C. Thomas 1979; 197–212.

7. Beecher HK. The first anesthesia records. Surg Gynecol Obstet 1940; 71:689–93.

8. Beneken JEW, Blom JA, Meijler AP, et al. Computerized data acquization and display in anesthesia. In Prakash O (ed): Computing in Anesthesia and Intensive Care. The Hague: Martinus Nijhoff, 1983; 25–43.

9. Block FE Jr, Burton LW, Rafal MD, et al. Two computer based anesthetic monitors; the Duke automatic monitoring equipment (DAME) system and the micro DAME. J Clin Monit 1985; 1:30–51.

10. Cook CL, Mc Donald JS, Nunziata E. Differences between handwritten and automatic blood pressure records. Anesthesiology 1989; 71:385–90.

11. Edsall DW. Computerization of anesthesia information management—USERS' perspective. J Clin Monit 1989: 7:351–358.

12. Eichhorn JH. Disadvantages of automated anesthesia records. In Safety and Cost Containment in Anesthesia Boston: Butterworths, 1988; pp223–32.

13. Gravenstein JS. The uses of anesthesia record. Presentation at Massachusetts General Hospital, March 30, 1989.

14. Gravenstein N, Feldman J. Anesthesia records and automation. Semin anesthesia 1989; 8(2):119–29.

15. Lerou JGC, Dirksen R, van Daele M, et al. Automated charting of physiological variables in anesthesia; a quantitative comparison of automated versus handwritten anesthesia records. J Clin Monit 1988; 4:37–47.

16. Noel TA. Computerized anesthesia records may be dangerous [letter]. Anesthesiology 1986; 64:300.

17. Paulus DA, van der Aa J, Mc Laughlin G, et al. A more accurate anesthesia record: the electronic clipboard [abstract]. Anesthesiology 1988; 69:A33.

18. Trosty S. In: Automated anesthesia records aid risk management. Hosp Risk Manage 1989; 11(8):99–101.

19. Zollinger RM, Kreul JF, Schneider AJL. Malt-made versus computer generated anesthesia records. J Surg Res 1977; 22:419–24.

20. Westenskow DR. In: Viewpoint-should the user be able to alter the computerized anesthesia record? Med Innov Quarterly Report 1989; 1(6):6.

Chapter 21
The Role of Smart Medical Systems in the Space Station

Reed M. Gardner, David V. Ostler,
Brent D. Nelson, and James S. Logan

Introduction

Historically, the United States has assigned minimal priority to "complex" medical care in space, largely because most space flights have been of short duration. The Space Station currently being designed presents new challenges [1–5]. The design calls for crew to be transported by shuttle, but to then remain isolated in the Space Station for 45 to 180 days, a much longer period of time than most previous flights. The shuttle can be in space for approximately 7 days; it was designed to be a "space truck" and cannot carry large supplies of fuel, rations, and oxygen for longer flights. For the first time in the space program, an "ambulance" may not be called to return sick or injured crew members. Such a call, were it even feasible, would be very expensive (about $300 million) and slow (14 to 45 days). As a result, the Space Station must be equipped with a self-sufficient medical unit, and to this end, NASA engineers are designing a computerized Health Maintenance Facility [1–5].

Space Station Health Maintenance Facility

There are eight design guidelines for the Space Station Health Maintenance Facility (HMF) [5]:

1. Capacity to accommodate a single critical care patient, or four to six patients with minor injury or illness, for 45 days.
2. Capacity for two medical officers with expertise comparable to that of paramedics or emergency medical technicians.
3. Equipment and supplies occupying 3 m³ and weighing 950 kg.

Adapted from an article published in the *Int J Clin Monit Comput* 6:91–98, 1989. Reprinted with permission of Kluwer Academic Publishers.

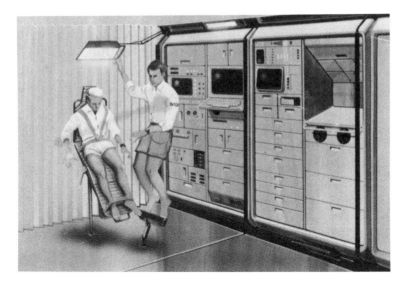

Figure 21.1. Conceptual drawing of the Space Station Health Maintenace Facility with a patient in a "restraint"—the microgravity analog of a bed. See text for description of the equipment modules.

4. Ability to perform minor emergency medical and surgical procedures.
5. Ability to communicate with NASA flight surgeons at medical support centers on earth.
6. Protocols to prioritize medical procedures and algorithms for specific methodologies.
7. Commercial technologies that are functional in the Space Station's microgravity environment.
8. Medical instruments which automatically communicate data to the HMF computer through a Medical Information Bus.

An artist's conceptual layout of the Space Station Health Maintenance Facility is shown in Figure 21.1. The patient is held in a restraint and is surrounded by support equipment. The bank of equipment behind the medical officer (standing) contains a dental instrument module, a pulse oximeter, a ventilator, suction and air fluid separator, IV pumps, a patient monitor, and defibrillator. The second bank (with the large screen) includes an intravenous (IV) fluid production and support system, a computer terminal, and a medical information system. The third bank contains an x-ray and imaging system [4] and medical supplies storage space. The fourth bank (right side of the photo) includes a microbiology workstation, clinical laboratory system, and pharmacy module.

Figure 21.2 shows the major support modalities of the Space Station Health Maintenance Facility: prevention, diagnosis, and therapy [5]. Crucial to the operation of the HMF is the computerized medical decision

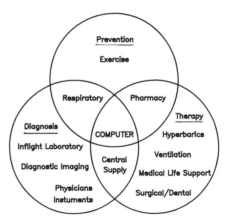

Figure 21.2. Combining the capabilities or the Space Station showing computer system at the center of prevention, diagnosis, and therapy.

support system which integrates data from all three care support modalities (center of the diagram).

An exercise facility will be used to minimize cardiovascular decompensation caused by deconditioning in microgravity. Diagnostic capabilities will include clinical laboratory facilities such as chemistry, hematology, and microbiology, as well as radiographic imaging. Medical care in the Space Station will include physiological monitoring, cardiac defibrillation, IV fluid support, pharmacy, capabilities for minor surgery, and a support ventilator.

Which Medical Problems to Expect

The Health Maintenance Facility will function as physician's office, pharmacy, hospital, clinical laboratory, and exercise station. Instrumentation and computer facilities will utilize ground-based technology. To determine the requirements of such a facility, a careful estimation of potential medical problems was needed. Extensive studies have been made of the physiological changes associated with microgravity, but only limited data existed for inflight disease and injury incidence. There was well-documented medical information concerning Antarctic crews, nuclear submarine crews, and US military populations, but these comparable populations were imperfect models and the data required extrapolation to be useful.

Using anonymous computerized hospital records for calendar year 1985, researchers studied more than 1.2 million US Army and Navy personnel. The records contained the International Classification of Diseases 9th Edition Clinical Modification (ICD-9-CM) categories, length of illness, mortality, and disability retirement information [6, 7]. These data were adapted to the Space Station environment by taking the following

Table 21.1. Top 15 Categories of Medical Problems Expected on Space Station*

Rank	ICD-9 code	Category
1	427	Cardiac dysrhythmias
2	410	Acute myocardial infarction
3	780	General symptoms
4	724	Disorders of back, other and unspecified
5	717	Internal derangement of knee
6	733	Disorders of bone and cartilage, other
7	718	Derangements of joint, other
8	722	Intervertebral disc disorders
9	296	Affective psychoses
10	135	Sarcoidosis
11	695	Erythematous conditions
12	719	Disorders of joint, other and unspecified
13	070	Viral hepatitis
14	592	Carculus of kidney and ureter
15	728	Disorders of muscle, ligament, and fascia

*Based on evaluation of hospitalization records for the US Army and Navy (1.2 million population) for the year 1985 [6,7].

facts into consideration: 1) that microgravity would reduce traumatic injuries; 2) that crew members would be placed in isolation several days before the mission, and therefore only microorganisms brought on board would colonize; 3) that there would be cardiopulmonary and musculoskeletal deconditioning as well as bone demineralization; 4) that stricter selection criteria would be applied to the Space Station crew than had been operative with military personnel.

A Medical Impact Score was used to rank the diseases and injuries by incidence rate and consequence to the crew. Results of this analysis are shown in Table 21.1 [6, 7]. The fact that cardiac dysrhythmias and acute myocardial infarction rank at the top of the categories clearly indicates a need for monitoring capabilities similar to those in a coronary care unit. Note also that joint and bone disorders have projected frequent occurrence, which clearly suggests a need for an x-ray imaging system on board the Space Station.

Design Requirements of Medical Decision Support System

The Health Maintenance Facility Medical Decision Support System must meet the following requirements [5]:

1. Provide an on-board integrated computerized medical record. Since conventional paper medical records are heavy and cannot be easily shared with ground-based flight surgeons and consultants, the medical records will be computerized.

2. Provide preventive, diagnostic, and therapeutic management algorithms. In case communications with ground-based medical experts is unavailable, computerized diagnostic and treatment protocols will be self-contained in the support system.
3. Provide electronically retrievable NASA contingency checklists and procedures and indexed medical references. References such as the *Physicians' Desk Reference* (PDR) will be available in electronic form.
4. Transmit measurement data, images, medical monitoring alarms, and charted information to ground-based flight surgeons and medical consultants as necessary.
5. Provide two-way air-to-ground "private" and "public" electronic mail and voice communications. The "private" medical conference is essential for confidentiality among crews and ground staff and family.
6. Provide computer-assisted inventory management of medical supplies and pharmaceuticals, since the Space Station will be in continuous use and will continually need to be resupplied.

In addition to these requirements, the Space Station has several other constraints:

a. All physiological and laboratory data will be processed by "smart" monitors on board the Space Station.
b. Medical storage space will be limited.
c. Only clinically validated medical methodologies will be practiced.
d. All systems software must be written in the Ada computer language.
e. Computer processing support must be based on software and hardware components common to the remainder of the Space Station Data Management System.

Hardware Design

The Space Station represents a major technological advance in computing capability, compared with that used in former manned space flight. The network supporting the Space Station, of which the Medical Decision Support System is one node, will consist of distributed 4-million-instruction-per-second (mips) computers, known as Standard Data Processors, connected via a 100 mips fiber optic network. Both fixed and portable workstations will be supported from a global network and mass storage system. Each component in the network will have a redundant backup and will provide reliable service to all Space Station systems including the HMF.

Medical Information Bus (MIB)

Technology in intensive care unit (ICU) patient monitoring is just beginning to address the problem of how to collect data centrally from a wide variety of bedside instruments [9, 10]. A Medical Information Bus (MIB) has been designed to allow different medical instruments, from different manufacturers, to communicate with a host computer over a common communications link [9]. Proposed standards for the MIB are being developed by the Institute of Electrical and Electronic Engineers (IEEE) and designated P1073. The existence of an MIB standard will allow manufacturers to integrate standardized hardware and software into their monitoring devices. LDS Hospital has begun to integrate prototype MIB hardware and software into a wide variety of medical devices. Clinical experience with the MIB on IVAC 960 IV pumps in the Thoracic Intensive Care Unit has provided insight into problems associated with the application of this communications strategy. For example, an IV pump can report changes in infused volume every 0.1 ml, but clinicians do not require that level of detail; recording such information is like adding "noise" rather than "signal" to the record. It was therefore necessary to develop methods of recording only relevant information in the clinical record.

Further hardware and software in interfaces now undergoing clinical testing include the Ohmeda 370 Pulse Oximeter, the Siemens 900C Ventilator, the Dinamap Vital Signs Monitor (Models 1846 and 8100), the Puritan-Bennett 7200A Ventilator, the Spacelabs 90600A Series Monitors, the Oximetrix 3 venous SO_2 monitor and several blood gas instruments.

Clinical experience has revealed important strategies regarding use of the MIB: 1) Better methods to identify mechanical or electrical disturbances must be designed and validated, so that, medical devices will transmit only "representative" information. 2) MIB systems must be able to collect information at several levels; for example, at certain times it may be appropriate to measure 0.1 ml volume changes from an IV pump, while at other times 10 ml changes would be sufficient. 3) The host computer must be capable of presenting meaningful information from the MIB.

The MIB has proven valuable for reporting, record keeping, and decision-making at LDS Hospital. Detailed charting during crisis situations, almost impossible with manual methods, is now convenient and accurate. Furthermore, with the MIB it is possible to integrate data from diverse instruments and laboratories. Such data integration is crucial for medical decision making, for the provision of information to medical officers in the Space Station, and for communication to flight surgeons and consultants on earth.

NASA actively supports the IEEE MIB committee and is committed to interface its instruments to the host computer on board the Space Station.

Communications Systems

The Space Station crew will be in constant contact with earth via a complex communication system which will link four Telecommunications and

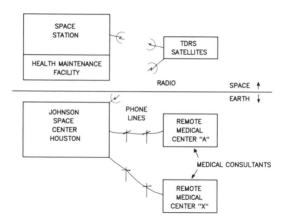

Figure 21.3. Block diagram of the communications network of the Space Station decision support system with the linkage to computers and flight-surgeons at Johnson Space Center in Houston, Texas. TDRS = Telecommunications and Data Relay Satellites.

Data Relay Satellites (TDRS), all in high geosynchronous orbit. Since the Space Station will be in low earth orbit (the same orbital path as the shuttle), communications will be made to earth via the TDRS communications system. This will avoid the current problem on shuttle flights where segments of the orbit have no radio contact with earth stations.

The Space Station communications system will have video, voice, and data transmission. These two-way air-to-ground links can be "public" (i.e., new conferences) or "private" (i.e., conversations and pictures transmitted to flight surgeons and family members).

The Medical Decision Support System will have both "down-link" and "up-link" communications with NASA control on earth. To supplement the on-board decision support, ground-based medical experts will be on-line consultants. Figure 21.3 shows the conceptual design of the ground network for the Health Maintenance Facility. The ground consultants will have workstations with video, radiographic imaging, audio, and data review capabilities. Thus, if NASA ground-based flight surgeons at Johnson Space Center need other medical expertise, such as from remote medical centers or clinics, the ground-based consultants will be able to quickly access the flight crew's medical data through the communications capability of the Health Maintenance Facility.

Decision Support System

Shortliffe has defined a Medical Decision Support System as "any computer program designed to help health professionals make clinical decisions" [11]. He also notes that *any* computer system that deals with clinical data or medical knowledge is intended to provide decision support. For example, each of the following programs can be considered a medical decision support system: 1) information retrieval, such as MEDLINE bibliographic searches; 2) focus of attention, such as drug alerts; and 3) patient-specific consultation, such as algorithms.

The Space Station Medical Decision Support System is similar to the HELP system operational at LDS Hospital [12–17]. Pryor and colleagues have programmed the HELP system to provide the following types of decision support [12–17]:

1. Alerting—Automatic notification of time-critical or action-oriented events: for example, notification of abnormal laboratory values, vital sign trends, or medication contraindications.
2. Interpreting—Assimilation of data resulting in a conceptual understanding: for example, ECG interpretation for both morphology and rhythm, or interpretation of blood gas data.
3. Assisting—Use of decision support to speed or simplify some action: for example, assistance with clinical orders, or data collection during a history or physical exam.
4. Critiquing—Analysis and validation of decisions [18]: for example, critiquing drug prescriptions.
5. Diagnosing—Application of a medical "model" for the purpose of understanding the state of a physiological system: for example, diagnosing using a Bayesian strategy.
6. Managing—Algorithms for clinical treatment: for example, suggestions about ventilator management.

Figure 21.4 is a block diagram of the Medical Decision Support System. The Space Station system will have four major areas: 1) the medical record, 2) a medical knowledge base, 3) a medical textbook/checklist database, and 4) an inventory maintenance database.

The medical records and knowledge-base areas will simulate features of the HELP system [12–17]. Currently, many computerized medical decision support systems are passive, i.e., they require the physician or health care provider to recognize a need for the system and enter the data by hand. Conversely, the HELP system is active, i.e., medical decisions are automatically generated, based on patient-specific data contained in the database, without data entry by the physician. A similar design will be used on the Space Station, including using the MIB.

Shortliffe maintains that decision support programs operate at optimum effectiveness when they are integrated with routine data management functions [19, 20]. The HELP system has these capabilities since it integrates data from a wide variety of sources and can be both data and time driven [12–17]. A data-driven medical decision support system provides a tireless watch over the patients. It culls an enormous volume of low-yield clinical data to discover the occasional mistake if one occurs.

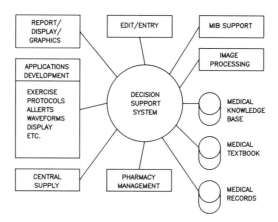

Figure 21.4. Block diagram of the computerized Medical Decision Support System, showing its interconnection to data gathering equipment, knowledge bases and reporting functions.

Data-driven systems can produce virtually errorless medicine by scrutinizing data and considering every possible inference—something human practitioners cannot achieve [21]. To realize this advantage, a decision-making system must be integrated into a comprehensive clinical database. Secondly, the execution of the decision logic must be an automatic consequence of data capture or the passage of time (i.e., time-driven), and not be dependent on the health care provider's conscious activation [11, 21].

Discussion

When the Space Station is launched and assembled in the 1990s, medical computer technology will be sophisticated enough to evaluate the Medical Decision Support System, and the requisite electronic medical record. McDonald and associated ascertain that over the next few years, on-line medical records will become technically and economically feasible [22]. Such technology will have three major advantages:

1. Improved logistics and organization of the medical record, to speed treatment and improve efficiency.
2. Automatic computer review of the medical record, to limit errors and control cost.
3. Systematic analysis of past clinical experience, to help guide future practice.

The methods of data collection and decision-making presented in this paper are clinically operational or have been tested in a prototype form.

The space program nurtured microcomputer technology so prevalent in modern sophisticated bedside monitors. Now, it is likely that the Space Station inhabitants will benefit from the medical computerized data collection and decision support systems developed with the aid of microcomputers.

Summary

NASA is developing a Health Maintenance Facility to provide medical equipment and supplies requisite for the Space Station to be launched in the late 1990s. An essential component of this medical facility is a computerized Medical Decision Support System which will expedite medical officers' efforts to maintain the crew's health. The computerized system includes four major functions:

1. A data collection and storage system with a self-contained medical expert scheme for performing treatment protocols. The expert system has "data-driven" and "time-driven" capabilities to facilitate automatic decision-making functions.
2. An integrated medical record and medical "reference" information management component.
3. An inventory management system for medical supplies and pharmaceuticals.
4. Video, audio, and data communications between the medical officer in the Space Station and ground-based medical personnel.

This paper discusses the design of such computerized data collection, communications, and expert medical systems as will be developed for use in a Space Station Health Maintenance Facility.

Acknowledgments

This work was supported in part by contracts from NASA 9-17425.

References

1. Logan JS, Stolle MF. Treatment capabilities of Space Station Health Maintenance Facility. Research and Technology Annual Report 1986. NASA Technical Memorandum 58227 pp8.
2. Logan JS, Jurmain MH. Considerations in the design of a Health Maintenance Facility for the Space Station. Research and Technology Annual Report 1986. NASA Technical Memorandum 58227 pp7.
3. Raymond CA. When medical help is *really* far away. JAMA 1988; 259:2313–4.

4. Raymond CA. Unearthly medicine demands special devices. JAMA 1988; 259:2514–5.
5. McKinley BA. Medical care aboard NASA's Space Station: A systems approach to critical care monitoring. IEEE-Engineering in Medicine and Biology Society 10th Annual Conference 1988; 10:1791–2.
6. Nelson BD. An analysis, prioritization, and simulation of space station medical care. Master of Science Thesis, University of Utah, August 1987.
7. Nelson BD, Gardner FM, Ostler DV, Schulz JM, Logan JS. Medical impact analysis for the Space Station. Aviation, Space Environ Med 1990; 61:169–175.
8. Gardner RM. Computerized management of intensive care patients. MD Comput 1986, 3:36–51.
9. Shabot MM. Standardized acquisition of bedside data: The IEEE P1073 Medical Information Bus. Int J Clin Monit Comput 1989; 6:197–204.
10. Hawley WL, Tariq H, Gardner RM. Clinical implementation of an automated medical information bus in an intensive care unit. SCAMC 1988; 12:621–4.
11. Shortliffe EH. Computer programs to support clinical decision making. JAMA 1987; 258:61–6.
12. Pryor TA, Warner HR, Gardner RM. Clayton PD, Haug PJ. The HELP system development tools. In Orthner H, Blum B (eds): Implementing Health Care Information Systems. New York: Springer-Verlag, 1989; 365–83.
13. Pryor TA, Gardner RM, Clayton PD, Warner HR. The HELP system. J Med Systems 1983; 7:87–102.
14. Evans RS, Gardner RM, Bush AR, Burke JP, Jacobson JA, Larsen RA, Meier FA, Warner HR. Development of a computerized infectious disease monitor (CIDM). Comp Biomed Res 1985; 18:103–13.
15. Evans RS, Larsen RA, Burke JP, Gardner RM, Meier FA, Jacobson JA, Conti MT, Jacobson JT, Hulse RK. Computer surveillance of hospital-acquired infections and antibiotic use. JAMA 1986; 256:1007–11.
16. Sittig DF. COMPAS: A computerized patient advice system to direct ventilatory care. PhD Dissertation. University of Utah, June 1988.
17. Bradshaw KB. CLAS: A computerized laboratory alerting system. PhD Dissertation, University of Utah. June 1988.
18. Miller PL. Expert Critiquing Systems: Practice-Based Medical Consultation by Computer. New York. NY: Springer-Verlag, 1986.
19. Rennels GD, Shortliffe EH. Advanced computing in medicine. Sci Am 1987; 257:154–61.
20. Shortliffe EH. Medical expert systems: Knowledge tools for physicians. West J Med 1986; 145:830–9.
21. Clayton PD. The AI Purists and the engineers—Editorial. MD Computing 1987; 4:5–6.
22. McDonald CJ, Tierney WM. Computer-stored medical records: Their future role in medical practice. JAMA 1988; 259:3433–40.

V
Conclusions

Chapter 22
The Why, What, and So What of Computers in the ICU

Reed M. Gardner and Stanley M. Huff

There is continued interest and determination to use "free text" recording for computerized ICU records. Recently Hohnloser and Purner [0] pointed out several advantages of using off-the-shelf text-processing software packages to support patient care. Such an ICU record-keeping system allows physicians to enter progress notes in a "free text" format. In addition, their system has the capability of coding (using ICD-9) the patient's admitting diagnosis and to gather data from a laboratory computer system. A useful innovation of these and other similar systems is the integration of "hypertext" software tools to manipulate free text notes in the patient record. However, many desirable features of ICU systems are precluded by systems that are mainly free-text-based. We have strong emotional and scientific support for our stand that coded and integrated computerized ICU systems are superior to "free text" systems. The development of computerized ICU charting has been underway for two decades. Therefore, we are reminded of philosopher George Santayana's (1863–1952) comment, "Those who fail to remember the past are condemned to repeat it."

Why?

Why are computers used in medicine and the data-rich area of ICU care? Although the specific answer to this question cannot yet be completely quantitated, much is known about the subject. Based on a broad literature review, it is clear that many factors are important. In the United States, the Institute of Medicine (IOM) of the National Academy of Sci-

Adapted from Gardner RM, Huff SM. Editorial: Computers in the ICU: Why? What? So What? Int J Clin Monit Comput 1992; 199–205, with permission.

ences recently declared that a computer-based patient record was an essential technology for health care [1, 2]. Information in the medical record should be easily retrievable and reviewable in a temporal relationship to other associated data. Records having these characteristics would facilitate the routine processing of data required for medical decisions [3–6]. Traditional manual medical records lack these attributes [1–8]. Data found in the medical record are central to all medical care. These data are used to make medical decisions, be they diagnostic or therapeutic. Since the mid-1960s computers have been used in intensive care units (ICU) [8–15]. These systems have been used for a variety of tasks.

An implicit assumption of free-text-only systems is that the physician can provide *all* the necessary intellectual analysis of the patient data. McDonald, Eddy, and others have clearly shown that humans are *not* perfect information processors [16–24]. The statement by Hohnloser and Purner that "(existing) systems may decrease patient contact time and do not necessarily improve patient care," stands in contrast to the literature, which shows the value of integrated clinical computing systems used for decision support [16–43].

With only *free-text-oriented* computerized systems, one gives up the ability easily to detect drug-drug interactions and drug-laboratory contraindications [25, 26], assistance with selecting appropriate antibiotics [27–31], laboratory and blood gas alerts and interpretations [32–34], assistance with blood ordering [35–37], and the ability to provide automated adverse drug event monitoring [38, 39]. In addition, computer-driven protocols for guiding complex patient care in the ICU are not possible [40–43].

What?

There are a host of ways computers can be used in the ICU: 1) to acquire signals; 2) to chart vital signs; 3) to chart medications; 4) to communicate data, for example from the clinical laboratory; 5) to store data; 6) to produce reports; 7) to generate alerts; 8) to implement computerized care protocols; 9) to code data, for example the ICD-9 Codes; 10) for patient care planning by nurses and physicians; 11) for review of dictated reports; 12) for recording of procedures; 13) for determination of acuity such as with TISS and APACHE scoring system; 14) quality assurance; 15) order entry and charge capture; 16) administrative needs; 17) educational needs, for example, doing MEDLINE searches.

A careful review of the field of medical informatics shows that all of these tasks need be to integrated. In 1982 the National Library of Medicine in the United States started funding Integrated Academic Information Systems (IAIMS) [44]. These centers were to be pilots of the "future" systems that would allow those in medical centers to have access to a variety of computer services. Several pilot IAIMS have now been established in the United States, for example, at Columbia-Presbyterian Medical Center in New York City [45]. The breadth of IAIMS is best illustrated by the 6 data resources they allow users to access:

1. *Scholarly information services* include library, electronic textbooks, knowledge frames, natural language processing.
2. *Administrative information service* encompasses space and facility availability, directory, grants management, personnel management, word processing, desktop publishing.
3. *Core services* include networking, electronic mail, and communications.
4. *Basic medical research* consists of items such as biomedical research tools, supercomputing, and graphics.
5. *Clinical research services* include epidemiology research, database statistical packages, clinical information services such as ancillary applications, admit, discharge and transfer (ADT) medical records, order entry, results review, and nursing.
6. *Medical information research* includes decision-making, knowledge base, work-stations, human interfaces, and education.

Some centers have chosen to provide only reference materials so MEDLINE searches could be done or medical texts could be easily accessed. Coding data with ICD-9 coding schemes and establishing acuity scores has been the emphasis of those who have developed the TISS and APACHE scoring schemes [46, 47]. Collection of charges and resource utilization data for the purposes of looking at financial and cost-effectiveness research has been important to many. The main consideration of others has been gathering only "monitoring" data by collecting and storing this data in coded format. Still others have tried to integrate data from many sources and of multiple types to augment physician decision making.

To gather statistics on what data were important for *physician decision-making* in intensive care, Bradshaw and colleagues observed physicians in ICU "teaching rounds" and also had them complete questionnaires when they had made bedside visits to determine what data were used [48]. Laboratory data made up 42% of the data used; observations (an area where free text is often used) were 21%; drugs, input/output, and IV data usage ranged from 13 to 23%; bedside monitor data usage was 13 to 22%; while the "other" miscellaneous data were used 3 to 5% of the time.

The complexity of answering the *what* data question is amplified by a recent article by Forsythe and colleagues [49]. These investigators used anthropologists' methods to observe physicians in four clinical settings in internal medicine at a university teaching hospital. They undertook the study because they found that 1) there was no explicit consensus on what the information needs of physicians were, 2) previous investigations had limited "information needs" to only bibliographic and textbook needs, and 3) previous research had been too narrow. They found that physicians expressed needs for information of many types, some of a formal nature such as the type found in libraries and national databases (literature), while questions about bureaucratic and logistical issues were also necessary. Some had need for information that tends to be codified in guide books and textbooks in the form of "rules," "laws," and "principles." Thus, computer systems cannot meet "information" requirements of care givers if we do not address the full range of information needed.

Clearly the definitions of what is "information" and what and how it should be accessed in medicine are complex and still open to question. Therefore, focusing on the narrow view of recording data in only a "free text" format is inappropriate.

Hohnloser and Purner said about coding, "no code is as accurate as free text" [0]. It may be true that free text is the most flexible and expressive representation for clinical data, but it does not follow that it is the most useful or desirable form. Natural language understanding is fraught with a major problem of *ambiguity* [50]. In fact, with coding systems the computer can manipulate and add structure to data. As Shortliffe and Barnett state:

> Scientific disciplines generally develop precise terminology or notation that is standardized and is accepted by all workers in the field. Consider, for example, the universal language of chemistry. . . . Medicine is remarkable for its failure to develop a standardized vocabulary and nomenclature, and many observers believe that a true scientific basis for the field will be impossible until this problem is addressed. . . . Imprecision and lack of standardized vocabulary are particularly problematic when we try to aggregate data recorded by multiple health professionals or to analyze trends over time. Without a controlled, predefined vocabulary, data interpretation is inherently complicated and the automated summarization of data may be impossible. . . . Given the lack of formal definitions of many medical terms, it is remarkable that medical workers communicate as well as they do [8].

An enormous amount of work has been done both on vocabulary and data structures for medicine. One of the most active areas involving data structures are the electronic data exchange standards groups [51–55]. Several efforts deal extensively with controlled vocabularies [56–61]. Another group of people are working to integrate vocabulary terms with data structures to make record structures that will retain all relevant information in a clinical database [62–67]. Thus, while free text offers ultimate freedom of expression, current research is providing more flexible and comprehensive medical coding mechanisms than have existed in the past.

Hohnloser and Purner give a perfect example of where data coding is important because they use ICD-9 coding for the purpose of statistical reporting and epidemiologic research [0]. In addition the coding process extends the usefulness of the reporting process. The value of using computerized extraction of coded findings from "free-text" radiographic dictation has been shown to be important in computerized nosocomial infection monitoring [68, 69].

So What?

Those developing computerized systems used in health care often postulate how a system ought to behave, build it, and say that if it works, "it works" [70–72]. If the system developed does not work, the system's complexity is such that developers may not learn why it does not work and their efforts may be wasted. When a new system does work, it may be difficult to separate the system from its physical and organizational operating environment to provide something useful to the scientific community at large. Therefore, careful study of applied medical informatics research is necessary if we are to increase the productivity of research.

Basic research in medical informatics can and should be designed according to methodologies developed for the natural and social sciences [70]. Applied medical informatics research presents unique problems which make it difficult directly to utilize these materials from other sciences. Therefore, it is important to formulate systems development in terms of testable hypotheses and divide and subdivide complex projects into modules, each of which can be developed and tested rigorously, and to utilize qualitative studies in situations where more definitive quantitative studies are impractical. The system development stages are specification, component testing, systems testing, integrated systems testing, and postimplementation analysis. And the evaluation strategies involve 1) the definition; 2) laboratory testing in either (a) benchwork or (b) fieldwork; 3) remote field testing; and 4) routine operations.

Then there is a bare bones set of questions that might be asked of the adequacy of studying advanced information systems. First, the purpose of studying a computerized medical system should be to evaluate whether there is a therapeutic, diagnostic, screening, prognostic, predictive, or a quality assurance emphasis. For many situations the emphasis seems to be for therapy and quality assurance. If the emphasis is therapy, then the following questions should be asked: 1) Is there an assignment of patients to an intervention and control group that is randomized? 2) Are clinically important outcomes assessed objectively? 3) Is the innovation feasible to implement in the usual clinical practice? 4) Are follow-up procedures adequate to insure at least 80% follow-up of participants? 5) Is the sample size based on a clinically important but realistic benefit? 6) Is the search for adverse effects and costs analyzed? Then there are quality assurance questions: 1) Is the assignment of patients to an intervention or control group really randomized? 2) Have the clinical actions under study been shown to do more good than harm? If not, does the study compare process to outcome? 3) Are clinical processes or acts measured in a clinically sensible and valid way? 4) Are follow-up procedures adequate to insure at least 80% follow-up of participants? 5) Are both clinical and statistical significance considered? 6) Are contamination or co-intervention and compliance dealt with adequately?

Conclusions

As Osborn stated so eloquently a decade ago:

> The great mass of useful numbers we generate by computer has got to be tamed and controlled. We have learned how to make the measurements. Now we must learn how to handle the resulting data and present them in understandable terms. Used right, automation can integrate these data, simplify them, scan and evaluate them. Automation is not a cold-blooded monster-machine between us and the patient. It is a tool to expand our medical power, to let us get closer to the patient, and take better care of him [9].

Projects that allow others to learn from the experience can be valuable even if the outcome is not as intended. Investigators should select the most rigorous measure suitable for the situation. Qualitative and quantitative assessments are needed. Thus we are like the small boy who is blindfolded and touches an elephant at different points and gets a different "feel" for what the animal is, whether he is touching the ear, the leg, the tail, or the tusk. The care of the intensive care patient is a complex and multi-faceted task. It includes nursing, therapists, laboratory, radiology, and data that comes from as many as 25 hospital locations. The idea of communicating and sharing data across all of these fields and integrating them into one data source is the objective of most information systems used in critical care. Those proposing use of only free text data usually only focus on a set of functions that can be accomplished with free-text user interface, but do not discuss the many desirable features of an ICU system that are *excluded* by using only a free text approach. Clearly free text that is machine readable (and can be read better than hand written scribbles) provides some interesting and innovative, potential.

Therefore, we feel the field of medical computing in general and specifically in the area of intensive care computer applications should develop much more carefully controlled strategies and methodologies for evaluating the effectiveness and value of care. These evaluations can be done in terms of qualitative methods such as interviews and questionnaires or they can be done in the form of time-motion studies or, still further, they can be done in the randomized controlled trials that might assess differences in patients' length of stay or long-term outcomes.

References

0. Hohnloser JH, Purner F. PADS (Patient Archiving and Documentation System): A computerized patient record with educational aspects. Int J Clin Monit Comput 1992; 9:71–84.
1. Shortliffe EH, Tang PC, Detmer DE. Patient records and computers [editorial]. Ann Intern Med 1991; 115:979–981.
2. Dick RS, Steen EB (Editors). The Computer-Based Patient Record. Institute of Medicine. Washington, DC: National Academy Press, 1991.
3. Fries JF. Alternatives in medical record formats. Med Care 1974; 12:871–881.
4. Whiting-O'Keefe QE, Simborg DW, Epstein WV. A controlled experiment to evaluate the use of time-oriented summary medical records. Med Care 1980; 8:842–852.
5. Shea S, Margulies D. The paperless medical record. Soc Sci Med 1985; 21:741–746.
6. McDonald CJ, Tierney WM. Computer-stored medical records. Their future role in medical practice. JAMA 1988; 259:3433–3440.
7. Hammond J, Johnson HM, Varas R, Ward CG. A quantitative comparison of paper flowsheets vs a computer-based clinical information system. Chest 1991; 99:155–157.
8. Shortliffe EH, Barnett GO. Medical Data: Their Acquisition, Storage, and Use. In Shortliffe EH, Perreault LE (ed): Medical Informatics: Computer Applications in Health Care. Reading, MA: Addison-Wesley Publishing Co., 1990; pp37–69.
9. Osborn JJ. Computers in critical care medicine: promises and pitfalls. Crit Care Med 1982; 10:808–810.
10. Gardner RM, West BJ, Pryor TA, Larsen KG, Warner HR, Clemmer TP, Orme JF Jr. Computer-based ICU data acquisition as an aid to clinical decision-making. Crit Care Med 1982; 10:823–830.
11. Gardner RM. Computerized management of intensive care patients. MD Comput 1986; 3(1):36–51.
12. Brimm JE. Computers in critical care. Crit Care Q 1987; 9:53–63.
13. Bradshaw KE, Sittig DF, Gardner RM, Pryor TA, Budd M. Computer-based data entry for nurses in the ICU. MD Comput 1989; 6(5):274–280.
14. Gardner RM, Bradshaw KE, Hollingsworth KW. Computerizing the intensive care unit: Current status and future directions. J Cardiovasc Nurs 1989; 4:68–78.
15. Gardner RM, Shabot MM. Computerized ICU Data Management: Pitfalls and Promises. Int J Clin Monit Comput 1990; 7:99–105.
16. McDonald CJ. Protocol-based computer reminders, the quality of care and the Nonperfectibility of man. N Engl J Med 1976; 295:1351–1355.
17. Eddy DM. Clinical decision making from theory to practice: The challenge. JAMA 1990; 263:287–290.
18. Eddy DM. Clinical decision making from theory to practice: Anatomy of a decision. JAMA 1990; 263:441–443.
19. McDonald CJ, Tierney WM. Computer-stored medical records. Their future role in medical practice. JAMA 1988; 259:3433–3440.
20. Berwick DM. Continuous improvement as an ideal in health care. N Engl J Med 1989; 320:53–56.

21. Kritchevsky BS, Simmons BP. Continuous quality improvement—Concepts and application for physician care. JAMA 1991; 266:1817–1823.
22. Kuperman GJ, James BC, Jacobsen JT, Gardner RM. Continuous quality improvement applied to medical care: Experience at LDS Hospital. Med Decis Making 1991; 11:(*Suppl*) S60–S65.
23. Elliott CG. Computer-assisted quality assurance: Development and performance of a respiratory care program. QRB 1991; 17:85–89.
24. Edsall DW. Quality assessment with a computerized anesthesia information management system (AIMS). QRB 1991; 17:182–193.
25. Hulse RK, Clark SJ, Jackson JC, Warner HR, Gardner RM. Computerized medication monitoring system. Am J Hosp Pharm 1976; 33:1061–1064.
26. Gardner RM, Hulse RK, Larsen KG. Assessing the effectiveness of a computerized pharmacy system. SCAMC 1990; 14:668–672.
27. Evans RS, Larsen RA, Burke JP, Gardner RM, Meier FA, Jacobson JA, Conti MT, Jacobson JT, Hulse RK. Computer surveillance of hospital-acquired infections and antibiotic use. JAMA 1986; 256:1007–1011.
28. Evans RS, Burke JS, Pestotnik SL, Classen DC, Menlove RL, Gardner RM. Prediction of hospital infections and selection of antibiotics using an automated hospital data base. SCAMC 1990; 14:663–667.
29. Evans RS, Burke JP, Classen DC, Gardner RM, Menlove RL, Goodrich KM, Stevens LE, Pestotnik SL. Computerized identification of patients at high risk for hospital acquired infections. Am J Infect Control 1992; 20:4–10.
30. Evans RS, The HELP System: A review of clinical applications in infectious diseases and antibiotic use. MD Comput 1991; 8:282–288.
31. Classen DC, Evans RS, Pestotnik SL, Horn SD, Menlove RL, Burke JP. The timing of prophylactic administration of antibiotics and the risk of surgical-wound infection. N Engl J Med 1992; 326:281–286.
32. Shabot MM, LoBue M, Leyerle BJ, Dubin SB. Inferencing strategies for automated ALERTS on critically abnormal laboratory and blood gas data. SCAMC 1989; 13:54–57.
33. Bradshaw KE, Gardner RM, Pryor TA. Development of a computerized laboratory alerting system. Comp Biomed Res 1989; 22:575–587.
34. Tate KE, Gardner RM, Weaver LK. A computerized laboratory alerting system. MD Comput 1990; 7(5):296–301.
35. Gardner RM, Laub RM, Golubjatnikov OK, Evans RS, Jacobson JT. Computer Critiqued Blood Ordering Using the HELP System. Comp Biomed Res 1990; 23:514–528.
36. Lepage E, Gardner RM, Laub RM, Golubjatnikov O. Optimizing medical practice using a computerized hospital information system. Example of blood transfusions. Nouv Rev Fr Hematol 1990; 32(5):301–302.
37. Lepage EF, Gardner RM, Laub RM, Golubjatnikov OK. Improving blood transfusion practice: Role of a computerized hospital information system. Transfusion 1992; 32:253–259.
38. Evans RS, Pestotnik SL, Classen DC, Bass, SB, Menlove RL, Gardner RM, Burke JP. Development of a computerized adverse drug event monitor. SCAMC 1991; 15:23–27.
39. Classen DC, Pestotnik SL, Evans RS, Burke JP. Computerized surveillance of adverse drug events in hospital patients. JAMA 1991; 266:2847–2851.
40. Sittig DF, Pace NL, Gardner RM, Beck E, Morris AH. Implementation of a

computerized patient advice system using the HELP clinical information system. Comp Biomed Res 1989; 22:474–487.

41. East TD, Morris AH, Clemmer TP, Orme JF Jr, Wallace CJ, Henderson S, Sittig DF, Gardner, RM. Development of computerized critical care protocols—a strategy that really works! SCAMC 1990; 14:564–568.

42. Henderson S, Crapo RO, Wallace CJ, East TD, Morris AH, Gardner RM. Performance of computerized protocols for management of arterial oxygenation in an intensive care unit. Int J Clin Monit Comput 1992; 8:271–280.

43. Morris AH. Use of monitoring information in decision making. In: Contemporary Management in Critical Care #4: Respiratory Monitoring. London: Churchill Livingston Inc., 1991; pp 213–229.

44. Matheson NW, Cooper JAD. Academic information in the academic health science center: Roles for the library information management. J Med Education 1982; 57(10):part 2.

45. Hendrickson G, Anderson RK, Clayton PD et al. The integrated academic information management system at Columbia-Presbyterian Medical Center. MD Comput 1992; 9:35–42.

46. Cullen DJ, Civetta JM, Briggs BA et al. Therapeutic intervention scoring system: A method for quantitative comparison of patient care. Crit Care Med 1974; 2:57–60.

47. Knaus WA, Draper EA, Wagner DP, Zimmerman JE. APACHE II: A severity of disease classification system. Crit Care Med 1985; 13:818–829.

48. Bradshaw KE, Gardner RM, Clemmer TP, Orme JF Jr, Thomas F, West BJ. Physician decision-making—Evaluation of data used in a computerized ICU. Int J Clin Monit Comput 1984; 1:81–91.

49. Forsythe DE, Buchanan BG, Osheroff JA, Miller RA. Expanding concept of medical information: An observational study of physicians' information needs. Comp Biomed Res 1992; 25:181–200.

50. Carbonell JG, Hayes PJ. Natural language understanding. In: Encyclopedia of Artificial Intelligence, 2nd ed. 1992; 2:997–1016.

51. Shabot MM. Standardized acquisition of bedisde data: The IEEE P1073 medical information bus. Int J Clin Monit Comput 1989; 6:197–204.

52. Harrington JJ. IEEE P1157 Medical Data Interchange (MEDIX): Application of open systems to health care communications. Top Health Rec Manag 1991; 11(4):45–58.

53. Digital Imaging and Communications. ACR-NEMA Standard Publication 300–1985. Washington, DC: NEMA, 1988.

54. DeMoor G (ed). Euclides, a European standard for clinical laboratory data exchange. In: Readings in Medical Informatics, pp373–75.

55. Health Level Seven. Health Level Seven: An application protocol for electronic data exchange in healthcare environments. Version 2.1. American Medical Assoc, Chicago: HL7, 1990.

56. Clauser SB, Fanta CM, Finkel AJ (eds). CPT–1984: Physicians' Current Procedural Terminology. Chicago: American Medical Assoc, 1984.

57. Cote R. SNOMED—The Systematized Nomenclature of Medicine, College of American Pathologists, Illinois, 1979.

58. ICD-9-CM, The International Classification of Diseases, 9th Revision, Clinical Modifications, Vols. 1–3, 2nd edition. DHHS Pub No. (PHS) 80-1260, Washington DC, 1980.

59. Lindberg DAB, Humphreys BL. The UMLS knowledge sources: Tools for building better user interfaces. SCAMC 1990; 14:121–125.
60. Gabrielli ER. A new electronic medical nomenclature. J Med Sys 1989; 13:355–373.
61. Read JD. The Read clinical classification. Proc. MIE 88, Oslo, Norway, August 1988. Heidelberg: Springer-Verlag, 1988; pp587–591.
62. Stead, WW. Systems for the year 2000: The case for an integrated database. MD Comput; 1991; 8(2):103–110.
63. Linnarsson R, Wigertz O. The data dictionary—A controlled vocabulary for integrating clinical databases and medical knowledge bases. Meth Info Med 1989; 28:78–85.
64. Rossi-Mori A, Thorton AM, Gangemi A. An entity-relationship model for a European machine-dictionary of medicine. SCAMC 1990; 14:185–189.
65. Rector A, Nowlan WA, Kay S. Unifying medical information using an architecture based on descriptions. SCAMC 1990; 14:191–194.
66. Friedman C, Hripcsak G, Johnson SB, Cimino JJ, Clayton PD. A generalized relational schema for an integrated clinical patient database. SCAMC 1990; 14:335–339.
67. Stahlhut RW, McCallie DP, Waterman DM, Margulies DM. A relational model for clinical objective results. SCAMC 1990; 14:354–358.
68. Haug PJ, Ranum DL, Frederick PR. Computerized extraction of coded findings from free-text radiology reports. Radiology 1990; 174:543–548.
69. Evans RS, Gardner RM, Bush AR, Burke JP, Jacobson JA, Larsen RA, Meier FA, Warner HR. Development of a computerized infectious disease monitor (CIDM). Comp Biomed Res 1985; 18:103–113.
70. Stead WW, Haynes BR, Fuller S, et al. Designing medical informatics research and library resource projects to increase what is learned. JAMIA 1994; 1:(in press)
71. Clayton PD, Anderson RK, Hill C, McCormack M. An initial assessment of the cost and utilization of the integrated academic information system (IAIMS) at Columbia Presbyterian Medical Center. SCAMC 1991; 15:109–113.
72. Pace NL. Technology assessment of anesthesia monitors. J Clin Monit 1992; 8:142–146.

Chapter 23
A Strategy for Development of Computerized Critical Care Decision Support Systems

Thomas D. East, Alan H. Morris,
C. Jane Wallace, Terry P. Clemmer,
James F. Orme, Jr., Lyndall K. Weaver,
Susan Henderson, and Dean F. Sittig

Introduction

It is not enough merely to manage medical information. It is difficult to justify the cost of hospital information systems (HIS) or intensive care unit (ICU) patient data management systems (PDMS) on this basis alone. The real benefit of an integrated HIS or PDMS is in decision support. We recently went to the bedside of a critically ill patient and counted the current information categories (not repeated measures) that were reviewed for physician decision-making. The total was in excess of 236! Dr. Eddy summarized it best: 'It is simply unrealistic to think that individuals can synthesize in their head scores of pieces of evidence, accurately estimate the outcomes of different options, and accurately judge the desirability of those outcomes for patients . . . All confirm what would be expected from common sense: The complexity of modern medicine exceeds the inherent limitations of the unaided human mind" [1]. Although there are a variety of HIS and ICU PDMS systems available, there are few that provide ICU decision support.

The HELP systems at the LDS Hospital [2–4] is an example of an HIS which provides decision support on many different levels. In the ICU there are decision support tools for antibiotic therapy, nutritional management, and management of mechanical ventilation. Computer protocols for the management of mechanical ventilation (respiratory evaluation, ventilation, oxygenation, weaning and extubation) in patients with adult respiratory distress syndrome (ARDS) have already been developed and clinically validated at the LDS Hospital.

Adapted from an article in the *Int J Clin Monit Comput* 8:263–269, 1992. Reprinted with permission of Kluwer Academic Publishers.

Our initial goal was to develop protocols to meet four basic investigative needs of our current Clinical Trial [5], "Extracorporeal CO_2 Removal for ARDS" (ECCO$_2$R, NIH grant HL36787):

1. Use of uniform logic in decision-making.
2. Examination of a uniform database for decision-making.
3. Equal frequency of monitoring (i.e., interrogation of the database).
4. Equal intensity of care for all patients (both those randomized to traditional positive pressure ventilation and those randomized to new therapy which includes extracorporeal CO_2 removal). This requires equal time intervals and equal increments between changes in therapy.

These protocols had to be designed to be followed by the routine clinical care staff around-the-clock at the bedside. A review of the literature revealed that there was no existing set of protocols which would meet the four goals of our research trial. Over the next three years we developed computerized protocols to meet these four goals. An unexpected outcome from this work has been the tremendous success of the protocols. The protocols have not only been religiously applied by the ICU clinical staff, but the staff have actively pursued the generation of new and more extensive protocols in other areas of critical care. The purpose of this paper is to describe the techniques which we use to generate critical care protocols which have good physician acceptance and are used around-the-clock by the routine clinical staff.

Methods

Over the last four years we have refined the process which we use for generating computerized protocols. This six-step process is outlined in Fig. 23.1. The protocol logic is developed using our existing consensus-generating physician group (step 1). The paper flow diagram is then used at the bedside to test the logic initially (step 2). Once the logic is complete and reasonably correct, the protocol logic is computerized (step 3). Once a protocol is computerized, it is validated with archival data (step 4). As the protocols have become more and more complex, the use of paper flow diagrams at the bedside has become extremely difficult. In this case, the logic is computerized and tested first (steps 3 and 4) and then evaluated at the bedside (step 2). If the protocol logic handles the archival data successfully, it is then validated, alone or in combination with already clinically validated protocols, in a clinical trial (step 5). Once the protocol is refined and tested at the bedside it is prepared as a routine clinical protocol and put into routine clinical use (step 6).

Step 1: Develop Protocol Logic by Consensus

A key element of the whole protocol development process was a driving desire to integrate the clinical environment into the logic-generation proc-

OVERVIEW OF PROTOCOL DEVELOPMENT METHODS

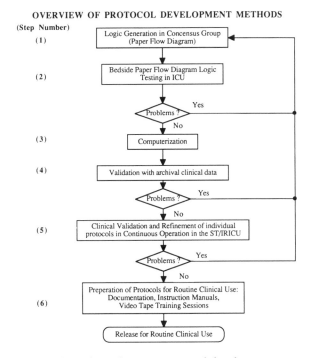

Figure 23.1. Overview of current protocol development process.

ess. It was felt that this was the only way to generate a successful protocol which would handle the majority of circumstances encountered and be acceptable to the clinical care staff. A therapy consensus committee of fourteen physicians, three nurses, one respiratory therapist and one Ph.D. was formed to develop and refine protocol logic further. The committee members came from the departments of Pulmonary, Respiratory Care, Critical Care Medicine, and Anesthesia at LDS Hospital and the University of Utah and included two research associate physicians from the University of Milan (Dr. Gattinoni's group). The composition of this group has changed over time with normal personnel changes as well as the evolution of new areas for protocol development. All physicians agreed to forego personal bias and style and accept the consensus recommendations for ARDS therapy which were incorporated into the protocol logic.

The consensus committee meets once a week. There is a chairperson and someone taking minutes. The general format for the meetings is as follows:

a. Presentation of clinical staff protocol logic challenges (problems) which occurred during the previous week.
b. Presentation of new or modified logic in paper flow diagram form.
c. Defense of new or modified logic based on physiology, literature, clin-

ical experience, and the results of bedside protocol testing. Logic was not defensible based on personal bias or style issues. If there was no scientific evidence that the proposed logic was better than existing logic then it was not changed.

d. Discussion/Criticism of the new logic.
e. Minor modifications suggested by the group.
f. Vote on acceptance.

Any member of the committee may propose new or modified logic. In general, development of modified logic is prompted by problems encountered clinically with the existing logic. New protocols are initiated by the realization that there is another area of critical care which could benefit from protocol controlled therapy. The majority of the committee time is spent in steps d and e. As new logic is presented and critiqued, many heated discussions ensue. It is often very difficult for a physician who has been giving quality patient care for years to realize that many of his decisions are based not on scientifically proven superior therapies but on the theory, "I have always done it that way and it works!" It becomes obvious that decision criteria fluctuate from day to day. Physicians' decisions are influenced by many different things, including the journal article that they read yesterday, the research meeting they attended, the colleague they spoke to last week, the last drug representative that visited, and the current patient that they just spent the whole night trying to save. A fundamental philosophy of this committee was to enforce the KIS principle (Keep It Simple). The committee focused on defining the minimal data set necessary to make decisions and the simplest logic. The fundamental belief was that if the logic was too constrained that it would become rapidly evident during testing at the bedside. If persistent problems were encountered at the bedside, the logic could always be made more complex to deal with them. This philosophy resulted in simple logic which focused on just a handful of the myriad of variables available at the bedside. Despite their simplicity these protocols have been found to work in most situations and have received great physician acceptance.

Step 2: Bedside Logic Testing

If protocol logic is approved by the committee, the paper flow diagrams are used by the consensus team to do some initial logic concept testing at the bedside in the Shock-Trauma Intermountain Respiratory ICU (ST/IRICU). This not only increases the interaction with the clinical environment but also rapidly uncovers major logical flaws or other stumbling blocks. In this phase of clinical testing there is usually a protocol team member as well as a physician at the bedside interpreting the validity of each therapy decision. Any decision which is not followed is carefully documented, and the reasons for not following the decision are recorded.

These results are then used to modify the logic which will then be brought to the next consensus committee meeting for review.

Step 3: Computerization of Protocol Logic

Step 3a. Computerize protocols. Computerization of protocol logic is achieved through close collaboration between medical informatics and clinical staff members. A weekly computer protocol meeting is held between members of the medical informatics and clinical staff, which assures close collaboration. At this meeting problems with the computer implementation of the protocols are discussed. In addition, this meeting has become a forum for preparation of new or modified protocol logic proposals. This allows new logic proposals to be critically reviewed in a small group before presentation to the consensus committee. It also allows the medical informatics staff to critique the proposed logic from the point of view of computer implementation. It is not always feasible to implement the proposed medical logic because of the inherent structure of the HELP system and its user interface [6].

The computerized protocols were implemented in the HELP system, a comprehensive, hospital-wide, integrated data and decision support system [2–4]. The arterial hypoxemia protocols required knowledge of the past history of events over time. Expert system tools such as EMYCIN [7], KAS [8], and EXPERT [9] provide no mechanism to represent the passage of time explicitly. The computerized protocols [6,10–12] are written in modular form using PAL (PTXT Application Language) on the HELP system. PAL allows the retrieval of a temporal sequence of patient data thus providing the past history of events necessary to operate the protocols.

Step 3b. Debug computer protocols. To test the accuracy of the computerization of the protocols, a HELP system program was developed to generate sets of data which look like actual patient data. This simulator allows the user to enter data in a tabular form with a text editor. Each column is a different variable needed by the protocols. The first column specifies the elapsed time between the current data entry and the last. Each row represents one full data set at a particular time. The simulator program reads this file and stores the simulated patient data in the HELP system, one data set at a time, in real time (if the protocol requests a 2 hr wait before a new blood gas is drawn, the simulator will wait 2 hr before placing the next set of data into the patient file). From the computer-protocol point of view this simulator appears to be exactly like a "real" patient. Since the HELP system is a multitasking environment, many of these simulated patients can be running simultaneously.

The user does not need to be concerned about the physiologic appropriateness of the simulation data. The purpose of this simulator was to test all possible logic branches of the protocol methodically. Therefore, the simulated patients may represent extremely unlikely as well as commonly encountered clinical scenarios. For example, a simulation may be written with the PaO_2 less than 30 torr for 24 hr and a pH less than 7.0. It is extremely unlikely that this temporal chain of events would be allowed to occur naturally, but it allows a thorough evaluation of the extremes of the hypoxemia and ventilation-acid/base protocols.

Each protocol was put through 500 hr (approximately 250 decisions) of different simulations to test methodically each branch of the protocol and guarantee that it was accurately computerized. In addition, these simulations provided information on the response time of the HELP system (e.g., the time between input of the arterial oxygenation, ventilation or acid/base categorization and the generation of an instruction at the bedside).

A library of 27 simulated data sets was developed to test the protocols. As new protocols are developed, new simulated data sets will be designed to test them. Once in place, this library of simulated data sets can be used whenever a new version of the computer protocols is introduced as a means to evaluate their accuracy quickly.

Step 4: Validate Protocols with Archival Computerized Data

As part of the protocol logic development, large sets of data from previous ST/IRICU patients are retrieved from the HELP system database and used as a basis for comparing protocol logic decisions with actual therapy decisions. Each protocol is tested with ten real patient data sets. These patient data sets will be selected from at least five different patients. The suggested therapy decisions and the actual therapy decisions are evaluated by members of our research medical staff and the consensus committee. This process helps to clarify the necessary protocol logic as well as to detect gross logic errors.

Step 5: Clinically Validate and Refine Protocols

Individual protocols or small groups of protocols are tested at the LDS Hospital using the Shock Trauma/Intermountain Respiratory ICU (ST/IRICU) that has been the site of previous protocol evaluation for 3.5 years. We complete development of the routine clinical protocols through bedside evaluation and around the clock application. Previous experience has shown that testing in approximately 20 patients is required for adequate refinement of each major protocol. Each patient is in the protocols for at least 96 hr. The computer is used to generate protocol therapy suggestions. The therapy suggestion, actual therapy decision, and reason for any discrepancy are recorded automatically in the HELP system. Our protocol development research staff assists clinical staff in around-the-clock protocol performance evaluation. Variables assessed are—

a. Accuracy of computer prompting: Therapy instructions generated by the protocols are reviewed and manually compared to the protocol logic to determine their accuracy.

b. Computer response time: The time between entry of patient data and the appearance of the therapy instruction is determined from the patient data file.

c. Clincian response time: The time between placing the therapy instruction in the patient file and the next therapy change is measured from the information in the patient data file.

d. Percentage of time protocols were followed: The therapy change implemented is compared with the therapy instruction and data contained in the patient data file. If the therapy instruction was not followed, the reason is retrieved from the patient data file and used to generate a table of reasons for protocol suspensions and logic violations.

e. Percentage of time protocols were suspended: Elapsed time during protocol suspension is calculated. This is expressed as a percentage of total time the protocol was used or attempted to be used in each patient.

f. Reasons for protocol suspension: The reasons for suspension were obtained from the patient data file and stratified according to a hierarchy to characterize the severity of the event which led to the suspension.

This data is then summarized and presented to the consensus group for use in revising protocol logic.

Step 6: Preparation of Routine Clinical Protocols

Annotated copies of the flow diagrams, detailed instruction manuals, and videotape training sessions are prepared to introduce the use protocols effectively to the clinical environment. In-service training sessions are held with physicians. nurses, and respiratory therapists prior to the introduction of major new protocols into routine clinical use.

Results

The protocols (in paper flow diagram and computerized form) have been used for over 40,000 hr in more than 125 adult respiratory distress syndrome (ARDS) patients. The protocols controlled care for 94% of the time. The remainder of the time patient care was not protocol controlled

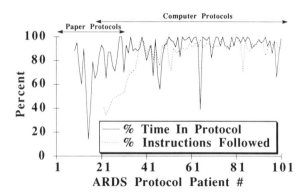

Figure 23.2. Percentage of total hours during which protocols controlled patient care and the percent of total instructions followed by the clinical staff.

was a result of the patients' being in states not covered by current protocol logic (e.g., hemodynamic instability, or transport for x-ray studies). Fifty-two of these ARDS patients met extracorporeal membrane oxygenation (ECMO) critieria. The survival of the ECMO criteria ARDS patients was 41%, four times that expected (9%) from historical data ($p < .0002$) [13]. The success of these computer protocols and their acceptance by the clinical staff clearly established the feasibility of controlling the therapy of severely ill patients.

The computerized protocols have been used for over 30,000 hr in more than 95 ARDS patients [2, 10]. There were a total of 19,802 computer protocol instructions generated; 17,670 out of the 19,802 (90%) computer decisions were actually followed clinically. Figure 23.2 illustrates that the computer performance has improved dramatically over time. The performance has been improved by reduction of incomplete, erroneous, and unrepresentative patient data (database errors), improvement of the protocol logic and its interpretation (clinical staff logic errors), and elimination of many of the software errors. Each value is expressed as a percentage of the total computer instructions as a function of the ARDS patient number in chronological sequence. The remainder of the instructions which were not followed were a result of the patients' being in states not yet adequately covered by the protocol logic (i.e., hemodynamic instability, or transport to the CT scanner).

Discussion

The assurance of uniformity of care for patients in a clinical trial was an unprecedented challenge. We have, in fact, achieved this goal of uniformity of care with the successful application of the protocols in our ST/

IRICU. This has not been an easy process. It took approximately two years to get the first paper-based flow diagram protocols into a form which was accepted by the clinicians for routine use at the bedside. A large part of this time was spent in careful review of the performance of the early protocols. It took a long time for the clinical staff to become convinced that protocols could successfully manage these critically ill patients. It took an additional year to initiate the computer implementation of these protocols. As shown in Fig. 23.2, there were many challenges to the successful implementation of these computerized protocols. Despite these problems, clinical acceptance has slowly improved. After two years and about 36 patients we went over a "hump" in acceptance and performance of the computer protocols. Physicians began to request that their patients be cared for by computer protocol, and the consensus committee became more willing to try new logic and modifications of existing logic. It is unclear exactly what was responsible for this change in acceptance of the protocols; however, it was closely related to reduction in computer protocol errors and observed clinical success in several key patients. The protocol development which had once been driven by the need to do a carefully controlled clinical trial had now swung to being driven by clinical needs. As more people began to be convinced that protocols would work in the ICU environment, more and more new ideas and opportunities for protocol development become apparent. We are now working on new critical care protocols for oxygenation and ventilation for a wide variety of ventilatory modes, hemodynamics, acid/base balance, coagulation therapy, sedation, and paralysis.

In the future, these protocols could be transported to other hospitals; however, there are several key points which would need to be addressed to assure success. The most important ingredient is the willingness of the physicians to support the protocols. It can be very difficult for physicians to forgo personal style in order to adhere to the protocol. The second issue is the implementation of the protocols. Paper protocols can be used; however, they can be confusing and difficult to follow at the bedside. A computerized version assures accurate interpretation of the logic even in crisis situations. The simplest method for transferring the computer protocols would be to install them on a HELP system at another hospital. Since only a small number of hospitals currently use the HELP system, the most realistic implementation would be a small standalone PC version of the protocols. We have currently developed one section of the protocols that operate independently on a PC and are considering conversion of the rest of the protocols in the future. The third issue is the proper training and introduction of the protocols to the nursing, respiratory therapy, and physician staff. We have found that acceptance improves dramatically with good education and in-service programs prior to the introduction of a protocol into routine clinical use.

Summary

It is not enough merely to manage medical information. It is difficult to justify the cost of hospital information systems (HIS) or intensive care unit (ICU) patient data management systems (PDMS) on this basis alone. The real benefit of an integrated HIS or PDMS is in decision support. Although there are a variety of HIS and ICU PDMS systems available, there are few that provide ICU decision support. The HELP system at the LDS Hospital is an example of an HIS which provides decision support on many different levels. In the ICU there are decision support tools for antibiotic therapy, nutritional management, and management of mechanical ventilation. Computer protocols for the management of mechanical ventilation (respiratory evaluation, ventilation, oxygenation, weaning, and extubation) in patients with adult respiratory distress syndrome (ARDS) have already been developed and clinically validated at the LDS Hospital. These protocols utilize the bedside ICU computer terminal to prompt the clinical care team with therapeutic and diagnostic suggestions. The protocols (in paper flow diagram and computerized form) have been used for over 40,000 hours in more than 125 adult respiratory distress syndrome (ARDS) patients. The protocols controlled care for 94% of the time. The remainder of the time patient care was not protocol controlled was a result of the patient being in states not covered by current protocol logic (e.g., hemodynamic instability, or transport for x-ray studies). Fifty-two of these ARDS patients met extracorporeal membrane oxygenation (ECMO) criteria. The survival of the ECMO criteria ARDS patients was 41%, four times that expected (9%) from historical data ($p < .0002$). The success of these computer protocols and their acceptance by the clinical staff clearly establishes the feasibility of controlling the therapy of severely ill patients.

Acknowledgments

This work was supported by NIH grant HL 36787 "Extracorporeal CO_2 Removal for ARDS," the Deseret Foundation (LDS Hospital), and the Respiratory Distress Syndrom Foundation.

References

1. Eddy DM. Clinical decision making. JAMA 1990; 26:1265–75.
2. Gardner RM. Computerized management of intensive care patients. MD Comput 1986; 3(1):36–51.
3. Gardner RM, Sittig DF, Budd MC. The computer in the ICU. Match or mismatch? In Textbook of Critical Care Medicine. 2nd ed. Philadelphia: WB Saunders, 1989: 248–58.

4. Pryor TA. The HELP medical record system. MD Comput 1988; 5(5): 23–33.
5. Morris AH, Menlove RL, Rollins RJ, Wallace CJ, Beck E. A controlled clinical trial of a new 3-step therapy that includes extracorporeal CO, removal for ARDS. Trans AM Soc Artif Intern Organs 1988; 11(1):48–53.
6. East TD, Henderson S, Morns AH, Gardner RM. Implementation issues and challenges for computerized clinical protocols for management of mechanical ventilation in ARDS patients. Proceedings Symposium on Computer Applications in Medical Care (SCAMC), Nov 5–8. 1989. New York: IEEE Computer Soc Press, 1989; 583–7.
7. Musen MA. Automated Generation of Model-Based Knowledge-Acquisition Tools. San Mateo, CA: Morgan Kaufmann, 1989.
8. Rebon R. Knowledge engineering techniques and tools in the Prospector environment Technical report 243. Menlo Park. CA: SRI International, 1981.
9. Weiss SM, Kulikowski CA. EXPERT, A system for developing consultation models. Proceedings of the Sixth International Joint Conference on Artificial Intelligence. Tokyo (Japan), 1979: 942–7.
10. Henderson S, East TD, Morris AH, Gardner RM. Performance evaluation of computerized clinical protocols for management of mechanical ventilation in ARDS patients. Proceedings Symposium on Computer Applications in Medical Care (SCAMC), Nov 5–8. New York: IEEE Computer Soc Press. 1989; 588–92.
11. Henderson S, Crapo RO, East TD, Morris AH, M GR. Computerized clinical protocols in an intensive care unit; How well are they followed? Proceedings of the Fourteenth Annual Symposium on Computer Applications in Medical Care. New York: IEEE Computer Soc Press, 1990; 248–8.
12. Sittig DF, Pace NL, Gardner RM, Beck E, Morris AH. Implementation of a computerized patient advice system using the HELP clinical information system. Comp Biomed Res 1989: 77:474–97.
13. Morris AH, Wallace CJ, Clemmer TP, et al. Extracorporeal CO_2 Removal therapy for adult respiratory distress syndrome patients. A computerized protocol controlled trial. Réan Soins Intens Méd Urg 1990; 6(7):485–90.

Chapter 24
The Role for Artificial Intelligence in Critical Care
Michael C. Higgins

The other chapters in this book have discussed the variety of data used in the care of critically ill patients. Bedside monitoring equipment, ventilators, radiographic and other imaging procedures, laboratory tests, blood gas measurements, input and output record-keeping, drug administration, physical examination, and numerous other sources all contribute to the large volume of data that must be collected, processed, displayed, and interpreted in the ICU. Some of this work is being transferred to computers. Electronic patient information systems are now available from several vendors. Hospital-wide data networks and the use of computers in other departments are becoming commonplace. The automation of ICU data management most likely will accelerate with the adoption of communication standards like those discussed in chapters 8 and 9.

This chapter describes an emerging group of technologies that will help to automate the integration and synthesis of information. Collectively, these technologies compose the field called *artificial intelligence* (AI). The focus here will be the potential applications of AI in critical care medicine.

The ICU provides AI with a challenging arena. Critically ill patients often undergo rapid changes during the progression and treatment of their illnesses. The physiologic and pathophysiologic mechanisms causing these changes cannot always be monitored directly. Moreover, the models that might be used to infer the patient's condition often are incomplete. The analysis of dynamic systems based on limited data and incomplete models has long been the focus of the more established fields of biostatistics, applied probability, control theory, signal processing, and mathematical modeling. In part this chapter will present AI as the adaptation, extension, and integration of these more traditional tools so that they can support critical care decision-making.

The sections in this chapter are organized according to the following outline. AI systems must encode the medical knowledge that is used to derive new information from the available data. Section 1 discusses several of the most widely used approaches to knowledge encoding. The interpretation of ICU data usually involves some degree of uncertainty. Section 2 shows how this uncertainty can be reflected in the derived information. Section 3 describes how AI systems can respond to the changes that an ICU patient is undergoing. Mathematical models of critically ill patients have been developed. Section 4 shows how these models can be incorporated into AI systems. Finally, Section 5 shows how several different approaches to data interpretation can be integrated.

Section 1: Representation of Medical Knowledge

Processing the data used to manage a critically ill patient typically involves a variety of medical knowledge. This knowledge is used to relate the observable data to the possible physiologic mechanisms and ultimately the diagnostic or therapeutic endpoints of the clinical problem. All AI systems rely on some form of knowledge representation to organize the relevant medical facts into a collection of smaller, more manageable relationships. Several representation schemes are discussed in this chapter. The current section begins by showing how knowledge can be encoded as if-then expressions or rules. This rule-based approach is the oldest and probably still the most widely used form of knowledge representation. The remainder of the section presents several important extensions to this basic approach.

Rule-Based Knowledge Representation

A rule is a statement that relates a premise to a conclusion. For example, the rule listed in Figure 24.1 might be used to derive etiology from the available data in a system that evaluates acid-base balance. A complete acid-base evaluation system will include rules for the other clinically meaningful combinations of low, normal and high pH, CO_2 partial pressure, and bicarbonate concentrations. As formulated in this discussion, these rules assume that the relevant laboratory data will be expressed as *low, normal, or high*. The numeric data can be translated into these levels by rules like that shown in Figure 24.2. A system called PONJAB has

IF: (1) arterial pH is low AND
        (2) arterial CO_2 partial pressure is high AND
        (3) arterial bicarbonate ion concentration is high

THEN: respiratory acidosis

Figure 24.1. A rule that derives etiology from observable data.

IF: arterial pH < 7.35

THEN: arterial pH is low

Figure 24.2. A rule that converts numeric data into categories.

IF: (1) gram stain of the organism is gram negative AND
         (2) morphology of the organism is rod AND
         (3) aerobicity of the organism is anaerobic

THEN: there is suggestive evidence that the identity of the organism is
         bacteroides.

Figure 24.3. MYCIN rule that relates the characteristics of an organism to its identity.

been built using rules. PONJAB is connected directly to the instruments that measure pH, CO_2 partial pressure and bicarbonate concentration [1]. Therefore, several steps in the collection and interpretation of this data are automated.

Rules can be used to build complex medical knowledge bases. For example, MYCIN, the system that pioneered the use of rules in medicine, contains several hundred rules [2]. This experimental system was designed to assist in the diagnosis and treatment of bacterial infections. Some of the rules used by MYCIN relate the characteristics of an organism to its identity (see Fig. 24.3). Other rules used by MYCIN relate the identity of an organism to the recommended treatment (see Fig. 24.4).

The modularity of rules simplifies the construction of large knowledge bases like that used in MYCIN, since each rule can be developed independently. For example, the two MYCIN rules shown in Figures 24.3 and 24.4 are related in that the conclusion for the rule that identifies the organism is contained in the premise for the rule that recommends treatment. However, neither rule makes any assumptions about how the other

IF: identity of the organism is bacteroides

THEN: recommend that therapy is chosen from among the following
         drugs:
         (1) clindamycin
         (2) chloramphenicol
         (3) erythromycin
         (4) tetracycline
         (5) carbenicillin

Figure 24.4. MYCIN rule that relates the identity of an organism to its recommended treatment.

rule is organized. The treatment rule does not specify how the organism is identified. Nor does the logic of the identification rule specify how the identity of the organism will be used. The organism could be identified as the conclusion of a rule, as is the case in MYCIN. Alternatively, the identity of the organism could be supplied directly by the doctor using the system. Formulating the knowledge base as a collection of independent rules simplifies the work involved in building and maintaining a system since each logical step can be formulated and tested in isolation.

In principle, rules can be used to express virtually any form of medical knowledge. The only theoretical limitation is that the conclusion of a rule cannot be used directly or indirectly to imply its premise. Otherwise the evaluation of the knowledge base will require circular reasoning. For example, the abstract knowledge base shown in Figure 24.5 contains three rules. Rule 1 concludes that B is true if A is true; Rule 2 concludes that C is true if B is true; and Rule 3 concludes that A is true if C is true. Therefore, the evaluation of Rule 1 would indirectly require the evaluation of itself.

Different system behavior can be achieved by varying the design of the mechanism that controls rule evaluation. PONJAB, the acid-base system mentioned earlier, uses what is called *data-driven* evaluation. The availability of new data from the instruments triggers the evaluation of the rules that classify the measurements into levels. The conclusions of these classification rules trigger the evaluation of the rules that determine etiology. In general, data-driven evaluation propagates through the knowledge base, starting with the data sources and ending with the clinical endpoints of the system. In effect, data-driven evaluation extends the output of the data sources by automatically deriving the implications of new data as it

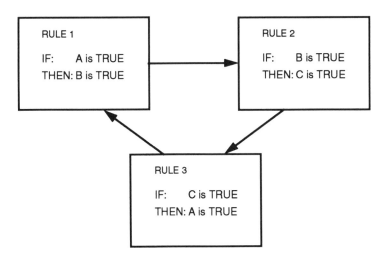

Figure 24.5. Abstract knowledge base illustrating circular logic.

becomes available. This form of rule evaluation is also called *forward chaining*, since the order of rule evaluation proceeds through the knowledge base in the direction of logical implication.

The alternative to data-driven evaluation is called *goal-driven* evaluation, or *backward chaining*. The evaluation of rules in a goal-driven system begins with a rule that will resolve the clinical endpoint and proceeds backward through the knowledge base until the data sources are reached. Goal-driven evaluation is economical in that only the rules needed to resolve a specific clinical endpoint are evaluated. This advantage is particularly important for systems like MYCIN in which the user is the data source. Backward chaining assures that the user will be required to enter the minimum amount of information needed to resolve the specified clinical endpoint. The efficiency of goal-driven evaluation is also important if the rules are difficult to evaluate. The shortcoming of goal-driven evaluation is that the system must be triggered by events like a user request. These events do not always coincide with the arrival of new data. The resulting delay in the interpretation of the data stream can be unacceptable in a monitoring system.

The languages used to write rule-based systems often incorporate the special terminology required for application areas like cardiology. These languages simplify the formulation of rules that cannot be easily expressed in simple logic statements. For example, the waveform interpreter in the Hewlett-Packard ECG Management System (Model 5600C) uses a rule-based classifier. The data source in this system is a module which uses adaptive filters to derive a set of parameters for individual ECG waveforms. The rules, which define waveform categories based on these parameters, are written in a language called ECG Criteria Language (ECL) [3]. The premise

Positive P waves greater than 0.25mV in two of leads 1,2 and aVR

can be expressed as the ECL statement

(P:AMPLITUDE IS POSITIVE AND GT .25) IN 2 OF L1 L2 AVR

The conclusion of a criteria rule in this system can assign a waveform to a category or trigger the evaluation of other criteria rules that will identify more specific categories.

Typically, the rules in a knowledge base are intended to reproduce the reasoning strategies that would be used by human experts faced with the same problem. For example, ECL statements express the logic that a cardiologist would use to interpret ECG data. A group at MIT has built an experimental system, called CALVIN, which encodes the expert knowledge used to recognize ventricular premature beats (VPBs), normal sinus rhythm, and artifact in noisy ECG data [4]. CALVIN functions as the post-processor to an arrhythmia detector. The arrhythmia detector quantifies the noise level in the signal while identifying and classifying indi-

IF.   (1) the time interval between N and B1 is within the distribution for intervals that start with a normal beat and end with a VPB AND

        (2) the time interval between N and B2 is within the distribution for intervals that start and end with normal beats AND

        (3) the time interval between B2 and B3 is within the distribution for intervals that start with a normal beat and end with a VPB
AND

        (4) the time interval between B3 and X is within the distribution for intervals that start with a VPB and end with a normal beat AND

        (5) the time interval between B1 and B2 is less than the distribution for intervals that start with a VPB and end with a normal beat AND

        (6) the time interval between B3 and X is greater than the distribution for intervals that start and end with normal beats AND

        (7) no previous interpolated VPB's have been observed

THEN: (1) B1 is an artifact AND

        (2) B2 is a normal beat AND

        (3) B3 is a VPB

Figure 24.6. Example of a CALVIN rule that classifies consecutive beats B1, B2, and B3 which follow beat N, which has been classified as normal, and precede beat X, which is unlabelled.

vidual beats [5]. CALVIN accumulates the lengths of the intervals between the beats that are detected in the data segments which have low noise levels. When the noise level in the data becomes large CALVIN uses a knowledge base of approximately 150 rules to reclassify the beats that have been identified by the detector. The premises in these rules are relationships between the time intervals and morphology for sequences of beats. An example of a rule that will classify sequences of beats in CALVIN is shown in Figure 24.6. The knowledge base in CALVIN was formulated by asking a cardiologist to describe the logic that could be used to classify beats in noisy data. When tested on eight selected cases, the performance of CALVIN with the arrhythmia detector is significantly better than the performance of the arrhythmia detector alone.

Trends in data often are used to detect critical events like the onset of shock. Recognizing trends in noisy clinical data can be difficult. Trend detection and other topics related to the dynamics of variables are the focus of a later section in this chapter. However, the following two examples show how rules can be used to isolate trends in ICU data.

An experimental system called VM monitors the data collected from a patient on a mechanical ventilator [6]. The goal of VM is to assist in the

IF: (1) ventilator mode is:
            (a) constant volume OR
            (b) controlled mandatory ventilation OR
            (c) patient initiated assist OR
            (d) T-piece bypass of ventilator AND
        (2) heart rate is acceptable AND
        (3) pulse rate does not change by 20 bpm in 15 minutes AND
        (4) mean arterial pressure is acceptable AND
        (5) mean arterial pressure does not change by 15 torr in 15
            minutes AND
        (6) systolic pressure is acceptable

THEN: hemodynamics are stable

Figure 24.7. VM rule that interprets hemodynamic status [6].

management of postoperative patients. VM's knowledge base consists of rules that reach three types of conclusions: 1) interpretations, 2) expectations, and 3) suggestions. An *interpretation* is an assessment of the patient's clinical state. Figure 24.7 contains a rule that interprets the patient's hemodynamic status. An *expectation* defines the target ranges for the data. The definition of these ranges depends on the patient's clinical state and current ventilator management mode. Figure 24.8 shows two rules that conclude different expectations for heart rate data. Some of the rules used by VM conclude *suggestions* that should be brought to the attention of the doctors and nurses caring for the patient. Figure 24.9 contains two rules that conclude diagnostic and therapeutic suggestions. A state transition model underlies the reasoning used by VM. Ventilator management normally proceeds through a sequence of modes that reflect the progression of the patient's recovery after surgery. The interpretations, expectations and suggestions concluded by VM are largely derived from this model.

IF: (1) ventilator mode is constant volume AND
        (2) mode has changed from T-piece bypass of ventilator

THEN: the acceptable range for heart rate is 60 bpm to 110 bpm

IF: (1) ventilator mode is patient initiated assist AND
        (2) mode has changed from:
            (a) constant volume OR
            (b) controlled mandatory ventilation

THEN: the acceptable range for heart rate is 60 bpm to 120 bpm

Figure 24.8. Two VM rules that conclude expectations for heart rate [6].

IF: (1) ventilator mode is:
               (a) constant volume OR
               (b) controlled mandatory ventilation OR
               (c) patient initiated assist OR
               (d) T-piece bypass of ventilator
               AND
      (2) mean arterial pressure is very low AND
      (3) systolic pressure is low

THEN: there is severe hypotension

IF: (1) ventilator mode is controlled mandatory ventilation AND
      (2) patient is on controlled mandatory ventilation for more than
           30 minutes AND
      (3) there is no hypoventilation AND
      (4) hemodynamics are stable

THEN: expect that the patient will be assisting the ventilator

Figure 24.9. Two VM rules that conclude suggestions about the patient's diagnosis and treatment. [6].

A project at Tokyo Denki University has used a similar approach to detect trends in noisy hemodynamic data [7]. The goal of this project is a closed-loop system for regulating blood pressure. Their prototype varies the infusion rate for sodium nitroprusside, a vasodilating drug, based on hemodynamic data. Artifacts due to catheter flushing and movement by the patient can be mistaken for fluctuations in these data. Therefore, state transition rules are used to differentiate between artifacts and actual changes in the underlying variable. Figure 24.10 contains one of their rules. Similar rules identify when the state for heart rate changes from *decreasing* to *stable* or *stable* to *increasing*. In general, these rules detect a state change based on the validity of a statement for a percentage of the measurements collected over a time interval. The percentage and the length of the time interval can be adjusted to make rules that distinguish between the rapid changes that are artifacts and the slower changes due to actual fluctuations in physiology. Other groups have explored similar approaches to reducing false-positive rates in operating room monitors [8, 9].

IF: (1) the current heart rate state is *stable* AND
      (2) the heart rate data has been decreasing for 90% of the
           measurements in the last ten minutes

THEN: the heart rate state has changed to *decreasing*

Figure 24.10. A rule for detecting trends in noisy heart rate data [7].

Frame-Based Knowledge Representation

This subsection describes a design which organizes all of the knowledge related to a specific concept, such as a diagnosis, into a single *frame*. For example, a frame-based system that evaluates acid-base balance might include an acidosis frame, an alkalosis frame, and a normal frame. Each frame would consist of the relationships that define the corresponding acid-base state. In this simple system, these relationships could be encoded as logical statements about pH, CO_2 partial pressure, bicarbonate concentrations, and assessments of respiratory and renal status. Frames can also be used to capture the hierarchical concepts in a clinical problem. Respiratory acidosis and metabolic acidosis are two types of acidosis. Therefore, an acid-base evaluation system would also contain frames for each of these more refined classifications.

Figure 24.11 contains the frames for four acidotic disorders. The top frame in this figure corresponds to the most general of these disorders. The bottom frame corresponds to the most specific classification. This abbreviated knowledge base would be applied to a given patient by determining the most specific frame that most closely fits the available data. Notions of "fit" are discussed in Section 2 of this chapter.

The information in a frame usually is organized according to templates. The frames shown in Figure 24.11 use a template consisting of two slots. Each slot contains a property of the concept defined in the frame. One slot indicates the next most general classification of the disorder. The other slot lists the findings associated with the disorder. Slots can be used to include other types of information. For example, a slot can be used to include the possible treatments for the disorder. A slot can be added that lists the other frames that should be evaluated. Slots can also used to define the output generated when the patient matches a frame. Several diagnostic systems have been built based on frames. The next section will use INTERNIST, which is probably the largest frame-based system, to illustrate how inexact knowledge can be managed.

Noncategorical Approaches to Knowledge Representation

So far this discussion has focused on methods for deriving categorical information about a patient. A rule typically concludes with an etiologic category such as *respiratory acidosis* or a descriptive category such as *stable*. This derived categorical information usually is used in the premises for rules that derive additional categorical information. However, some data interpretation in the ICU involves arithmetic and therefore requires numbers. For example, a value like shunt fraction cannot be calculated if measurements are restricted to categories. In these cases values must be represented by numbers. A rule can be thought of as a function that computes a category from the values referenced in its premise. Numeric values must be derived from functions that compute numbers.

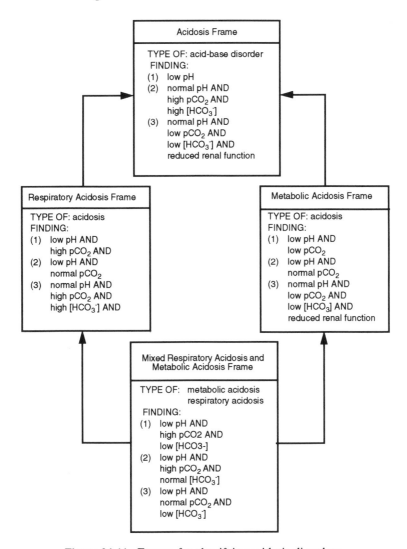

Figure 24.11. Frames for classifying acidotic disorders.

NAIVE, an experimental monitoring system under development in the corporate research labs of the Hewlett-Packard Company, uses both categorical and numerical relationships to interpret ICU data. NAIVE obtains data from intermittent sources to derive higher level information about the patient [10, 11]. For example, the distribution of fluids in the patient is derived from serum chemistry data, body weight measurements, and fluid input and output records. The numeric values used in these derivations typically must be extrapolated since the data are not collected continuously. The extrapolation procedures used in NAIVE are discussed in the third section of this chapter.

The knowledge base in NAIVE consists of nodes corresponding to the observed and derived variables of interest. The definition of each node includes a procedure that can determine the value of its variable at a given time from the values of the other variables represented in the knowledge base. In the case of an observable variable, this evaluation procedure attempts to retrieve the value from the patient's database. The evaluation procedures for the other nodes directly or indirectly depend on the data retrieved by these source nodes. Categorical results are derived from logical expressions that resemble the if-then structure in rules. Numeric results are derived from the appropriate mathematical equations. A node also can condition its evaluation method according to the availability of data. The value of a node is used in the evaluation methods for another node. Section 2 discusses how the uncertainty due to missing data is taken into account in this process.

Figure 24.12 contains a portion of the knowledge base in NAIVE that relates to serum osmolality and serum sodium. The evaluation procedure for the serum sodium node is a ranking of four alternative methods. First, the procedure attempts to use the value for the observed serum sodium

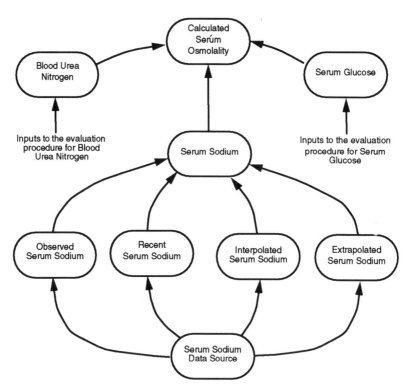

Figure 24.12. Portion of knowledge base used by NAIVE to determine serum osmolality and serum sodium concentrations.

node at the time of interest. Second, the procedure attempts to use the value for the recent serum sodium node if the database query generated by the observed serum sodium node is unsuccessful. Third, the procedure attempts to interpolate a value for serum sodium if a recent serum sodium value is not available. Fourth, the procedure resorts to extrapolation if the value can not be interpolated.

The time needed to evaluate complex equations involving large amounts of data can be excessive, especially when the uncertainty is taken into account. Therefore, a group at Yale has implemented a similar knowledge base design in a computer architecture that distributes the computation over several computer processors [12]. They have used this design to build an Intelligent Cardiovascular Monitor (ICM) [13]. The nodes in ICM use sophisticated signal processing algorithms to remove artifacts and identify the significant events in the data channels. Despite the complexity of these algorithms, the current prototype is able to monitor nine channels of data in real time. The design of ICM is described more fully in a Sections 3 and 5 of this chapter.

Summary

This section has described several methods for representing the knowledge that is used to interpret clinical data in the ICU. Modularity is a feature that is common to all of these methods. In principle, rules, frames and numeric evaluation procedures organize the relevant medical knowledge into separate structures. This modularity can reduce the complexity in building and maintaining a system. A large number of programming tools are commercially available for using these designs. The exploration of knowledge representation systems for use in critical care medicine continues to be a very active research area.

This section has deferred the discussion of several important topics. In particular, no mention has been made of how incomplete or contradictory data and medical knowledge can be processed by AI systems. The next section shows how these issues can be addressed. Later sections discuss the incorporation of temporal knowledge and the use of models that more directly describe the progression of diseases and the effects of treatments.

Section 2: Working with Incomplete Data and Inexact Knowledge

Uncertainty is an integral part of decision-making in the ICU. The data used to care for a critically ill patient seldom are complete. Artifacts frequently obscure the measurements made by bedside monitors. The data obtained from intermittent sources, such as laboratory procedures, invariably describe the patient in the past. The process of collecting clinical data can be unreliable. Moreover, doctors and nurses must reason about

IF: body temperature > 99.0 degrees Fahrenheit

THEN: the evidence is suggestive (CF = 0.5) that the patient has an
           infection

IF: body temperature > 37.2 degrees Celsius

THEN: the evidence is suggestive (CF = 0.5) that the patient has an
           infection

Figure 24.13. Redundant rules relating elevated body temperature to the presence of infection.

these data using models that only approximate the full complexity of an ICU patient. These models can also be inconclusive. For example, recall the MYCIN rule used to identify an infecting organism (Fig. 24.13). This rule concludes that the findings in its premise are only *suggestive* of bacteroides rather than the basis for a definite identification. Therefore, a system that expects to derive something about an ICU patient must work with approximate or even missing values. Accordingly, the representation and management of uncertainty is an essential component in most medical AI systems. This section discusses several of the approaches that can be used.

Categorical Representation of Uncertainty

Ordered categories provide a partial solution to the problem of uncertainty representation. For example, a trend is represented as *increasing, stable*, or *decreasing* in the closed-loop blood pressure regulation system discussed in the previous section. Each of these categorical values includes a wide range of numeric values. Nevertheless, the precision of these inexact values is adequate to determine the proper infusion rate for the vasodilating drug. The discussion of qualitative models in a later section will show how categories may provide the basis for fairly complex data interpretations.

The use of ordered categories to represent uncertainty provides only a partial solution. Even broad categories like *low, normal*, and *high* cannot capture the incompleteness of the data and medical knowledge in some problems. The available data may only imply a range of possible conclusions. The relative likelihood for each of these possibilities must be reflected in subsequent inferences made about the patient.

Informal Representations of Uncertainty

In MYCIN the likelihood of a statement is expressed as a number between -1 and $+1$ called a *certainty factor* (CF) [14]. A positive CF is assigned to a statement that is more likely to be true. For example, the rule in Figure 24.3 assigns a CF of 0.7 to the conclusion that the organism is bacteroides. A statement that is definitely true is given a CF of $+1$. A negative CF is assigned to a statement that is more likely to be false. A statement that is definitely false is given a CF of -1. The evaluation of a rule determines a CF for the conclusion based on the certainty factors for each of the clauses in the premise.

More than one rule can have the same conclusion. In this case a single CF is obtained by combining the certainty factors for each rule. This is done by the following equation in which CF1 and CF2 are the certainty factors for two rules that have the same conclusion:

$$CF(CF_1, CF_2) = \begin{cases} CF_1 + CF_2 - (CF_1 \times CF_2) & \text{if } CF_1 \geq 0 \text{ and } CF_2 \geq 0 \\ \dfrac{CF_1 + CF_2}{1 - min(-CF_1, CF_2)} & \text{if } CF_1 < 0 \text{ and } CF_2 > 0 \\ \dfrac{CF_1 + CF_2}{1 - min(CF_1, -CF_2)} & \text{if } CF_1 > 0 \text{ and } CF_2 < 0 \\ CF_1 + CF_2 + (CF_1 \times CF_2) & \text{if } CF_1 \leq 0 \text{ and } CF_2 \leq 0 \end{cases}$$

For example, if two rules both support a conclusion with a certainty factor of 0.50, then the CF derived by combining these two rules is

$$CF(0.50, 0.50) = 0.50 + 0.50 - (0.5 \times 0.5) = 0.75$$

If one rule strongly supports a conclusion with a CF of 0.90 and the other rule strongly contradicts the same conclusion with a CF of -0.80, then the CF derived by combining these two rules is

$$CF(0.90, -0.80) = \frac{0.90 - 0.80}{1 - min(0.90, 0.80)} = 0.50$$

If one rule strongly contradicts a conclusion with a CF of -0.80 and the other rule weakly contradicts the same conclusion with a CF of -0.20, then the CF derived by combining these two rules is

$$CF(-0.80, -0.20) = -0.80 - 0.20 + (0.80 \times 0.20) = -0.84$$

There is no objective basis for assigning a CF to a statement. Rather, these numbers are subjective measures of the opinions of the experts who help to build the system. Moreover, the equation used to combine certainty factors is an expediency rather than a relationship that can be derived from first principles. It was chosen because it combines certainty factors in a reasonable way. Nevertheless, one study found that the conclusions derived by MYCIN are comparable to the performance of experienced physicians [15].

INTERNIST-I, and the follow-up project QMR, are frame-based systems that use a different approach to represent uncertainty. The INTERNIST systems are designed to identify the differential diagnosis for a patient [16]. The current knowledge base correlates more than 600 diseases with more than 4,300 clinical findings [17]. This knowledge is organized into disease frames that list the corresponding patient history, signs, symptoms, and laboratory values. The uncertainty in the correlation between a finding and a disease is measured by two numbers:

Evoking strength: number between 0 and 5, representing the likelihood that the disease will be found in patients with the finding
Frequency value: number between 1 and 5, representing the likelihood that the finding will be found in patients with the disease

In addition every finding is assigned a number between 1 and 5 which measures its *clinical importance*. Low clinical importance values are assigned to nonspecific findings that can be easily disregarded by a valid diagnosis. High clinical importance values are assigned to findings that must be explained by a final diagnosis.

The INTERNIST systems use the evoking strengths, frequency values, and clinical importance values to score each of the diseases associated with the findings that are present in the patient. This scoring function favors a disease that assigns high evoking strengths to the findings that are present. A disease that assigns a high frequency value to an absent finding is penalized. The scoring function also penalizes any disease not associated with the findings that are present and which have a high clinical importance value. The diseases with scores that exceed a threshold are included in the final diagnosis.

The approaches to uncertainty representation in MYCIN and INTERNIST are intended as mathematical approximations of how experts reason. Certainty factors, evoking strengths, frequency values and clinical importance values quantify the relative likelihoods an expert assigns to various statements. The scoring functions mimic how an expert might balance these likelihoods while interpreting equivocal evidence. The favorable results of the evaluation studies suggest that both systems are reasonable approximations of expert behavior.

However, building systems in this manner is an open-loop process in which the validity of each design decision can only be judged based on the entire system's performance. There is no objective bases for determining if a particular CF should be 0.1 or 0.9. In addition, the validity of the combination function depends on the interactions between the rules that have been included in the knowledge base. For example, suppose that the MYCIN knowledge base contains the two rules shown in Figure 24.13. The first of these rules encodes the opinion that a minimally elevated temperature suggests the presence of an infection. The second rule encodes the same knowledge about the relationship between fever and infection except that temperature is expressed in different units. The premise of the second rule is always true if the premise of the first rule is true. Therefore, the CF for the statement that the patient with a low fever has an infection would be increased to 0.75 by including the redundant second rule. Of course, the builders of systems like MYCIN try to avoid this type of redundancy. However, these types of interactions between rules can be difficult to recognize or even define when the premises are more complicated and the linkages less direct.

Representing Uncertainty with Probabilities

Interest in more formal approaches to representing uncertainty has led to the use of traditional probability theory. The probability of a statement is a number between 0 and 1 that measures the likelihood that the statement is true. Statements that are definitely true have probability 1 and statements that are definitely false have probability 0. By definition, the probability that a statement is true equals 1 minus the probability that the same statement is false. Symbolically,

$$P(X) = 1.0 - P(not\,X)$$

An expert's opinion about a rule typically is encoded in terms of the following three probabilities:

True-positive rate: probability that the premise is true if the conclusion is true
False-positive rate: probability that the premise is true if the conclusion is false
Prior Probability: probability that the conclusion is true if the validity of the premise is not known

The true-positive rate is the same as the sensitivity for the rule. The false-positive rate is the same as 1 minus the specificity for the rule. The true-positive and false-positive rates are *conditional probabilities*. Let Y denote the premise and Z the conclusion for a rule. The true-positive rate for this rule is the probability of Y conditioned on Z, denoted $P(Y|Z)$. Similarly, the false-positive rate for this rule is the probability of Y conditioned on not Z, denoted $P(Y|not\,Z)$. The prior probability for Z is denoted $P(Z)$.

Probabilities are used in a rule-based system as subjective measures of the expert's uncertainty. However, unlike certainty factors and the measures used in the INTERNIST systems, probabilities can also be interpreted as frequencies. Therefore, the opinion encoded in a probability can be tested empirically.

Probability theory also provides combination functions that are derived from first principles. For example, suppose that X and Y are the premises for two rules which have the same conclusion, denoted by Z. The probability of Z if both X and Y are true can be computed by the following relationship:

$$P(Z|X, Y) = \frac{P(Z)P(X|Z)P(Y|Z)}{P(Z)P(X|Z)P(Y|Z) + P(not\,Z)P(X|not\,Z)P(Y|not\,Z)}$$

This relationship is called *Bayes' formula*.

Like the combining function used in MYCIN, the validity of Bayes' formula depends on the interactions between the rules in the knowledge base. Probability theory provides a formal definition for this relationship which is called *conditional independence*. Two rules that relate X and Y to conclusion Z are conditionally independent if

$$P(X, Y|Z) = P(X|Z) \times P(Y|Z)$$

$$P(X, Y|\,not\,Z) = P(X|\,not\,Z) \times P(Y|\,not\,Z)$$

For example, recall the two hypothetical rules that relate body temperature and infection mentioned in the discussion of certainty factors. Suppose that

$$P(temp > 99.0°F|infection) = 0.8$$

Then it is also true that

$$P(temp > 37.2°C|infection) = 0.8$$

from which it follows that

$$P(temp > 99.0°F|infection) \times P(temp > 37.2°C|infection) = 0.64$$

However,

$$P(temp > 99.0°F, temp > 37.2°C|infection) = P(temp > 99.0°F|infection)$$
$$= 0.8$$

Therefore, these two rules are not conditionally independent.

Conditionally dependent rules can be combined into a single rule. The premise for this new rule is the intersection of the premises for the two dependent rules. For example, suppose that the following two rules are not conditionally independent:

IF: X

THEN: Z

and

IF: Y

THEN: Z

These two rules can be replaced by the following rule:

IF: X and Y

THEN: Z

Therefore, conditional independence is a test that can be used to guide the organization of a knowledge base.

The knowledge bases in probabilistic AI systems typically are implemented as collections of conditional probabilities. Suppose that variable Y can be derived from variable X. Denote the n possible values for

X by $x_1, x_2, \ldots, x_n$ and denote the m possible values for Y by y_1, $y_2, \ldots, y_m$. The relationship between these two variables can be encoded in the following matrix of conditional probabilities:

$$\begin{bmatrix} p_{11} & p_{12} & \cdots & p_{1n} \\ p_{21} & p_{22} & \cdots & p_{2n} \\ \vdots & \vdots & & \vdots \\ p_{m1} & p_{m2} & \cdots & p_{mn} \end{bmatrix}$$

where

$$p_{ij} = P(Y = y_i | X = X_j)$$

In effect, this matrix encodes a collection of $m \times n$ rules that relate the value of X to the value of Y. The complete representation of X and Y in this knowledge base will also include the list of prior probabilities for X, which will be denoted by $q_1, q_2, \ldots, q_n$, where

$$q_j = P(X = x_j) \quad for \quad j = 1, \ldots, n$$

One advantage to using these matrices to represent the relationships between variables is that the implications can be reversed. For example, suppose that the value of X is known to be x_j. The probability that Y equals a particular value, say, y_i, is the conditional probability p_{ij}, which can be gotten directly from the matrix. Conversely, suppose that Y is known to be y_i. The probability that X is equal to x_j can be computed by the following version of Bayes' formula:

$$P(X = x_j | Y = y_i) = \frac{q_j \times p_{ij}}{(q_1 \times p_{i1}) + \cdots + (q_n \times p_{in})}$$

$$= \frac{q_j \times p_{ij}}{\displaystyle\sum_{k=1}^{n} q_k \times p_{ik}}$$

The value for Y may also be uncertain given what else is known about the patient. Let

$$r_i = P(Y = y_j | E) \quad for \quad i = 1, \ldots, n$$

where E represents everything else that is known about the patient. Then

$$P(X = x_j | Y = y_i) = \frac{(q_j \times p_{1j} \times r_1) + \cdots + (q_j \times p_{mj} \times r_m)}{(q_1 \times p_{i1}) + \cdots + (q_n \times p_{in})}$$

$$= \frac{q_j \times \displaystyle\sum_{k=1}^{m} p_{kj} \times r_k}{\displaystyle\sum_{k=1}^{n} q_k \times p_{ik}}$$

An experimental system called VENTPLAN uses probabilities to determine the optimal management for a patient on a mechanical ventilator [18]. This system identifies ventilator management problems by interpreting the current ventilator settings and measurements of the patient's oxygen carrying capacity, cardiac output, stroke volume, heart rate and pulmonary function. Part of the knowledge base in VENTPLAN is organized as a probabilistic *belief network* that contains nodes for each of the variables interpreted or derived by the system. These nodes are connected by directed arcs which correspond to the dependencies between variables.

VENTPLAN belief network is shown in Figure 24.14. For example, cardiac output (CO) depends on stroke volume (SV) and heart (HR). The possible values that a variable can have are grouped into ranges. The uncertainty in how the value of one variable affects the values of another variables is expressed as conditional probabilities of the form:

$$P(3.5 < CO < 6.5 | 30 < SV < 80, 50 < HR < 100)$$

The belief network in the current version of VENTPLAN contains about 40 nodes. Seven of these nodes correspond to the diagnoses that are recognized by the system. The remaining nodes correspond to the variables that are observed and the variables that are derived.

Traditional probability theory can be applied to numeric calculations. For example, the serum osmolality can be calculated from serum sodium (Na), serum glucose (Gluc) and blood urea nitrogen (BUN) concentrations by the well-known formula:

$$Osmolality = (2 \times Na) + \frac{Gluc}{18} + \frac{BUN}{2.8}$$

These three concentrations are not always measured at the same time, so osmolality often must be calculated using extrapolated and therefore uncertain values. The probability that serum osmolality equals a given value can be determined from the probabilities for the possible values of the three concentrations. For the sake of illustration, suppose that these extrapolated values have the following probabilities at time t:

$$P(Na = 145 \ mEq/L) = 0.5 \text{ and } P(Na = 146 \ mEq/L) = 0.5$$
$$P(Gluc = 72 \ mg/dl) = 0.5 \text{ and } P(Gluc = 90 \ mg/dl) = 0.5$$
$$P(BUN = 12 \ mg/dl) = 0.5 \text{ and } P(BUN = 15 \ mg/dl) = 0.5$$

Of course, in a real case each concentration would have more than two possible values. Also, the probabilities would not all be equal. The next section will discuss how probabilities for extrapolated values can be determined. However, proceeding with this simplified example, if the serum sodium is 145 mEq/L, the serum glucose is 72 mg/dl and the BUN is 12 mg/dl then

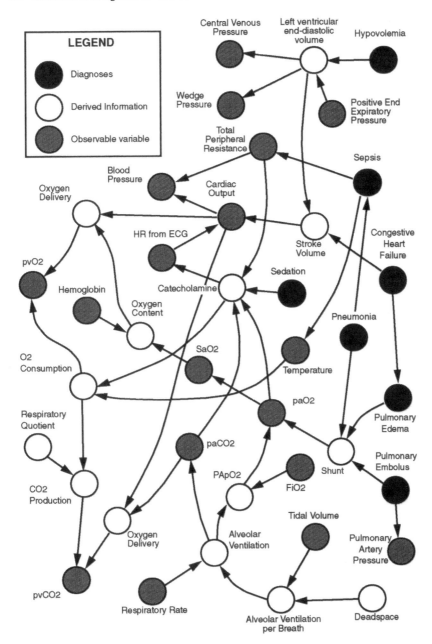

Figure 24.14. The VENTPLAN belief newtwork [19].

$$Osmolality = (2 \times 145) + \frac{72}{18} + \frac{12}{2.8} = 298 \; mOsm$$

Assuming independence, the probability of that these three concentrations occur is

$$P(Na = 145) \times P(Gluc = 72) \times P(BUN = 12) = 0.5 \times 0.5 \times 0.5 = 0.125$$

The following table of probabilities for the possible values of osmolality at time t can be computed by proceeding through the other seven possible combinations:

$$P(\text{osmolality} = 298 \text{ mOsm}) = 0.125$$
$$P(\text{osmolality} = 299 \text{ mOsm}) = 0.250$$
$$P(\text{osmolality} = 300 \text{ mOsm}) = 0.250$$
$$P(\text{osmolality} = 301 \text{ mOsm}) = 0.250$$
$$P(\text{osmolality} = 302 \text{ mOsm}) = 0.125$$

The principle in this simple example can be generalized to determine the probabilities for virtually any transformation of uncertain data. NAIVE, the experimental monitoring system discussed in the previous section, uses this approach to represent the uncertainty in its derivations. The data sources for NAIVE are mostly intermittent. Therefore, the current value for a variable usually must be obtained by extrapolating the last available observation. Section 3 of this chapter describes some of the extrapolation procedures that can be used. The result of these procedures typically is a range of possible values for the variable. Probabilities are paired with each value. The current value for a derived variable, like serum osmolality, can be then be calculated using methods like those described above.

Summary

Several methods can be used to represent the uncertainty in the interpretation of ICU data. The methods discussed in this section range from the partial solution provided by categorical values to formal probability theory. In practice, the uncertainty in derived information can only be approximated. Certainty factors, evoking strengths and probabilities are only opinions that will differ from expert to expert. Nevertheless, these methods can be used to make systems that function even when the knowledge and data are incomplete.

Section 3: Representation of Temporal Events

Time complicates the processing of ICU data. First, the patient's condition changes over time. In order to be useful an AI system must be able to track these changes. Second, the changes themselves can provide critical information. Events like the onset of shock, changes in body temperature, or shifts in acid-base balance can be important clues to how the patient is progressing. Third, the available data will change with time. Test results are returned by the lab. The effects of treatments are learned. Additional symptoms are observed. A system must be able to incorporate these new data as they are reported. Finally, the urgent nature of ICU medicine can limit the time available to meet these requirements.

This section discusses the approaches that are used in AI systems to detect interpret and manage temporal events. The discussion is organized around two topics: 1) detecting trends and the other temporal properties of the data, and 2) the incorporation of new data as they become available.

Detecting Temporal Events

A system like MYCIN provides a snapshot of the patient that summarizes the available data at a given moment. In principle, the sequence of snapshots obtained by periodically reevaluating MYCIN would depict the time course of the patient's state. However, this approach was not designed to take advantage of history as it interpreted the patient's state. Changes in variables are ignored so that, in effect, MYCIN assumes a static patient model. This simplification is reasonable given the intended role of MYCIN as a one-time consultation system. Nevertheless, the result is a system that cannot recognize and interpret temporal events.

VM, the rule-based system that monitors patients on ventilators, works with a more dynamic view of the patient. The rules in VM's knowledge base consider changes in the data and ventilator mode when deriving new information. These rules are based on values that reflect the temporal behavior of the variables. For example, the rule shown in Figure 24.7 determines that the patient's hemodynamics are *stable*. The therapy rule in Figure 24.9 includes this temporal value in its premise. The blood pressure regulation system discussed in earlier applies a similar approach to the monitoring of hemodynamic variables.

Both VM and the blood pressure regulation system obtain most of their data from sources that continuously sample the patient. On the other hand, ICU data also comes from sources that provide a more intermittent view of the patient. Laboratory values, physical findings, and the other data used by these systems are collected at irregular and often widely spaced intervals. The knowledge base must include interpolation and extrapolation procedures in order to provide a continuous patient assessment based on this type of data.

The portion of the knowledge base in NAIVE that pertains to the extrapolation of serum sodium levels is shown in Figure 24.15. An extrapolated value is less certain than an observed value. The knowledge base

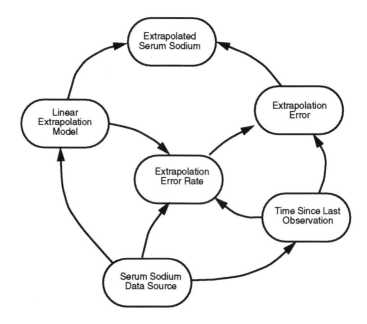

Figure 24.15. The NAIVE knowledge base nodes that determine extrapolation uncertainty.

measures this uncertainty by comparing an extrapolated value with the observed value whenever new data is obtained. The difference between an extrapolated value and observed value is divided by the time that has elapsed since the previous observation. The accumulation of the resulting errors characterizes how the uncertainty in an extrapolation increases with time since the last observation. NAIVE uses this error rate distribution to compute an error term that is combined with the extrapolated value. The current version of NAIVE relies on first order linear models; however, this approach can be extended to more sophisticated extrapolation methods.

Patient monitoring is based on the detection of temporal events like the crossing of a threshold or a change in a trend. In principle, any system that provides a continuous assessment of the patient can be used to recognize these events. For example, the closed-loop blood pressure regulation system mentioned earlier determines whether a variable is decreasing, stable or increasing. The appropriate change in the infusion rate for the vasodilating drug is based on this derived information.

In practice, the detection of trends is more complicated for systems that must take uncertainty into account. Ideally the trend in a variable would be determined by its current value with its value at some time in the recent past. However, the probability distributions for these two values will not be independent if they are both derived by extrapolating the same data points. The comparison of these two dependent distributions must take into account the covariance between the two extrapolations.

ICM, the monitoring system that distributes computation over several computer processors (see above), detects trends with a type of Kalman filter. A Kalman filter is a data analysis technique that has been used extensively in signal processing. The Kalman filter used in ICM matches a collection of models to the data [20]. These models correspond to the different trends that may be present in segments of the data. For example, the following four models might be used to categorize the behavior of an observation in a data stream:

1. Continuation of a linear trend.
2. Change in slope for a linear trend.
3. An abrupt change in level.
4. The observation is an outlier.

These four models are illustrated in Figure 24.16. The temporal behavior of the data will switch between these alternatives as the physiologic mechanisms controlling the underlying variable change. Kalman filters provide statistical estimates of the probabilities for each model at a given

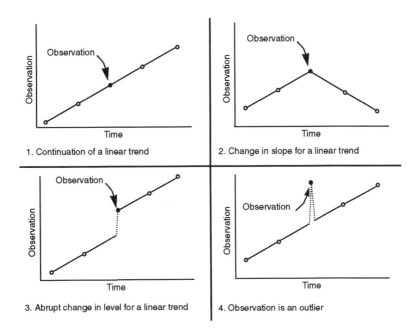

Figure 24.16. Four models that can be used to classify the behavior of an observation in a data stream.

observation. The result is an intermittent assessment of the trends that are present in the data. Each trend assessment coincides with the reporting of an observation. A monitor can use these assessments to determine if there has been a change in the variable's trend. This information can also be used to derive other information about the patient.

Incorporating New Data

VM and the closed-loop blood pressure regulation system (above) respond to the arrival of new data by reassessing the patient's current state. However, monitoring can also require the assessment of the patient's state over a wider time window. For example, a system might be used to derive and display the history for a variable during the past 24 h. In principle, a monitor could also derive future values for variables in order to decide if the patient is headed for trouble.

A system that limits its assessments to current time can use the forward chaining mechanism discussed earlier (see above) to incorporate new data. The arrival of a new observation will trigger the corresponding source node in the knowledge base. This source node will in turn trigger the nodes that use the new data in their evaluation procedures. This process propagates through the knowledge base until all of the affected values are reevaluated.

On the other hand, a system that assesses the patient's state over a wider time interval requires a more selective response to the arrival of new data since the number of affected values can be very large. For example, the most recent serum sodium level implies the current serum sodium value. However, that same piece of data can be used to estimate the serum sodium level one hour ago, two hours ago, three hours ago and so forth into the past. That single observation also can be used to predict the future serum sodium values. Moreover, all of the current, past and future values for the variables that are derived from serum sodium levels can be affected.

One solution is to select the values that should be reevaluated according to what is required by the parts of the system that use the derived information. For example, a monitor might include a predictive alarm mechanism. This mechanism compares the values projected for a variable to a threshold. An alarm is sounded if the projected values will cross the threshold during the next 30 min. The values that should be reevaluated when new data arrives are the values that are required by this predictive alarm mechanism.

NAIVE uses this approach selectively to reevaluate the nodes in its knowledge base when new data arrives. A forward chaining mechanism notifies all of the nodes that may be affected by the new data. The nodes in the knowledge base normally do not reevaluate themselves when this notification is received. Instead a node simply passes the notification onto

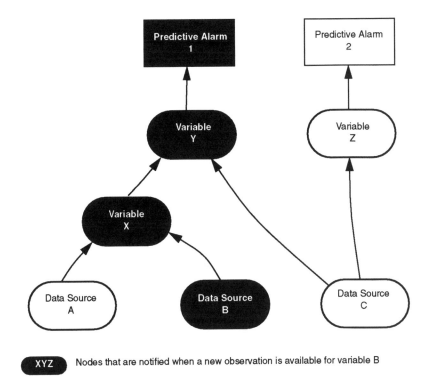

Figure 24.17. Abstract knowledge base illustrating the propagation of new data in NAIVE.

the other nodes that use its value in their evaluation procedures. Eventually the notification is received by a part of the system that uses the information derived from the new data to generate a display or determine if an alarm should be generated. These terminal nodes force the reevaluation of the nodes that supply the required values.

Figure 24.17 shows an abstract knowledge base that illustrates this process. The nodes labelled *A*, *B*, and *C* are data sources. The evaluation procedure for the node labeled *X* combines the data provided by *A* and *B*. The evaluation procedure for the node labeled *Y* combines the values provided by *X* and *C*. The data provided by *C* is also used in the evaluation procedure for the node labeled *Z*. The terminal nodes in this example are the predictive alarms labeled *1* and *2*. These alarms monitor the values for nodes *Y* and *Z* at 10, 20, and 30 min into the future. The availability of new data at a source node *B* will result in the notification of nodes *X*, *Y*, and the first predictive alarm. Predictive alarm *1* responds to this notification by obtaining the values for *Y* at 10, 20, and 30 min into the future. Node *Z* and the second predictive alarm are not affected.

This approach is an improvement over simple forward chaining, since the affected variables are only reevaluated at the times required by how the derived information is used. However, it is possible that a node will be reevaluated unnecessarily. For example, referring to the system shown in Figure 24.17, suppose that a change in an old value for node B is reported. In theory this "new" data will affect the values that are projected for Y. However, in practice the effect of a very old value for B may be negligible. Nevertheless, the reporting of any new information about the value of B ultimately causes the reevaluation of Y.

A design for monitors has been proposed at MIT which can further improve the efficiency of how new data is incorporated. This design is called the Temporal Control Structure (TCS). In effect, the other designs discussed in this chapter represent the dependencies between the *variables* defined in the knowledge base. TCS represents the dependencies between *values*. This information about value dependencies is used to determine which values are affected with the availability of new data.

TCS determines the time intervals during which the value of a variable is constant. These intervals are determined from the intervals during which the values for the other variables represented in the system are constant. The notion of "constant value" is very general in TCS. For example, a variable like serum sodium level is constant over an interval during which it equals a particular numeric value. However, a variable is also constant over an interval during which its value is determined by the same function of time. Virtually any programmable function can be used to represent the procedure that identifies the extent of an interval.

For example, suppose that the serum sodium level was reported to be 140 mEq/L at 9:00 A.M. and 3:00 P.M. These two observations might be used to infer the following interval for serum sodium:

$$0900 \text{ to } 1500: \text{value} = 140 \text{ mEq/L}$$

Similarly, suppose that the serum glucose and blood urea nitrogen levels were reported to be constant over the same time interval. Recalling the formula used earlier, we can use these three intervals to define a fourth interval over which calculated serum osmolality is constant. The definition of this serum osmolality interval depends on the definitions of the corresponding intervals for the other three concentrations. Now suppose that a serum sodium level of 146 mEq/L is reported for noon on the same day. This new data implies that the original constant interval for serum sodium should be divided into two intervals:

$$0900 \text{ to } 1200: \text{value} = 140 + (2 \times (t - 9.00)) \text{ mEq/L}$$

$$1200 \text{ to } 1500: \text{value} = 146 - (2 \times (t - 12.00)) \text{ mEq/L}$$

where t is time measured in hours. In other words, the data now implies two intervals over which serum sodium is "constant." In this case the values for the variable are functions of time. This redefinition of the serum sodium interval would trigger a redefinition of the dependent interval for calculated serum osmolality. The other intervals for serum sodium and serum osmolality would not be affected. Similarly, the intervals for serum glucose and blood urea nitrogen levels would not be changed, provided that no other data is reported.

Keeping track of the value dependencies and the generalization of constant values in TCS require a fair amount of computational overhead. Whether or not this added complexity results in a net improvement in system performance depends on the complexity of the evaluation procedures and the rate at which new data arrives. The management of arrhythmias has been used to illustrate the discussion of TCS in the literature [21].

Summary

This section has described the design of AI systems that can monitor the rapid changes encountered in the care of critically ill patients. These systems detect and interpret the temporal patterns found in a data stream. A continuous assessment of the patient can be derived using the data obtained from intermittent sources. Reevaluation of this derived information can be triggered when new data becomes available.

The next section presents the designs for what are often called "model-based systems." These systems contain mathematical representations of physiologic or pathophysiologic mechanisms. To a large degree, the goal of these systems is to represent the dynamics in critically ill patients. Therefore, the next section will, in part, be a continuation of the discussion that has been started in this section.

Section 4: Model-Based Systems

So far the discussion has focused on what might be thought of as models of reasoning. For example, recall the rules in Figures 24.1 and 24.2. These rules represent a line of reasoning that might be used to deduce the validity of one true-false statement from the validity of other true-false statements. This section describes an approach to knowledge representation based on models of physiology rather than reasoning. These physiological models encode the behavior of and interactions between the components in a body system. A model based system uses knowledge of these interactions to derive unmeasured characteristic of the patient from the available data.

In principle a physiological model implies the knowledge that would have to be stated explicitly if a traditional knowledge representation system is used. The explicit statement of these rules can be infeasible except for limited medical domains. Moreover, the representation of knowledge in a model based system more closely matches how health care providers organize their understanding of the patient. Some researchers also believe that model based systems are more robust than systems based on more traditional forms of knowledge encoding.

This section begins by describing the use of numeric models to represent physiology. The discussion then turns to the use of nonnumeric, or *qualitative*, models.

Numeric Models

VENTPLAN, the system designed to assist in the management of patients on mechanical ventilation, uses a numeric model of pulmonary function [22]. This model is a system of differential equations that represents the diffusion and circulation of O_2 and CO_2 in the arterial, venous, tissue, pulmonary and alveolar compartments. For example, the following differential equation describes the dynamics of the venous O_2 content:

$$\frac{dVO_2}{dt} = \frac{CO \times (TO_2 - VO_2)}{V_v}$$

where

$$VO_2 = \text{Venous } O_2 \text{ content}$$
$$V_v = \text{Venous volume}$$
$$CO = \text{Cardiac output}$$
$$TO_2 = \text{Tissue } O_2 \text{ content}$$

According to this differential equation, the rate of change of venous O_2 content is inversely proportional to venous volume and proportional to cardiac output and the difference between the tissue O_2 content and the venous O_2 content. The other equations in the model represent similar relationships between the O_2 and CO_2 content in the other compartments used in the model. VENTPLAN uses this system of differential equations to predict the steady-state response of the patient to changes in ventilator settings and changes in the other variables under the control of the physician.

Differential equation systems have been used for many years to aid in the general understanding of physiology. However, the goal of VENTPLAN is the application of a numeric model to a specific patient. Parameter estimation is the fundamental challenge to achieving this goal. VENTPLAN uses a Bayesian estimation technique to determine probability distributions for the model parameters. This technique begins with a prior distribution for each parameter. These prior distributions are updated by comparing the values predicted by the model with the actual values observed for the patient.

Parameter estimation is inherently inexact. VENTPLAN uses probability distributions to represent this inexactness. Qualitative models, which are described next, uses a different approach to represent the inexactness in patient modeling.

Qualitative Models

The formulation of a numeric model requires fairly complete knowledge of the physiology that is being represented. In addition, it must be possible to determine the values for the parameters used in the model. Clinical applications require that this estimation process fit the model to a specific patient. On the other hand, the formulation of qualitative models may be less difficult. Qualitative models describe the corresponding physiology in nonnumeric terms such as *low, medium*, and *high*. The relationships between model components are also represented nonnumerically, such as *causes increase* or *causes decrease*. The inexactness in this qualitative representation reflects the limitations in our understanding of the corresponding body system.

A group at MIT used this approach to model the causal relationships in cardiovascular physiology [23]. Their goal was a system that could reason about the treatment of cardiovascular diseases. Figure 24.8 shows an excerpt from one of their models. The large circles in this diagram represent the various cardiovascular variables such as *heart rate* and *myocardial ischemia*. Variables like cardiac output and heart rate are fairly concrete and could be represented by numbers. Other variables, like myocardial perfusion and beta state are more conceptual and can only be represented by levels, like *low, medium*, and *high*. The arcs connecting variables represent how the level of one variable affects the level of other variables. The small circles represent the direction and relative strength of these causal relationships. For example, the model excerpt shown in Figure 24.18 represents a strong positive relationship between *heart rate* and *myocardial O_2 consumption* and a weak negative relationship between *heart rate* and *diastolic time*.

The portion of the MIT model shown in Figure 24.18 is selected to represent the effects of beta adrenergic blocking drugs on *myocardial ischemia*. These drugs lower the *sympathetic beta state*. The primary effect of this change is a reduction in *inotropy* state and *heart rate* which, in turn, lowers the *myocardial O_2 consumption* and *myocardial ischemia*. A secondary effect is that the heart rate reduction causes a small increase in the diastolic time, which increases the *coronary flow* and *myocardial perfusion*. The later change further reduces the level of *myocardial ischemia*. Similarly, Figure 24.19 shows one of the feed-back loops represented in the MIT model. A drop in the *sympathetic beta state* causes a drop in the *heart rate* which lowers the *cardiac output*. A drop in *cardiac output* lowers the *blood pressure*, which eventually increases the *sympathetic beta state*.

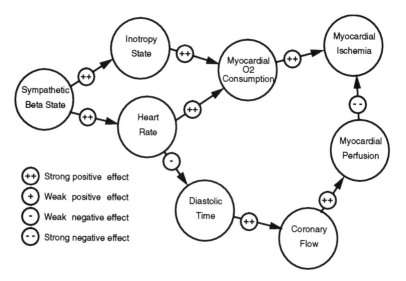

Figure 24.18. Excerpt from the MIT model representing the effects of beta-blockers [23].

The interactions discussed so far for the MIT model are purely qualitative. However, some of the relationships between variables require a quantification of these interactions. For example, consider the model fragment shown in Figure 24.20. The direct effect of a decrease in *heart rate* is a decrease in *cardiac output*. However, a decrease in *heart rate* also causes an increase in *left ventricle stroke volume*, which, in turn, causes an increase in *cardiac output*. Therefore, the net result on *cardiac output* depends on the relative magnitude of two effects.

The MIT model uses the following algorithm to quantify the magnitude of the interactions between two variables. Weak interactions are assigned a magnitude of 0.5, and strong interactions are assigned a magnitude of 1.0. The cumulative effect of an indirect interaction between two

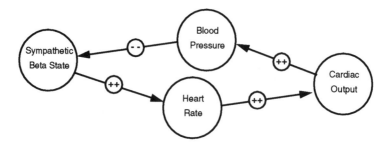

Figure 24.19. Excerpt from the MIT model representing a feed-back loop [23].

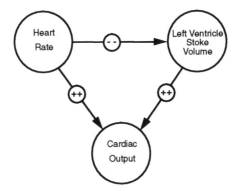

Figure 24.20. Excerpt from the MIT model representing the direct and indirect effects of changes in heart rate on changes in cardiac output [23].

variables is computed by multiplying the magnitudes for each of the arcs comprising the path connecting these two variables. For example, referring to Figure 21.18, the magnitude for the secondary effect of *heart rate* on *myocardial ischemia* is

$$0.5 = (-0.5) \times (1.0) \times (1.0) \times (-1.0)$$

⟶ Effect of *myocardial perfusion* on *myocardia ischemia*
⟶ Effect of *coronary flow* on *myocardial perfusion*
⟶ Effect of *diastolic time* on *coronary flow*
⟶ Effect of *heart rate* on *diastolic time*
Cumulative magnitude for secondary effect of *heart rate* on *myocardia ischemia*

Similarly, the net effect from multiple variables is computed by summing the individual magnitudes. For example, referring to Figure 24.20, the magnitude for the total effect of *heart rate* on *cardiac output* is

$$0.0 = ((-1.0) \times (1.0)) + 1.0$$

⟶ Direct effect of *heart rate* on *cardiac output*
⟶ Effect of *left ventricle stroke volume* on *cardiac output*
⟶ Effect of *heart rate* on *left ventricle stroke volume*
Total magnitude for effect of *heart rate* on *cardiac output*

This algorithm is somewhat arbitrary. Moreover, cardiovascular diseases can alter the interactions between variables. Therefore, the application of the MIT model to a specific patient may require the adjustment of the magnitudes on the various arcs to reflect that patient's condition. Nevertheless, the MIT group used their model to predict the effects of various drugs, such as beta-blocking agents, on variables that can be measured. They compared these predictions with the effects described in the literature for these drugs. The predicted effects and the reported effects were in good agreement [23].

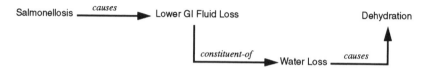

Figure 24.21. Excerpt from the ABEL model relating salmonellosis with dehydration [24].

The relationship between variables in the MIT model is limited to causality. The ABLE project, also at MIT, modelled electrolyte and acid-base physiology using four additional relationships [24]:

Relationship	Examples
Constituent-of	The *loop of Henle* is a constituent-of the *tubule*
	The *tubule* is a constituent-of the *nephron*
Connected-to	The *glomerulus* is connected-to the *tubule*
	The *tubule* is connected-to the *collecting duct*
Contained-in	The *glomerular space* is contained-in the *cortex space*
	The *cortex space* is contained-in the *kidney space*
Erect-below	The *abdominal cavity* is erect-below the *thoracic cavity*

ABEL uses these relationships, together with causality, to describe the anatomy and physiology of electrolyte and acid-base regulation.

For example, Figure 24.21 shows the portion of the ABEL model that relates *salmonellosis* to *dehydration*. According to this model, *salmonellosis* causes *lower GI fluid loss*, *lower GI fluid loss* is a constituent of *water loss*, and *water loss* causes *dehydration*.

Qualitative models have been used in several medical AI research projects. One example is a physician's workstation project underway in the corporate research labs of the Hewlett-Packard Company [25]. This workstation uses a causal model to derive the patient context for data queries. The patient context derived by this model is used to interpret the data query and to organize the presentation of the results.

The SIMON project at Vanderbilt University provides another example of how medical information systems are using qualitative models [26]. This project has built an experimental patient monitoring system for use in a neonatal ICU. The goal is a system that can assist in the management of ventilator therapy for premature infants with respiratory distress syndrome. The qualitative model in the SIMON prototype determines the patient's pathophysiologic state and assesses the effects of therapy. The model also makes qualitative predictions about trends in the patient's variables.

SIMON uses 30 numeric variables to represent the patient. The independent variables in this set are arterial bicarbonate concentration ($[HCO^-_3]$), arterial partial pressures for oxygen (PaO_2), and carbon dioxide ($PaCO_2$), and five ventilator settings. The other numeric variables used in SIMON are derived from these eight independent variables.

SIMON expresses the patient's status in terms of *views* and *processes*. A *view* is defined according to value ranges for a group of variables. For example the *respiratory acidosis* view is defined by low pH and high $PaCO_2$. The more complicated *corrected metabolic acidosis* view is defined by pH and $[HCO^-_3]$ values that currently are normal and low, respectively, with previous pH and $[HCO^-_3]$ values that were both low implying uncorrected metabolic acidosis. SIMON recognizes approximately 40 different views.

A *process* is a mechanism that affects the relationships between variables. For example, the *assisted ventilation* process is a therapeutic intervention that can be represented by the following qualitative proportionality relationships:

> alveolar ventilation $\propto$ (tidal volume + dead space) $\times$ rate
> tidal volume $\propto$ lung compliance $\times$ (PIP − PEEP)
> oxygenation $\propto FIO_2$
> oxygenation $\propto$ MAP
> MAP $\propto$ ((PIP − PEEP) $\times$ I:E ratio) + PEEP

These proportionality relationships are similar to the causality relationships used in the MIT cardiovascular model. For example, the fourth relationship listed above implies that an increase in the mean airway pressure causes an increase in the oxygenation level.

The *assisted ventilation* process also is defined by the following qualitative differential relationships:

$$\Delta PaO_2 \propto O_2 \text{ uptake rate}$$

$$\Delta PaO_2 \propto -O_2 \text{ consumption rate}$$

$$\Delta PaCO_2 \propto CO_2 \text{ production rate}$$

$$\Delta PaCO_2 \propto -CO_2 \text{ elimination rate}$$

For example, the change in PaO_2 is proportional to the oxygen uptake rate and inversely proportional to the oxygen consumption rate. It is important to note that these four relationships describe the direction of the change but not the magnitude of the change.

Qualitative differential relationships are similar to the ordinary differential equation used in VENTPLAN to model the dynamics of the venous O_2 content. The important difference is that the former represents differential relationships in qualitative rather than numeric terms. The methods used to solve qualitative differential equations are analogous to the methods applied to ordinary differential equations. Solutions are generated by simulation in which a sequence of values are generated by integration [27].

The qualitative model in SIMON assesses the patient's situation by deciding which of the views and processes are active. SIMON also uses a scoring system to nominate additional hypotheses that may provide a

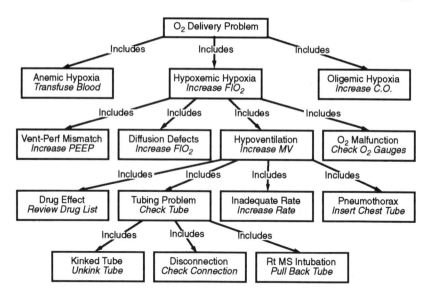

Figure 24.22. Excerpt from the clinical knowledge base in Guardian [28].

more complete explanation for the observed values. This scoring system assigns numeric values to each of the views and processes based on discrepancies between actual values and the values predicted from the previous patient assessment. A hypothesized view or process is activated when it reduces the overall score. However, this activation algorithm ignores the possibility that a combination of views or processes may provide the best explanation.

A research group at Stanford University has also built a patient monitoring system based on a qualitative modelling. They call their prototype Guardian [28]. The clinical knowledge in the current version of Guardian is limited to the management of hypoxia in patients on mechanical ventilators. However, the goal is a system that can be extended to assist in the general care of ICU patients.

Guardian contains several knowledge bases. Figure 24.22 contains part of the clinical knowledge base describing the management of hypoxia problems. The clinical knowledge base is a taxonomy of the problems relating to oxygen delivery. Therefore, the relation between the diagnoses in this model is *includes*.

The clinical knowledge base is supported by several physiology models, including a model of the oxygen transport mechanism. A portion of this knowledge base is shown in Figure 24.23. This knowledge base uses several qualitative relationships. For example, *ventilator inhalation* includes the *tube in-flow* process and *machine inspiration*. The *tube in-flow process* occurs in the *tube* and delivers to the *respirator air supply process*. *Ventilator inhalation* is measured by the *inspired air flow* which has an O_2 content and a N_2 content.

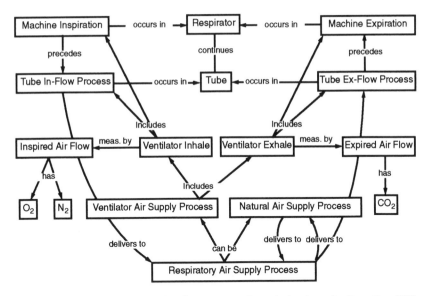

Figure 24.23. Excerpt from the O_2 transport knowledge base in Guardian [28].

The physiology models in Guardian are supported by a collection of models which describe the principles underlying fluid and gas flow, gas diffusion, gas exchange, equilibrium and metabolism. The application of this first-principle knowledge is supported by models describing the general principles used to form diagnoses, make predictions, and so forth.

Therefore, Guardian is based on a layered knowledge representation scheme. Each layer corresponds to a different type of reasoning. The top layer contains the knowledge that is specific to the clinical application. The next layers contain the knowledge pertaining to the corresponding physiologic systems. The layers below that describe of the physics of the problem. The bottom layers describe the general principles of classification and prediction.

Both SIMON and Guardian represent innovative approaches to knowledge representation. On the other hand, these two prototypes, like the other systems discussed in this section, have not been subjected to anything that approaches a clinical trial. Therefore, the long term clinical significance of the technology they apply remains to be seen.

Summary

This section has described the use of models to encode medical knowledge. The discussion started with a system based on a traditional mathematical representation of cardiopulmonary physiology. The discussion then introduced qualitative models. The simplest qualitative models represent knowledge as a collection of causal links. More elaborate qualitative models make use of a number of relationships in addition to causality. Qualitative modelling can be extended to represent dynamics. The discussion concluded with a system that contains multiple qualitative models. Each of these models represent a different level of generality in the patient monitoring process.

Building a system that make use of multiple knowledge bases involves an architectural challenge in which the evaluation of the different knowledge bases must be coordinated. The final section of this chapter describes how this challenge can be met.

Section 5: System Integration

The previous sections have described different approaches to automating the processing of information in the critical care setting. No one of these approaches represents a complete solution. Most likely the construction of a comprehensive system will be a hybrid that combines several of the knowledge representation schemes that have been discussed. VENT-PLAN, the system designed to assist in the management of ventilator patients, illustrates this strategy. Recall that this system combines a probabilistic belief network (see above) with a numeric simulation model (see above). This final section will describe two different approaches to building systems that integrated different knowledge representation schemes.

The challenge in building an integrated system is coordinating the behavior of the components. For example, both SIMON and Guardian, the two model-based monitoring systems discussed in the previous section, use feature extraction modules to process the raw data. These modules detect the significant features in the data obtained from the patient. The extracted features are passed on to the various reasoning modules that perform the higher level analysis of the data. The feature extraction modules typically must handle relatively high data rates. On the other hand, the features extracted by these modules are relatively infrequent thereby allowing the other modules to use more computationally intensive algorithms. The overall system must provide an interface between these disparate components.

Dependency Networks

NAIVE and the Temporal Control Structure discussed earlier illustrate one approach to building integrated systems. These two systems organize their components into dependency networks. For example, recall Figure 24.17. This figure depicts the propagation of a new data, starting with the source and ending with an alarm. Each of the nodes visited in this graph corresponds to a different step in the analysis of the data. An arc connecting one node with another corresponds to how the output of one step in the analysis is the input for another step.

Dependency graphs have two important disadvantages. First, the design of a component must reflect the behavior of the components with which it interacts. For example, referring again to Figure 24.17, the analysis in the node labelled *Variable X* must be able to process the output of the nodes labelled *Data Source A* and *Data Source B*. Or conversely, the two data source nodes must provide outputs that can be processed by the node labelled *Variable X*. In order to minimize the difficulty in designing modules so that they can interact, dependency networks usually implement a communication protocol. For example, NAIVE requires that probability density functions are used to communicate data between nodes.

Another potential disadvantage of dependency graphs is the lack of a central control mechanism. As discussed earlier, the activation of a module is triggered by the modules upon which it depends. However, suppose in Figure 24.17 that the evaluation of *Predictive Alarm 1* is more urgent than the evaluation of *Predictive Alarm 2*. The availability of a new value from *Data Source C* will trigger the evaluation of *Variable Y* and *Variable Z*. These two nodes in turn will trigger the evaluation of the two alarm nodes which must then compete for the available computational resources. This decentralized mechanism is unable to favor the evaluation of *Predictive Alarm 1* over the evaluation of *Predictive Alarm 2*.

Blackboard Architecture

The blackboard architecture, developed at Stanford University, is an approach to building integrated system that addresses the need for centralized control [29]. The essential parts of a blackboard architecture are a collection of *agents* that provide and make use of information, a *communication mechanism* and a *scheduler*. Agents use the communication mechanism to announce the need for information. Agents can also use the communication mechanism to announce the availability of information. Normally an agent is activated by the announcement of the need for the information it provides or when the information it uses becomes available. The scheduler uses global knowledge about the system to regulate when an agent responds to a request for information. Conversely, an agent which needs information suspends its evaluation until the required information becomes available. The suspended status of various agents is reflected in the decisions made by the scheduler.

The Guardian project, with its multilayered design, is implemented using the blackboard architecture. The COMPAS project at the LDS Hospital and the University of Utah also uses the blackboard architecture to build an integrated system [30]. The goal of the COMPAS project is an advice system that can assist in the management of patients with adult respiratory distress syndrome (ARDS). The data used in the COMPAS prototype is obtained directly from the HELP clinical information system at the LDS hospital [31].

The knowledge bases in the COMPAS prototype are organized as the following four components:

Data processing programs: Calculates cardiopulmonary values from the raw data.

Classification programs: Converts the numeric values into qualitative values.

Patient management protocols: Specifies the management stage according to the mode of ventilator therapy and the patient's condition.

General rule sets: Specifies patient management advice according to the available data and the protocol stage.

These components are implemented as blackboard agents. The *data processing programs* are activated by the raw data and produce the processed data which, in turn, activates the *classification-programs*. The *classification programs* produce the classified data which activates the *patient management protocols*. The *patient management protocols* and the *general rule sets* generate the therapeutic suggestions. The scheduler, which regulates the activation of the *patient management protocols* and *general rule sets*, uses the classified data to assess the patient's situation and the adequacy of the current mode of therapy.

The COMPAS prototype is unusual because of the extent of its clinical evaluation. The system was applied to all ARDS patients treated in a 12-bed ICU over a six-month period. Five patients involving a total of 624 h of care and 407 decision-making opportunities were studied. COMPAS generated 379 therapeutic suggestions. The average time between the recording of a blood gas measurement and the generation of a therapeutic suggestion based on that measurement was 2.3 min. The medical staff complied with 84.4% of these suggestions. (See Chapter 23 for update)

Conclusions

This chapter has described a group of technologies that will help to automate the integration and synthesis of information. Several schemes for representing the medical knowledge used to process data were presented. The management of incomplete or contradictory data was discussed. Methods that can be used to detect, interpret and manage temporal events were outlined. The use of models of physiology was described. Finally, an architecture that can be used to build integrated systems was defined.

The introduction to this chapter described the application of these technologies to critical care medicine as *emerging*. All of the examples that have been presented are experimental and for the most part incomplete. With few exceptions, these demonstration systems have seen little, if any, clinical testing. At the same time, the application of AI to critical care medicine must also be seen as *inevitable*. The need to automate more of the information processing task in the ICU is growing. The hardware and software technology that can be used to build automated systems is improving. Both commercial and academic researchers are actively working to extend these technologies. One might conclude that the only uncertainty is when a practical system will be built.

References

1. Leng QW, Pau LF, Andersen OS, Gøthgen IH. PONJIP: A blood gas expert system for intensive care units. *Working Notes for the Symposium on AI in Medicine*, Stanford, 1990; pp 122–124.
2. Shortliffe EH. Details of the consultation system. In Buchanan BG, Shortliffe EH (eds): *Rule-Based Expert Systems. The MYCIN Experiments of the Stanford Heuristic Programming Project*. Reading: Addison-Wesley, 1984; pp 78–132.
3. Doue JC, Vallance AG. Computer-aided ECG analysis. *Hewlett-Packard J* 1985; 36(9):29–34.
4. Muldrow KW, Mark RG, Long JL, Moody GB. CALVIN: A rule based expert system for improving arrhythmia detector performance during noisy ECGs. *Comput Cardiol* 1987; pp 21–26. IEEE, New York
5. Mark RG, Moody GB, Olson WH, Peterson SK, Schluter PS, Walters JB. In *Comput Cardiol* 1979, pp 57–62. IEEE, New York
6. Fagan LM. VM: Representing time-dependent relations in the clinical setting. Ph.D. dissertation, Computer Science Department, Stanford University, 1980.
7. Fukui Y, Masuzawa T. Knowledge-based approach to intelligent alarms. *J Clin Monit* 1989; 5:211–216.
8. Garfinkel D, Matsiras PV, Lecky JH, Aukburg SJ, Matschinsky BB, Mavrides TG. PONI: An intelligent alarm system for respiratory and circulation management in the operating rooms. *Proceedings of the 13th Annual Symposium on Computer Applications in Medical Care*, Washington, DC, 1988; pp 13–17.
9. Beech M, Todd S, Tombs V. Knowledge-based techniques for alarm rationalization in patient monitoring. *Proceedings of the Colloquium on AI in Medical Decision Making*, 1990.
10. Higgins MC. NAIVE: A method for representing uncertainty and temporal relationships in an automated reasoner. *Proceedings of the Third Workshop on Uncertainty in Artificial Intelligence*, Seattle, 1987; pp140–147.
11. Higgins MC, Goodnature D, Lindauer JM, Pering RD. An architecture for combining alternative reasoning strategies in real-time patient monitoring. *Working Notes for the Symposium on AI in Medicine*, Stanford, 1990; pp 74–76.
12. Factor M, Sitting DF, Cohn AI, Gelernter DH, Miller PL, Rosenbaum S. A parallel software architecture for building intelligent medical monitors. *Proceedings of the 14th Annual Symposium on Computer Applications in Medical Care*, Washington, DC, 1989; pp11–16.
13. Sittig DF, Factor M. Physiologic trend detection and artifact rejection: A pa-

rallel implementation of a multi-state Kalman filter algorithm. *Proceedings of the 13th Annual Symposium on Computer Applications in Medical Care*, Washington, DC, 1989; pp 569–574.

14. Shortliffe EH, Buchanan BG. A model of inexact reasoning in medicine. *Math Biosci* 1975; 23:351–379.

15. Yu VL, Fagan LM, Wraith SM, Clancey WJ, Scott AC, Hannigan JF, Blum RL, Buchanan BB, Cohen SN. Antimicrobial selection by a computer: A blinded evaluation by infectious disease experts. JAMA 1979; 242(12):1279–1282.

16. Miller RA, Pople Jr HE, Meyers JD. INTERNIST-I, An experimental computer-based diagnostic consultant for general internal medicine. *N Engl J Med* 1982; 307:468–476.

17. Mabry ME, Miller RA. Distinguishing drug toxicity syndromes from medical diseases: A QMR computer-based approach. *Proceedings of the 14th Annual Symposium on Computer Applications in Medical Care*, Washington, DC, 1990; pp 65–71.

18. Rutledge G, Thomsen G, Beinlich I, Farr B, Sheiner L, Fagan LM. Combining qualitative and quantitative computation in a ventilator therapy planner. *Proceedings of the 13th Annual Symposium on Computer Applications in Medical Care*, Washington, DC, 1989; pp 315–319.

19. Chavez RM. Hypermedia and randomized algorithms for medical expert systems. *Proceedings of the 13th Annual Symposium on Computer Applications in Medical Care*, Washington, DC, 1989; pp 171–177.

20. Smith AFM, West M. Monitoring renal transplants: An application of the multiprocess Kalman filter. *Biometrics* 1983; 39:867–878.

21. Russ TA. Using hindsight in medical decision making. *Proceedings of the 13th Annual Symposium on Computer Applications in Medical Care*, Washington, DC, 1989; pp 38–44.

22. Thomsen G, Sheiner L, Fagan LM. SIMV: An application of mathematical modeling in patient monitoring and ventilator management. *Proceedings of the 13th Annual Symposium on Computer Applications in Medical Care*, Washington, DC, 1989; pp 320–324.

23. Long WJ, Naimi S, Criscitiello, MG, Kurzrok S. Reasoning about therapy from a physiological model. In *Medinfo* 1986; 86:756–760.

24. Patil RS. Causal representation of patient illness for electrolyte and acid-base diagnosis. Ph.D. dissertation, Department of Electrical Engineering and Computer Science, MIT, 1981.

25. Stanton WM, Tang PC. Knowledge-based support for a physician's workstation. *Proceedings of the 15th Annual Symposium on Computer Applications in Medical Care*, Washington, DC, 1991; pp649–653.

26. Uckun S. Dawant BM. Qualitative modelling as a paradigm for diagnosis and prediction in critical care environments. *Artificial Intelligence in Medicine* 1992; 4:127–144.

27. Forbus KD. Qualitative process theory. *Artificial Intelligence* 1984; 24:85–168.

28. Hayes-Roth B, Washington R, Ash D et al. Guardian: A prototype intelligent agent for intensive-care monitoring. *Artificial Intelligence in Medicine* 1992; 4:165–185.

29. Hayes-Roth B. A blackboard architecture for control. *Artificial Intelligence* 1985; 26:251–321.

30. Sittig DF, Pace NL, Gardner RM, et al. Implementation of a computerized patient advice system using the HELP clinical information system. *Comput Biomed Res* 1989; 22:474–487.

31. Pryor TA, Gardner RM, Clayton PD, Warner HR. The HELP system. *J Med Syst* 1983; 7:87–102.

Chapter 25
The Future of Computerized Decision Support in Critical Care
Reed M. Gardner and M. Michael Shabot

Prediction is very difficult, especially about the future.

Neils Bohr (1885–1962)

As we write this final chapter, there is a foot of new snow on the ground in R.G.'s backyard in Salt Lake City, and the snow continues to fall. Last night three local television weather forecasters predicted we would only have two inches of snow, and all they had to do was predict one day into the future! With some trepidation, and without the equivalent of weather satellites and 40 years experience with forecasting, the authors will try to predict the future of computers and decision support systems in critical care. Our projections are based on two decades of experience and a generally optimistic outlook. We believe that seven broad areas will determine the pace of the future of computerized decision support in critical care:

1. Human, cultural, and sociological issues relating to how computers will be used in the intensive care unit (ICU).
2. Standardization in medicine and the ability to share medical knowledge will be essential.
3. Expanded medical knowledge will lead to better patient care.
4. Hardware and software will continue to advance at a rapid rate.
5. Data acquisition methods and instrumentation will provide more accurate, timely, and less expensive measurements.
6. Sharing of computer and clinical knowledge in computer form will become common and encouraged by government and the clinical community.
7. Better methods for prognostic decision-making will enable medical practitioners and society to make better ethical decisions about health care.

Human, Cultural, and Sociological Issues

We believe that people, and not technology, will continue to be the major determinant of how quickly and successfully computers are applied to ICU decision making. To be successful at implementing computers in the ICU, everyone involved in patient care must be a participant in the design and implementation of the computerization process. Designing any human-computer interface is difficult. Designing computer applications for medical use is even more challenging.

Although the authors work with, encourage, and implore the medical products industry to start to work on the issues relating to medical computerization, it is not that easy. There are many human, cultural, and social interaction issues that must be resolved before we can achieve benefits of computerization. A recent book by Greenbaum and Kyng entitled *Design at Work: Cooperative Design of Computer Systems* offers several excellent suggestions that all designers should heed, be they hospital or industry based [1]. One of their contentions is that "We fail more often because we solve the wrong problem than because we get the wrong solution to the right problem. . . . The problems we select for solution and the way we formulate them depends more on our philosophy and world view than on our science and technology."

In addition, these authors provide six excellent guiding principles for designing computers for use by humans. The concepts are clear and filled with common sense, but a careful review by both Gardner and Shabot has humbled us both! We wondered why someone did not tell us this before we started. All of us must take these guidelines under advisement as we progress to future applications.

Guiding Principles of Greenbaum and Kyng

1. *Computer systems that are created for the workplace need to be designed with full participation from the users. Full participation, of course, requires training and active cooperation, not just token representation in meetings or on committees.*

    This statement means that one *must* have involvement of laboratory technicians, nursing staff, physicians, clerks, administrators, and medical informatics personnel in a cooperative, teamwork environment to be most successful. With this involvement, the systems developed will better meet the needs of the users and advance the state of the art of computer use in the ICU. With that cooperative spirit, looking at the applications of decision-making in the ICU will be a natural outcome. Patient care will be improved and communications and job satisfaction for all parties will be enhanced.

2. *When computer systems are brought into a workplace, they should enhance workplace skills rather than degrade or rationalize them.*

If teamwork and a collaborative spirit are developed, the work environment for physicians, nurses, therapists, and other clinical staff can be enhanced. By using the computer to better communicate and share data and patient concerns, the quality of patient care can be improved.

3. *Computer systems are tools, and need to be designed to be under the control of the people using them.*

Clearly computers should be used as tools and not as a mechanism to force a "round peg into a square hole." The tools must be developed as a joint venture to best meet the needs of all.

4. *Although computer systems are generally acquired to increase productivity, they also need to be looked at as a means to increase the quality of results.*

Quality of health care can be improved with the use of computers. Numerous examples of quality improvement have been presented in this book and demonstrated by several other groups. Since the main purpose of a medical record is to improve the quality of patient care, the computerized medical record has the same goal. Enhanced communications, alerting, alarming, advising, critiquing, and finally, consultation are primary areas where ICU computers can and should enhance patient care.

The ICU is the primary hospital location where "data overload" can occur. Patients in the ICU generate enormous amounts of data—from bedside monitors, lab tests, medications given, procedures performed, and care provided—yet attention to fine detail is crucial. The ICU computer, with its unresting eye and nearly prefect "memory" can help caregivers do the right thing, at the right time, every time.

5. *The design process is a political one and includes conflicts almost every step of the way. Managers who order the system may be at odds with the workers who are going to use it.*

These statements are particularly true for ICU. Many times physicians and administrators develop plans for computerization without involving nurses, therapists and clerks in the planning process. Institutional politics are never perfect, but involving as many people in the discussion of the future and ICU computer development will ensure that this will be carried out as a "team" activity rather than a dictatorship.

6. *Finally, the design process highlights the issues of how computers are used in the context of work organization. We see this question of focusing on how computers are used, which we call the use situation, as a fundamental starting point for the design process.*

One of the concepts the Japanese learned during the 1970s and 1980s was to have the entire organization learn to work together. For example, it is stated that the janitor in a Toyota plant in Japan knows why he is sweeping the floor in terms of how his task contributes to the production of better, higher-quality automobiles. On a recent visit to an ICU where computers were beginning to be installed at the bedside, the developers had not given much consideration to how the system would be used. Virtually every item of information about the patient required *manual* entry, including patient name, the vital signs, and all procedures performed by nurses and therapists. To establish patient billing, many of the procedures had to be *simultaneously and manually* entered into two or more systems. The engineers who designed this system had developed something that could be made to work, but they did not optimize the communications and integration capabilities of their system.

We have all too frequently observed the situation that Greenbaum and Kyng state: "When organizations don't 'make sense,' the people in them are aware of this, because they themselves work to create a framework of sensemaking." The work of Greenbaum and Kyng, and the example of Hewlett-Packard when the company was trying to develop a simple loading mechanism for a large scale plotter, clearly point out that we have MUCH to learn about the human interface and about solving the correct problem [2]. It is clear to Gardner and Shabot that a spirit of teamwork, a broad interest in sharing data and interface issues will be among the most important activities required to advance the state of the art of computerized medical decision making. We believe that the ICU will be the frontier upon which the practice of computerized medical decision making will occur.

Standardization

Everyone already expects that computers will be used in the grocery store check out line so that an itemized bill with the price and description of each item is provided. To do that, the grocery industry developed a universal product bar coding system and clever methods for scanning the bar codes as the product is swept across the scanner. We think nothing of having our travel agent book a seat for us on a trip three weeks in advance and at the same time giving us seat assignments. Both of these computer applications were developed at great cost and with careful integration of data and knowledge bases. Unfortunately, medicine is just starting the process that these two industries worked out almost two decades ago! In our opinion, standardization is crucial for implementation of computers in critical care, and only standardization will allow medicine to reap the benefits now enjoyed by so many other industries.

As Barnett and Shortliffe state so well in their chapter in the text *Medical Informatics*, lack of standardization of language and communications protocols is a major problem in medicine [3]. The practice of medicine has developed around a "free text" style of description and explanation. However, as medicine prepares to move into the 21st century, there is a need standardize data definitions and languages, data acquisition and communications technologies, and mechanisms to share medical knowledge in computer usable form, using a standard format. Today the effective practice of medicine is dependent on the ability of health professionals to locate relevant pieces of patient information and combine them with medical knowledge to interpret the data correctly [4, 5].

There are a number of forces at work that will increase the use of computerized information systems, enhancing the computer literacy of health professionals, including the development of user-friendly software that allows health professionals to search the medical literature; wider availability of machine-readable information sources; computerized diagnostic and therapeutic assisting systems; and the emergence of local, national, and international research communications networks; efforts to increase health professionals' awareness of currently available information services and the Unified Medical Language System (UMLS), a project of the National Library of Medicine in the United States [4–9].

Efforts are underway to have a common language that will hopefully be used by medical system developers to define the terminology used in the definition and description of diseases. This language can also be used to search the MEDLINE literature referencing system developed and maintained by the National Library of Medicine and used worldwide to allow clinicians and researchers to the medical literature. In addition there are coding systems used for classifying diseases, such as ICD-9-CM, the International Classification of Diseases version 9 with a Clinical Modification. ICD-9-CM codes are typically assigned and stored for each patient admitted to a hospital. The Diagnostic Related Groups (DRG) codes used to establish Medicare reimbursement were derived from the ICD-9-CM codes. A competing terminology is called the Systematized Nomenclature of Medicine, or SNOMED. This terminology has its roots in pathology and was developed to help pathologists classify their findings. The physician's Current Procedural Terminology (CPT) is used to define procedures performed by physicians, such as an appendectomy [4–9].

To illustrate the problems associated with categorizing and standardizing medical care, let us take a brief look at medications. By law in the United States, each medication has its own "drug code." Although this level of standardization is worthwhile and somewhat unique in the medical field, it still does not go far enough. For example, a medication containing aspirin will have its own unique drug code. If one wanted to develop a computerized medical knowledge-based system to prevent patients allergic to aspirin from having this medication prescribed, one would need to have knowledge of every drug's contents. As a result, several commercial firms, including First Databank, sell medication databases that detail the contents of each medication.

The UMLS is developing a strategy to enhance and standardize the communication of medical data. However, the UMLS was not designed to encompass the sharing of computer-based medical knowledge. In the past 15 years systems such as INTERNIST-1/QMR, ILIAD, DXplain, CARE, and HELP have been developed that encode medical knowledge [10]. In 1989 a group of medical informaticists assembled at Columbia University's Arden Homestead conference center to discuss sharing of computer-based knowledge. The group determined that there was a need for better ways to map terminology used from one setting or program to another; to catalogue a list of programs available to process medical knowledge; to develop a representational syntax and format for sharing computerized medical knowledge; to look into the possibility of developing standards for interfacing diverse program modules so that they could be shared; to develop methods of evaluating, validating, and testing knowledge-based computer systems; and finally to define the legal and financial aspects of sharing computerized medical knowledge with its implications to patient care [10]. As a result of this initial meeting at Arden Homestead, there has been a growing interest and series of developments that in the future will make sharing of computer-based medical knowledge not only possible, but essential [10–14].

Finally, standardization of methods and transport mechanisms to move medical data from one instrument or system to another are very important. As covered elsewhere in this book, the adoption and widespread use of specifications and standards such as Health Level 7 (HL7), the IEEE P1073 Medical Information Bus (MIB), and the IEEE P1157 Medical Data Interchange (MEDIX) standards are crucial to the implementation of ICU decision support systems.

Medical Knowledge

The acquisition of medical knowledge in a form that will be functional for computer-directed patient care will require a change in our operating paradigm. Medical scientists in general are not now prepared to put the required specificity and detail into the description and definition of the patient care process. For example, the statement "increase the FiO_2 if the pO_2 is low" seems clear when used in ordinary speech, but in terms of a computer algorithm what does "increase" mean, e.g., exactly how much of an increase? What does a "low" pO_2 mean? In addition there was no specification of time in these instructions nor was there an implied or stated indication of when or how often the pO_2 should be measured after the FiO_2 is increased. Thus, every physician and nurse "thinks" the other caregiver knows what to do, but in fact there is a large amount of variability in the patient care process. This variability is not the beneficial kind which may be related to thoughtful, personalized patient care.

Rather it involves a type of random variability which in other industries has been found to be at cross purposes to quality.

Recently at the LDS Hospital clinicians were developing protocols for the care of patients with Acute Respiratory Distress Syndrome (ARDS) a syndrome that when severe is fatal for about 90% of patients. As protocols were being developed, a computer scientist presented specific patient data to five physicians on a consensus panel. He then asked what treatment strategy each would use. To everyone's surprise, there were five different plans from a group of physicians who work together each day and thought they used the same treatment strategies!

Clearly if we are going to optimize patient care we must acquire and apply optimal treatment strategies. However, with each physician using his or her own "best" strategy, we do not have a scientific platform from which we can determine the most effective treatment plan. We are much like the electrical engineer who is trying to tease a "signal" from an overwhelming amount of "noise." With such "noisy" or variable medical treatment strategies, we will be a long time in determining optimal care. Therefore, we must develop strategies that will maximize the "signal" and minimize the "noise" in our care processes. Guidelines and critical pathways have recently been suggested as methodologies to help optimize patient care. However, many guidelines are outlined in very broad terms, much like our "increase the FiO_2" example above. Care processes must be standardized to a finer level of detail to allow improvement and eventual computerization.

Hardware and Software

Hardware

Hardware costs for computers have dropped dramatically in just the last decade, and it appears that in the next decade we will see further rapid hardware development. As stated in Chapter 14, if one compared computer systems' development with that of airplanes, a Boeing 767 in 1993 would be able to circle the globe in five minutes on one gallon of fuel! This represents a significant improvement from the 1985 projection in which the jet would circle the globe in twenty minutes and consume five gallons of fuel. Perhaps the largest change in hardware development has been the downsizing of mainframe and minicomputer systems to PCs and workstations.

Whereas ten years ago we might have projected that supercomputers would be ubiquitous, the market for large computers has been disrupted by technological progress and a paradigm shift in how work is done on computers. These changes, coupled with the move toward so-called "open systems" based on industry standard operating systems, allow smaller systems to be integrated into massive computing networks. The net result has been downsizing, with mainframes giving way to networks of personal computers anchored by mid-range "server" computers, while workstation clusters are substituting for supercomputers [15, 16]. Thus, we have computers on our desk or at the bedside that have the power of systems that in former times filled large computer rooms.

Mainframe vendors like IBM and DEC have finally realized that the era of mainframe dominance is over and that the market has shifted to networks and workstations. Personal computers and workstations which operate at 100 million instructions per second (MIPS) are readily available. A new interesting measure of processor capability will be in MIPS per milliwatt. Power consumption has always mattered in battery-powered laptops and palmtops, but it has become more important in general, as lower-voltage, lower-power, and longer-battery-life computers continue to be developed. These computers may push us to the point that we have very thin, very low power, very light portable computers that will allow nurses, physicians, and others to enter and review data from any place in a patient's room. At the same time we will be able to communicate quickly, efficiently, and accurately through optical or radio links to communication sites within the room. These computer and communications devices will not be as small and portable as a piece of paper, but they will be much more interactive and much more mobile than the terminals and workstations now used at the bedside.

Distributed databases and distributed access mechanisms are becoming widely available. During the past year, Hewlett-Packard announced a matchbox-sized magnetic disk drive with a diameter of 1.3 inches and a storage capability of 42 MB, which is projected to increase to 120 MB!

Although many have predicted that keyboards would disappear, this does not seem as clear to the industry as it did five years ago. Touch screens were not successful for data-intensive applications. Although pen-based systems and other types of devices are making progress, keyboards are still effective, and in our projections, will continue to be an effective method for data entry and retrieval. For pen-based systems to be widely accepted, they must be reasonably priced and have the ability rapidly to recognize any person's normal writing and translate it into computerized characters. It is a real challenge for computer systems to recognize hand scribbles and translate them into words when presently humans have great difficulty reading the handwriting of other humans. Indeed, this is one of the major problems of current-day medicine. Pointing devices such as mice and trackballs will remain crucial to graphically oriented systems.

Video displays will make dramatic improvements over the next decade. Currently 14–15-inch color displays are common and 21-inch color displays are available. Very high resolution color displays costing $4,000–$5,000 must be used to project x-ray images. In a "rounds room" which currently has 8 to 12 x-ray viewboxes, an investment of $50,000 would be required! Clearly this display technology must be made more cost-effective.

There are exciting prospects for the future with flat panel displays. These flat panel displays can be either in monochrome or color and have the advantage of being small, lightweight, low-power devices. Flat panels will typically be 0.5–1 inch thick and can be posted on the wall much like a framed picture, or they can be carried around as portable devices. Because these devices consume so little energy, there is no need for cooling. Space around the patient is usually quite limited, so we expect flat panel displays to have a major positive impact on adoption of bedside computer systems.

Software

Software development, debugging, and integration continues to be a major problem for the entire computer industry, not just in medicine or the ICU. Although software is becoming more standardized, the ability to exchange software is still a major problem. Clearly, the development of standards for data retrieval, display, and decision support will have to be universal. Medicine requires that local customization be available, but hopefully on a backbone of standardized data elements and display capabilities. Hospitals and ICUs in particular must place themselves in a position to take advantage of these developments [17].

Data Acquisition

The area of automated patient data acquisition is one that needs much more development and one where little progress has been made. Data acquisition of the physiological signals from patients is common for blood pressure, electrocardiogram (ECG), electroencephalograph (EEG), and a few other parameters such as oxygen saturation. There will be a dramatic improvement in our ability to acquire data from ventilators and other instruments. Exciting prospects are in the offing for promptly acquiring data that previously had to be sent out to distant locations such as clinical laboratories. The scenario in 1993 is to bring the clinical chemistry laboratory physically into the ICU in the form of a bedside "stat" lab. The scenario in the year 2000 will be that a major part of clinical laboratory services will be performed with implantable devices, typically catheter-tipped sensors. A number of companies have introduced instruments for measuring blood gases, pH, the PO_2, and the PCO_2 with catheter-tipped fiber optic sensors. Since flowing blood is a very difficult medium to work in, progress in this field has been long and difficult, but is steadily progressing. We project that over the next decade we will be able continuously to monitor serum electrolytes, glucose, and other chemistries, in addition to blood gases. Thus, rather than having to order laboratory results, which may take 10–15 min; then have a phlebotomist travel to the unit and draw the blood; transport the blood to another location; do the analysis; and transfer the results back, results will be "on-line" and continuous. The former delays caused instability in the care process because information was not immediately available [18, 19].

Having "real-time" data will require us to develop a new set of decision support strategies based on "decision–driven data collection." These strategies will allow us to use the computer to predict when certain data should be gathered. For example, if a physician decides to increase the inspired oxygen fraction from 40 to 50% and wants to see what the patient's response is, the computer will advise the caregiver to make additional measurements once the patient has stabilized from the step change in therapy. Once the measurements are made, the computer can then direct patient care through protocols.

The acquisition of timely and representative data, which seems like a trivial task but is really rather complex, will continue to develop. We clearly need to develop methodologies for acquiring timely and representative data from instruments such as ventilators, bedside monitors, pulse oximeters, IV pumps, and other instruments. However, some acquisition strategies have already been devised and are incorporated into commercially available instruments and ICU computer systems.

The sharing and the correlation of data measured by a variety of devices will become essential. To give an example, a patient may be connected to an electrocardiogram, a direct arterial blood pressure measurement, and a pulse oximeter. All three of these devices are capable of continuously measuring the heart rate. The heart rate determined from each of the devices for a normal patient should be identical. However, if a device is affected by noise or artifact, it may not be able to make the heart rate measurement. For example, if a patient moves the finger used for pulse oximetry measurement, artifacts are produced. At that time the heart rate from the pulse oximeter may be different from the heart rate derived from the ECG and direct arterial pressure sensor. Cross-correlating these signals and deciding which is "correct" is not a trivial problem, and thus this capability is not yet available in any patient monitoring system. However, from the example just given, one should be able to measure the heart rate from the other two signals and come up with a reasonable and rational estimate of what the heart rate is. However, if the patient has an arrhythmia and does not generate a reasonable stroke volume, the heart rate determined from the pulse oximeter and the direct arterial blood pressure may be quite different from that determined from the ECG. Thus, it is important to share and correlate data from multiple devices to gather real knowledge about the patient, rather than reporting different heart rates from each device. The same will be true for catheter-tipped sensors and other devices attached to patients. Integrating all of the data and making proper patient care decisions will be a crucial goal for the future.

Sharing of Knowledge

The development of practice guidelines and protocols for care is gaining importance in the medical field. David Eddy and others such as James Galligher [20–24] have shown that in the future, medicine will be practiced according to standards and guidelines. It is clear from the theory of continuous quality improvement that standardization of care is important to eliminate random variations and to enable us to determine what is appropriate care [25]. Physicians, nurses, and therapists are constantly subjected to an overload of data and need to use a standardized strategy to maximize the quality of care given to each patient.

If caregivers follow no guidelines and use different care strategies in the morning, at noon, and then in the evening, optimal practice can never be determined. The strategy that must be adhered to is to provide the *same* care each time. Even though the care may not be exactly the "optimal care," until we have standardized the care process, we will not be able to determine what optimal care is. Once care has been standardized, we can then by using scientific methods, perform experiments to determine what "optimal care" is. Measuring the effect of standardized changes will be the equivalent of clinical trials. Computerized ICU decision support will allow us to perform these tasks easily and rationally [26–29].

Most of us are faced with a huge information overload when we go to our office each day and sort through our mail. The problem is dealing with the incoming data contained in the envelopes. The equivalent happens to caregivers for critically ill patients. Information filtering has become a promising technology in the information age. Just as we must sort through what is important and unimportant in our "paper" mail and electronic mail, we must develop information filtering and retrieval methods that will allow us to care for critically in patients optimally [30–34]. Development of guidelines and specifically protocols for the care of the patients will allow us to use computer technology to maximize the information content from the flood of data emanating from the multiple devices and observers at the bedside.

Predictive Methods and Societal Decisions

A major focal point in United States today is putting a cap on the continued increase in the cost of health care. There are three major factors driving up the cost of health care today: quality waste, productivity waste, and provision of care with a limited cost-benefit ratio. The first two factors are well understood, but cost-benefit analysis is more difficult.

Quality waste could be considered having to reinsert a catheter because it became clotted, or having to repeat a laboratory test because a sample was inappropriately drawn. Inefficiencies can result from inefficient processes at all stages of the health care delivery system. The health care industry has within its capability the responsibility and need to eliminate quality waste and operating inefficiencies in the system.

However, cost-benefit is not a measurement that can be quickly and easily changed by the health care system by itself, rather it must involve the will of society. How does one decide whether or not to perform coronary artery bypass surgery on a 100-year-old male? And not only whether the surgery should be done, but at what cost and who should pay? These are questions that must be answered by *society*. However, the society is not anxious to make these decisions. Although it is relatively easy to theorize about society in general, for any given patient the family and physician are tempted to say, "Let's go for it." These issues are not easily resolved and will continue to grow as the "baby boomers" reach middle age and diseases such as AIDS continue to plague our society. The ethics of these issues are very complex and this represents another area that must clearly be defined so that caregivers can provide the best care for society and for the individual. Computers will not play a role in this kind of decision-making, beyond their ability to measure severity of illness and predict outcome, under certain circumstances.

Summary

Computer-assisted decision support for the care of critically ill patients is inevitable, but much more challenging than the use of computers in other industries. The need to deliver cost-effective and medically effective critical care will bring computers to the ICU bedside. In the end, this will become a simple business decision, one in which higher quality and lower cost are achieved through automation. The demands for these kinds of improvements in medical practice are converging on a computer industry that is beginning to deliver inexpensive, high-powered computer systems and networks to hospitals. Our patients will be the beneficiaries of this progress, which, though slow, remains inevitable.

References

1. Greenbaum J, Kyng M. Design at Work: Cooperative Design of Computer Systems. Hillsdale, NJ: Lawrence Erlbaum Associates, 1991.
2. Wield PJ. Design Jet plotter user interface design: Learning the hard way about human interactions. Hewlett-Packard Journal 1992; 43(6):12.
3. Shortliffe EH, Barnett GO. Medical data: Their acquisition, storage, and use.

In: Medical Informatics: Computer Applications in Health Care. Reading, MA: Addison-Wesley, 1990; pp37–69.

4. Humphreys BL, Lindberg DAB. Building a unified medical language system. SCAMC 1989; 13:475–480.
5. Humphreys BL, Lindberg DAB. The UMLS knowledge sources: Tools for building better user interfaces. SCAMC 1990; 14:121–125.
6. Huff SM, Warner HR. A comparison of Meta-1 and HELP terms: Implications for clinical data. SCAMC 1990; 14:166–169.
7. Humphreys BL, Lindberg DAB, Hole WT. Assessing and enhancing the value of the UMLS knowledge sources. SCAMC 1991; 15:78–82.
8. Masys DR. An evaluation of the source selection elements of the prototype UMLS information source map. SCAMC 1992; 16:295–298.
9. Chute CG, Yang Y. An evaluation of concept based latent semantic indexing for clinical information retrieval. SCAMC 1992; 16:639–643.
10. Clayton PD, Pryor TA, Wigertz OB, Hripcsak G. Issues and structures for sharing medical knowledge among decision-making systems: The 1989 Arden Homestead Retreat. SCAMC 1989; 13:116–121.
11. Clayton PD, Hripcsak, Pryor TA. Emerging standards for medical logic. SCAMC 1990; 14:27–31.
12. Hripcsak G, Clayton PD, Pryor TA, Haug P, Wigertz OB, Van der lei J. The Arden syntax for medical logic modules. SCAMC 1990; 14:200–204.
13. Shwe M, Sujansky W, Middleton B. Reuse of knowledge represented in the Arden Syntax. SCAMC 1992; 16:47–51.
14. Johansson BG, Wigertz OB. An object oriented approach to interpret medical knowledge based on Arden Syntax. SCAMC 1992; 16:52–56.
15. Bell TE. Annual Review—Technology 1993. IEEE Spectrum 1993; 30(1):24–25.
16. Comerford R. Technology 1993—PCs and workstations. IEEE Spectrum 1993; 30(1):26–29.
17. Comerford R. Technology 1993—Software. IEEE Spectrum 1993; 30(1):30–33.
18. Sarch R. Technology 1993—Data communications. IEEE Spectrum 1993; 30(1):42–44.
19. Stephenson J. Technology 1993—Medical electronics. IEEE Spectrum 1993; 30(1):76–79.
20. Eddy DM. Clinical decision making. JAMA 1990: 263:1265–1275.
21. Eddy DM. Practice policies—guidelines for methods. JAMA 1990; 263:1839–1841.
22. Eddy DM. Guidelines for policy statements: The explicit approach. JAMA 1990; 263:2239–2243.
23. Eddy DM. Designing a practice policy—Standards, guidelines, and options. JAMA 1990; 263:3077—3084.
24. Gallagher TJ. Guidelines for care: The time has come. Crit Care Med 1991; 19:138.
25. Scholtes PR. The Team Handbook: How To Use Teams To Improve Quality. Madison, WI: Joiner Associates, 1992.
26. East TD, Morris AH, Wallace CJ, Clemmer TP, Orme JF Jr, Weaver LK, Henderson S, Sittig DF. A strategy for development of computerized critical care decision support systems. Intl J Clin Monit Comput 1992; 8:263–269.

27. Guyatt G, et al. Guidelines for the clinical and economic evaluation of Health Care Technologies. Soc Sci Med 1986; 22:393–408.
28. Brook RH. Practice guidelines and practicing medicine—Are they compatible? JAMA 1989; 262:3027–3030.
29. Civetta JM. Critical care: How should we evaluate our progress? Crit Care Med 1992; 20:1714–1720.
30. Loch S, Terry D. Information filtering. Communications of the ACM 1992; 35(12):27–28.
31. Belkin NJ, Croft WB. Information filtering and information retrieval: Two sides of the same coin? Communications of the ACM 1992; 35(12):29–38.
32. Loeb S. Architecting personalized delivery of multimedia information. Communications of the ACM 1992; 35(12):39–50.
33. Foltz PW, Dumais ST. Personalized information delivery: An analysis of information filtering methods. Communications of the ACM 1992; 35(12):51–60.
34. Goldberg D, Nichols D, Oki BM, Terry D. Using collaborative filtering to weave an information tapestry. Communications of the ACM 1992; 35(12);61–70.

Index